Emergency Surgery

Emergency Surgery

EDITED BY

Adam Brooks, FRCS (Gen Surg), DMCC

Consultant in HPB Surgery
Major Trauma Pathway Lead
General Surgery Service Lead
Nottingham University Hospital NHS Trust
Nottingham, UK; and
Senior Lecturer
Academic Department of Military Surgery and Trauma
Royal Centre for Defence Medicine
Birmingham, UK

Bryan A. Cotton, MD, MPH

Associate Professor
Department of Surgery and the Center for Translational Injury Research
The University of Texas Health Science Center
Houston, Texas, USA

Lt Col Nigel Tai, MS, FRCS (Gen Surg), RAMC

Consultant in Trauma and Vascular Surgery, Defence Medical Services
Trauma Clinical Academic Unit
Royal London Hospital
Whitechapel
London, UK
and
Senior Lecturer
Academic Department of Military Surgery and Trauma
Royal Centre for Defence Medicine
Birmingham, UK

Col Peter F. Mahoney, OBE, TD, MSc, FRCA, RAMC

Defence Professor Anaesthesia and Critical Care
RCDM Birmingham Research
Park Vincent Drive
Birmingham, UK

Associate Editor

David J. Humes, BSc, MBBS, MRCS

Lecturer in Surgery
QMC Campus
University of Nottingham
Nottingham, UK

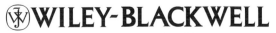

WILEY-BLACKWELL
A John Wiley & Sons, Ltd., Publication

BMJ|Books

This edition first published 2010, © 2010 by Blackwell Publishing Ltd

BMJ Books is an imprint of BMJ Publishing Group Limited, used under licence by Blackwell Publishing which was acquired by John Wiley & Sons in February 2007. Blackwell's publishing programme has been merged with Wiley's global Scientific, Technical and Medical business to form Wiley-Blackwell.

Registered office: John Wiley & Sons Ltd, The Atrium, Southern Gate, Chichester, West Sussex, PO19 8SQ, UK

Editorial offices: 9600 Garsington Road, Oxford, OX4 2DQ, UK

The Atrium, Southern Gate, Chichester, West Sussex, PO19 8SQ, UK

111 River Street, Hoboken, NJ 07030-5774, USA

For details of our global editorial offices, for customer services and for information about how to apply for permission to reuse the copyright material in this book please see our website at www.wiley.com/wiley-blackwell

The right of the author to be identified as the author of this work has been asserted in accordance with the Copyright, Designs and Patents Act 1988.

Wiley also publishes its books in a variety of electronic formats. Some content that appears in print may not be available in electronic books.

Designations used by companies to distinguish their products are often claimed as trademarks. All brand names and product names used in this book are trade names, service marks, trademarks or registered trademarks of their respective owners. The publisher is not associated with any product or vendor mentioned in this book. This publication is designed to provide accurate and authoritative information in regard to the subject matter covered. It is sold on the understanding that the publisher is not engaged in rendering professional services. If professional advice or other expert assistance is required, the services of a competent professional should be sought.

The contents of this work are intended to further general scientific research, understanding, and discussion only and are not intended and should not be relied upon as recommending or promoting a specific method, diagnosis, or treatment by physicians for any particular patient. The publisher and the author make no representations or warranties with respect to the accuracy or completeness of the contents of this work and specifically disclaim all warranties, including without limitation any implied warranties of fitness for a particular purpose. In view of ongoing research, equipment modifications, changes in governmental regulations, and the constant flow of information relating to the use of medicines, equipment, and devices, the reader is urged to review and evaluate the information provided in the package insert or instructions for each medicine, equipment, or device for, among other things, any changes in the instructions or indication of usage and for added warnings and precautions. Readers should consult with a specialist where appropriate. The fact that an organization or Website is referred to in this work as a citation and/or a potential source of further information does not mean that the author or the publisher endorses the information the organization or Website may provide or recommendations it may make. Further, readers should be aware that Internet Websites listed in this work may have changed or disappeared between when this work was written and when it is read. No warranty may be created or extended by any promotional statements for this work. Neither the publisher nor the author shall be liable for any damages arising herefrom.

Library of Congress Cataloging-in-Publication Data

Emergency surgery / edited by Adam Brooks ... [et al.].
    p. ; cm.
   ISBN 978-1-4051-7025-3
   1. Surgical emergencies.   I. Brooks, Adam, 1969–
     [DNLM: 1. Emergencies.   2. Surgical Procedures, Operative.   3. Emergency Medical Services. WO 700 E53 2010]
   RD93.E4496 2010
   617′.026–dc22

                                                                            2009026824

ISBN: 9781405170253

A catalogue record for this book is available from the British Library.

Set in 9.5/12pt Meridien by Aptara® Inc., New Delhi, India
Printed and bound in Singapore

1 2010

Contents

Contents

List of Contributors

Ian Beckingham
HPB and Laparoscopic Surgeon
Queens Medical Centre
Nottingham University Medical School
Nottingham, UK

Tracy R. Bilski
Assistant Professor
Mary Washington Hospital
Fredericksburg
VA, USA

Douglas M. Bowley
Consultant Surgeon
Heart of England NHS
Foundation Trust
Senior Lecturer
Royal Centre for Defence Medicine
Birmingham, UK

Nora Brennan
Specialist Registrar in Emergency Medicine
The Royal London Hospital
Whitechapel
London, UK

Adam Brooks
Consultant in HPB Surgery
Major Trauma Pathway Lead
General Surgery Service Lead
Nottingham University Hospital NHS Trust
Nottingham, UK; and
Senior Lecturer
Academic Department of Military Surgery and
Trauma
Royal Centre for Defence Medicine
Birmingham, UK

Matthew Button
Trauma Clinical Academic Unit
Royal London Hospital
Whitechapel
London, UK

C. Ross Carter
West of Scotland Pancreatic Unit
Glasgow Royal Infirmary
Glasgow, Scotland

Abeed Chowdhury
Department of Surgery
Queen's Medical Centre
Nottingham, UK

Bryan A. Cotton
Department of Surgery and the Center for
Translational Injury Research
The University of Texas Health Science Center
Houston, TX, USA

Ross Davenport
Trauma Research Fellow
Trauma Clinical Academic Unit
Royal London Hospital
London, UK

Euan J. Dickson
West of Scotland Pancreatic Unit
Glasgow Royal Infirmary
Glasgow, Scotland

Lesly A. Dossett
Division of Trauma and Surgical Critical Care
Vanderbilt University Medical Center
Nashville, TN, USA

J. Edward F. Fitzgerald
Department of Gastrointestinal Surgery
Nottingham University Hospital NHS Trust
Nottingham, UK

Aviram M. Giladi
Resident, Section of Plastic Surgery
Department of Surgery
University of Michigan Hospitals
Ann Arbor, MI, USA

John S. Hammond
Clinical Lecturer
Department of Surgery
Nottingham Digestive Diseases Centre
University of Nottingham
Nottingham, UK

Roland A. Hernández
Medical Student
University of Michigan
Medical School
Ann Arbor, MI, USA

David J. Humes
Lecturer in Surgery
QMC Campus
University of Nottingham
Nottingham, UK

Andrew McDonald Johnston
Specialist Registrar in Respiratory and Intensive
Care Medicine
Department of Military Medicine
Royal Centre for Defence Medicine
Birmingham, UK

Thomas König
Specialist Registrar in General Surgery
Defence Medical Services
Trauma Clinical
Academic Unit
Royal London Hospital
Whitechapel
London, UK

David Luke
Department of Colorectal Surgery
Heart of England NHS Foundation Trust
Birmingham, UK

Justin Manley
Resident in Surgery
University of Mississippi
Medical Center
Brandon, MS, USA

Gurminder S. Mann
Consultant Urological Surgeon
Nottingham University Hospitals NHS Trust
Nottingham, UK

Conor D. Marron
The Royal Victoria Hospital
Belfast Trust
Belfast, UK

Colin J. McKay
West of Scotland Pancreatic Unit
Glasgow Royal Infirmary
Glasgow, Scotland

Mark J. Midwinter
Professor of Military Surgery
Academic Department of Military Surgery and
Trauma
Royal Centre for Defence Medicine
Consultant Surgeon
Derriford Hospital
Plymouth, UK

A. Morris
Derriford Hospital
Plymouth, UK

Deborah Nicol
SpR General Surgery
West Midlands
Worcester, UK

Giles R. Nordmann
Specialist Registrar in Anaesthesia
Department of Military Anaesthesia
and Critical Care
Royal Centre for Defence Medicine
Birmingham, UK

Timothy C. Nunez
Department of Surgery
Division of Trauma and Emergency Surgery
Vanderbilt University Medical Center
Nashville, TN, USA

Tom Palser
Clinical Research Fellow
Royal College of Surgeons of England
London, UK

John Simpson
Lecturer in Surgery
Department of General Surgery
University Hospital
Nottingham, UK

J. Alastair D. Simpson
Academic Specialist Registrar
Nottingham University Hospital NHS Trust
Nottingham, UK

Stella R. Smith
Specialist Registrar
Department of Surgery and Anaesthesia
The Royal London Hospital
London, UK

Nigel Tai
Academic Department of Military Surgery
and Trauma
Royal Centre for Defence Medicine
Birmingham, UK

Mark Taylor
Consultant General and Hepatobiliary Surgeon
Mater Hospital
Crumlin Road
Belfast, UK

Jeff L. Tong
Reader in Anaesthesia
Department of Military Anaesthesia and
Critical Care
Royal Centre for Defence Medicine
Birmingham, UK

Igor V. Voskresensky
Department of Surgery
Division of Trauma and Emergency Surgery
Vanderbilt University Medical Center
Nashville, TN, USA

Thomas J. Walton
Specialist Registrar in Urology
Leicester General Hospital
Leicester, UK

Richard L. Wolverson
Consultant Colo-Rectal Surgeon
City Hospital Birmingham
Birmingham, UK

Paul Wood
Consultant Anaesthetist
University Hospital Birmingham
NHS Trust, Birmingham, UK

Victor Zaydfudim
General Surgery Resident
Department of Surgery
Vanderbilt University Medical Centre
Nashville, Tennessee
USA

1 Approach

1 The Initial Approach to the Emergency Surgery Patient

Adam Brooks & J. Alastair D. Simpson
Nottingham University Hospitals NHS Trust, Queen's Medical Centre Campus, Nottingham, UK

Introduction

Emergency surgical (ES) admissions in the UK are increasing. Between 1998 and 2006, there was an 18% increase in ES admissions resulting in more than half a million emergency general surgical admissions in the UK during the financial year 2005–2006. Many of these patients with relatively minor conditions were generally well and had short hospital admissions; however, a significant proportion were acutely unwell and required the full spectrum of surgical and critical care interventions and had prolonged hospital admission. In 2005–2006, there were more than 33,000 appendicectomies, more than 15,000 cases of acute pancreatitis and more than 3000 cases of diverticular perforation, taking up more than 300,000 hospital bed days. There were also a group of ES patients who were acutely unwell with sepsis and who progressed to severe sepsis and organ failure. In 2005–2006, 990 patients died of acute pancreatitis, 1671 patients died of either a perforated or bleeding duodenal ulcer and 1934 patients died of complications of diverticular disease.

Different models exist for the organisation of emergency surgery care both in the UK and internationally. Increasingly, US centres have integrated ES into the trauma service providing a single service for all acute surgical patients. In the UK, the Royal College of Surgeons of England (RCS) has long been advocating the separation of emergency and elective surgery in order to improve training and the efficiency of both work streams. Its 2007 publication 'Separating Emergency and Elective Surgical Care' contained recommendations about how services should be organised to maximise training of the future surgical workforce and, most importantly, improve patient care. Furthermore, in June 2007, the Association of Surgeons of Great Britain and Ireland (ASGBI) published a consensus document containing essential service standards. It also discussed separation of specialist services and some institutions now divide the general on call between upper and lower gastrointestinal (GI) surgeons.

Emergency Surgery, 1st edition. Edited by Adam Brooks, Peter F. Mahoney, Bryan A. Cotton and Nigel Tai. © 2010 Blackwell Publishing.

There are a wide range of conditions that present on the ES on call (Table 1.1–Table 1.2) and it is important that all emergency surgery patients are evaluated with a standard approach to avoid omissions, provide timely resuscitation, effective investigation and efficient surgical intervention.

ES patients may present through the emergency department, general practitioner surgical admission area, medical wards or as acute complications in elective patients on the surgical unit. An approach must be broad enough to be applicable in all these diverse situations. In many of these areas it is unlikely that the patient will be referred with an actual diagnosis but rather with a symptom, sign or physiological derangement.

Approach

The initial challenge in ES is to decide whether the patient is acutely unwell. With a little experience it is relatively simple to differentiate between the extremes; the patient who is comfortable, sitting up and talking, is not in extremis and a more measured approach can be adopted. Alternatively, some patients are clearly acutely unwell with significantly deranged vital signs and may have an altered level of consciousness; these patients require combined assessment and resuscitation, a coordinated approach and a greater degree of urgency. This is really an end of the bed evaluation of the airway, breathing and circulation (ABC) – as the patient who is well, talking and sitting up has an adequate ABC. Occasionally, differentiation between these extremes can be more challenging, as some early signs of impending deterioration can be subtle. It is better to fully evaluate rather than under-appreciate a patient who rapidly decompensates (Figure 1.1).

Recognition of the patient's severity of illness allows you to prioritise their clinical management, commence resuscitation, correctly focus investigations and appropriately communicate with seniors, theatres and critical care.

Within the first few minutes of meeting the ES patients, you should be able to develop a feeling of how unwell they are as well as begin to recognise patterns and non-verbal

3

Table 1.1 Emergency surgical conditions presenting to a teaching hospital.

Appendicitis	399
Obstruction	291
Pancreatitis	249
Abscess	226
Non-specific abdominal pain	225
Cholecystitis	177
Diverticulitis	167
PR bleed	157
Biliary colic	126
Trauma	98
Hernia	90
Perforation	82
Constipation	55
UTI	52
Stoma complication	42

A review of 2700 consecutive ES patients.

PR, per rectal examination; UTI, urinary tract infection.

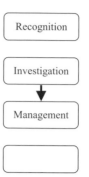

Figure 1.1 An approach to the emergency surgery patient.

signs that will assist in focusing the history, examination and investigations. For example, jaundice, fever and right upper quadrant pain would move you down a cholangitis pathway, the unwell patient who is lying rigidly on the bed with sudden onset of severe abdominal pain and a rigid abdomen suggests possible perforation and the well patient lying on their side with perianal pain is suggestive of a perineal abscess.

Resuscitation

All ES patients require some form of resuscitation, whilst this may only be intravenous (IV) fluid to replace intravascular

Table 1.2 ISCP mapping for emergency surgery.

- Manage patients presenting with an acute abdomen
  - Peritonitis
  - Acute appendicitis
  - Acute gynaecological disease
- Acute intestinal obstruction
- Manage infections of the skin including necrotising infections
- Strangulated hernia
- Manage the patient with multiple injuries
- Manage abdominal trauma
  - Especially splenic, hepatic and pancreatic injuries
- Manage perforated peptic ulcer
- Manage acute GI haemorrhage
- Manage acute HPB disease
  - Acute gallstone disease
  - Acute pancreatitis
- Recognise the acutely ischaemic limb

ISCP, Intercollegiate Surgical Curriculum Project; GI, gastrointestinal; HPB, hepato-pancreatic biliary.

losses, supplemental oxygen or appropriate analgesia, others will require full resuscitation, including airway management, central access and fluids.

Resuscitation can occur anywhere in the hospital and is not limited to the emergency room or the intensive care unit. The traditional ABC approach is tried and tested and is an appropriate pathway for the ES patient. Patients with small bowel obstruction or pancreatitis, for example, will have significant fluid losses and will require aggressive early fluid resuscitation, guided by measurement of urine output and/or central venous pressure. In the unwell or unstable patient, resuscitation must proceed at the same time as the evaluation and life-threatening conditions treated as they are discovered. It is vital to get senior help when looking after seriously ill patients and early referral to critical care and/or an outreach team will be valuable. Septic and peritonitic patients can decompensate rapidly and early involvement of critical care before surgery will be particularly valuable. The patient may need transfer to critical care before surgery for ventilatory and/or cardiovascular support. The surviving sepsis guidelines should be followed in septic patients and the sepsis care bundles commenced, however, the fundamental requirement is surgical drainage of the driving infection.

Investigations

It is important to focus the investigations towards the working diagnosis rather than to take a screening approach with the hope that a positive diagnosis will be thrown up. All investigations should be performed to either confirm or rule out the working diagnosis or as appropriate work up for anaesthesia. Investigations that do not add to the patient's care are inappropriate and add expense and can delay appropriate management. Investigations can be thought of as a ladder starting with basic urine and blood tests and progressing to advanced radiological investigations to confirm the diagnosis and plan surgery (Table 1.3).

Table 1.3 Investigations.

Urine	Blood	Radiology
Urobilinogen	Full blood count	Chest X-ray
White cells	Urea	Abdominal X-ray
Red cells	Electrolytes	Ultrasound
Microscopy and culture	Liver function tests	CT
	CRP	MRI
	Group and save	
	Cross match	

CRP, C-reactive protein; CT, computed tomography; MRI, magnetic resonance imaging.

Initial management

At each point in the patient's care pathway it is important to reassess the patient and if required to revise the management plan in light of changes in their physiological condition.

At each stage it is important to ask yourself the following questions:

Does the patient require?
- Further investigation
- Further resuscitation
- A different treatment strategy (conservative or surgical)

A management plan needs to be made on every ES patient and documented as well as discussed with your seniors and all those involved in the patient's care. This may be as simple as

Diagnosis	– Abdominal wall abscess
Plan	– Incision and drainage of abscess today
	– Nil by mouth until surgery
	– Analgesia

At other times the plan may be more complex and involved, e.g.

Diagnosis	– Acute severe pancreatitis
	– Severe sepsis and respiratory compromise
Plan	– Urgent referral/transfer to critical care
	– High flow oxygen
	– Arterial blood gases
	– Pancreatitis prognostic scoring
	– Full septic screen and cultures
	– Analgesia
	– IV fluid resuscitation
	– Urinary catheter – maintain urine output 0.5 mL/kg/hour

At each stage and after each set of investigations the plan needs to be revised and updated in the notes and changes communicated to staff.

Keep your seniors involved early and frequently. Do not be reluctant to ask for help. When talking to seniors make sure that you are clear and concise and that you know what you want to get out of the conversation. If it is simply to keep them informed tell them that; if you want them to come to assess the patient and help you, tell them directly.

Operative management

A significant proportion of ES patients will require surgical intervention to address their underlying pathology. The choice of procedure depends on a number of factors including the pathology, the skill set of the surgeons and equipment. It is important to ensure that a preoperative/pre-anaesthesia work up has been performed and the case discussed with the anaesthetists. Surgical issues in the preoperative period that need to be addressed include consent, marking of the operative side and stomas, informing the theatre coordinator of the procedure and urgency of the case and liaising with critical care regarding pre- and postoperative care.

Summary

Emergency surgery is an acute speciality where decisions often need to be made urgently. Information needs to be gathered quickly and appropriate management started. A standard approach to ES patients provides a framework upon which to base resuscitation, investigations and management decisions.

Communication is a key part of the ES approach as many people in numerous departments are involved in the acute management of these patients (Figure 1.2).

The chapters that follow in this book address the common diagnoses in ES and trauma. We hope that they will guide trainees in the assessment and management of these patients.

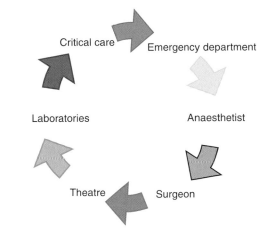

Figure 1.2 People involved in the acute care of the ES patient.

Preoperative Considerations

Paul Wood

University Hospital Birmingham, NHS Trust, Birmingham, UK

Introduction

This book considers emergency surgery and depending on the urgency of the situation, some of the considerations may become the responsibility of the operating theatre team. In particular, resuscitation will often need to be contemporaneous with surgery.

Your main responsibilities are:

1 Patient's history and physical examination.

2 Performing basic laboratory and clinical investigations as determined by the patient's medical history and current diagnosis.

3 Where necessary, initiating perioperative medical treatment including prescribing intravenous (IV) fluids and the patient's own medication when required.

4 To act as a coordinator between the various parties involved in the patient's overall care – this includes the theatre team and any other involved medical specialities.

5 Patient consent and listing of the patient on the appropriate theatre list.

6 Liaison with the high dependency or critical care units if these will be necessary postoperatively.

The preoperative pathway is described in Figure 2.1.

Clinical presentation

The medical preparation of a patient for an elective surgical procedure involves identifying actual or potential medical co-morbidity and where possible improvement before surgery. In a limb- or life-threatening emergency, these aims are often unachievable.

After taking a history and performing a physical examination, it is necessary to consider what is the potential impact of the patient's history and physiological condition on their subsequent surgical course and what further tests or investigations (if any) are required?

The essential purpose of any investigation is to identify and quantify physiological abnormality from which the patient can benefit by perioperative medical intervention.

Cardiovascular disease

In the Western world, ischaemic heart disease is common. Routine enquiry about the frequency of recent angina attacks and the response to the patient's usual treatment must be backed up with a 12-lead electrocardiogram (ECG). Patients at particular risk include those complaining of increasing frequency/severity of angina, and those who have sustained a recent (within 6 weeks) myocardial infarction.

Cardiac failure is also not unusual. The clinical history and examination should establish that this is well controlled. If not, unless the patient has a life- or limb-threatening surgical illness they present an unacceptable operative risk until modified by urgent medical treatment. If surgery is inevitable, postoperative admission to a critical care unit is likely. In these cases the intensive care team should be involved as early as possible. The potential morbidity associated with cardiac failure and ischaemic heart disease is easily appreciated by examining the relative risks given to various preoperative risk factors in Goldman's landmark study (Table 2.1).

A history or finding of an arrhythmia requires an ECG. Atrial fibrillation is a common problem in the elderly and a rapid uncontrolled rate needs correction prior to any non-emergency surgery.

Patients with valvular abnormalities are frequently aware that they 'have a murmur' and their old medical notes may document the cause and subsequent management. Beware of any new murmur found in patients aged 60 years or over – particularly so if the physical signs suggest *aortic stenosis*. Request for an anaesthetic review, following which surgery may well be delayed while echocardiography and/or a cardiology opinion is obtained.

Note any history of syncope, seizures or repeated falls. Such patients may have a bradycardia and any clinical

Emergency Surgery, 1st edition. Edited by Adam Brooks, Peter F. Mahoney, Bryan A. Cotton and Nigel Tai. © 2010 Blackwell Publishing.

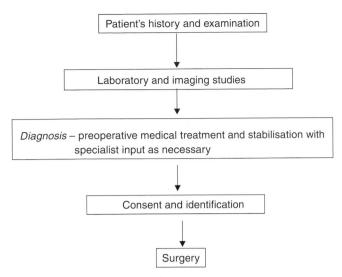

Figure 2.1 The preoperative pathway.

diagnosis must be supported by an ECG as some uncommon conduction defects will need cardiological intervention before surgery.

Unlike elective surgery, patients with undiagnosed or poorly controlled hypertension cannot be deferred for treatment. Recognise that pain and anxiety may be a factor. Measure the blood pressure in both arms, note any other cardiac risk factors and obtain an ECG.

The patient with a pacemaker

Most patients will be able to confirm that their pacemaker function is optimal and they may have details of the indications for pacing and the type of pacemaker. It is essential to perform a 12-lead ECG, chest X-ray (CXR) and attempt to obtain the relevant old notes. Ensure that the responsible anaesthetist and operating surgeon are aware of and annotate the patient's theatre listing with the phrase 'pacemaker in situ'.

Some of the modern pacemakers have a dual function as implantable defibrillators. These devices must be inactivated before surgery and then reactivated as soon as possible thereafter. This process normally requires the presence of a cardiology technician during the operative period, so an urgent cardiological opinion is mandatory.

Respiratory disease

Patients with chronic obstructive pulmonary disease (COPD) are frequent in the older population while younger patients with asthma are also not uncommon.

COPD patients can often be improved by attention to nebulised therapy and treating of any coexistent chest infection. A CXR will usually be required to ensure that a pneumothorax or pleural effusion is not present. In addition to the routine investigations assessment of these patients usually includes measurement of arterial blood gases (take the sample while the patient breathes room air).

Bronchospasm during general anaesthesia is potentially lethal and ideally before general anaesthesia the patient's condition needs to be at their personal best. Always enquire specifically about asthma as it is remarkable that many stable asthmatic patients do not regard themselves as having a medical condition. Conversely, in severe cases enquire specifically about current or recent steroid use. In patients describing recent deterioration there should be a low threshold for requesting a CXR as 'not all that wheezes is asthma'.

While the possible need for CXR and arterial blood gases have been stressed, note that in the acute setting formal assessment of lung function with spirometry or other techniques is rarely necessary. Also, note that with the exception of the oxygen partial pressure a venous blood gas will closely correspond to an arterial sample – thus it provides valuable information.

Table 2.2 lists preoperative features which are associated with postoperative respiratory failure in non-cardiac surgery.

Table 2.1 Cardiovascular risk factors – the Goldman index.

Risk factor and score
Third heart sound (11)
Elevated JVP (11)
Myocardial infarct in past 6 months (10)
ECG – ventricular ectopic activity or non-sinus rhythm (7)
Age >70 years (5)
Emergency procedure (4)
Intra-thoracic, intra-abdominal or aortic surgery (3)
Poor general status (3)

Patients with scores >25 had a 56% incidence of death, and a 22% incidence of cardiovascular complications.

Table 2.2 Risk factors for postoperative respiratory complications.

Old age >65 years
ASA class >II
Raised creatinine
Cachexia
Albumin <35 g/L
COPD and smoking
Cardiac failure
Reduced conscious level
Emergency surgery
Upper abdominal surgery and vascular surgery
General anaesthesia

Renal disease

Patients with vascular emergencies, not infrequently, have chronic renal impairment and should be closely monitored by the renal physicians. In patients who retain some degree of native renal function, it is imperative to maintain normotension.

Patients may have a restricted fluid intake but prolonged preoperative starvation is potentially harmful, and preoperatively IV fluids may be necessary. Remember to adjust or exclude doses of any drugs that are either nephrotoxic or largely renally excreted. Occasionally, dialysis-dependent patients may be referred for a general or vascular surgery opinion. If required, surgery will occur following optimisation of their renal condition and post-surgery they will return to the renal unit for continuing dialysis.

Ensure that you are central in all communication about the patient's preoperative preparation and be ready to discuss the case with the anaesthetist – make sure that you know the patient's target weight and their post-dialysis haemoglobin and potassium.

Endocrine disease

In practical terms, most often, this means being certain that steroid-dependent patients receive adequate dosage in the acute perioperative period than the management of diabetic patients.

Neurology

Patients may present with neurological deficits because of previous injury, or a medical condition. The extent of any problem needs careful documentation to alert the operating team to any regions of the body that require particular attention during general anaesthesia. Preoperative documentation also allows for comparison in the event that any postoperative neurological deterioration is attributed (correctly or otherwise) to the effects of surgery or anaesthesia.

Pregnancy

Pregnancy is a differential diagnosis in some acute abdominal emergencies. In these cases sensitive enquiry should be made as to the possibility of conception. If there is doubt, the woman should be advised to consent to a pregnancy test, particularly if there is a possibility of anaesthesia or exposure to X-rays.

Occasionally, surgery is necessary in a patient who is known to be pregnant. The anaesthetist should be informed as early as possible and depending on the stage of pregnancy obstetric advice should also be sought in respect of perioperative foetal monitoring.

Previous anaesthesia

Enquiries about previous surgery and anaesthesia may elicit a variety of responses but in the context of emergency surgery two special points to be noted are:

1 Suxamethonium apnoea is a prolonged paralysis following a single dose of the otherwise short-acting muscle relaxant suxamethonium. The patient or a family member may have experienced this problem, which is particularly relevant to patients who are not starved. Annotate the patient's notes and inform the anaesthetist at the earliest opportunity.
2 Rarely the patient may offer a history of a relative who died or nearly died following general anaesthesia for minor surgery. Several explanations are possible including the very rare malignant hyperpyrexia. In the emergency setting, there is little time for investigation – as soon as possible personally inform the anaesthetist who is responsible for this patient and in the meanwhile make determined efforts to obtain any hospital notes relevant to the incident in question.

Latex allergy

Allergy to the proteins found in natural rubber latex (NRL) seems increasingly common and is not infrequently claimed by patients despite repeated and uneventful surgical procedures. Once declared, you need to inform the ward nursing staff, the operating surgeon and the theatre team. If you are writing the operating list make sure that the patient's sensitivity is documented.

Routine clinical investigations

The baseline investigations are as follows: urinalysis, the measurement of haemoglobin, urea and electrolyte, a 12-lead ECG and plain CXR. In the UK, the National Institute for Clinical Excellence (NICE) has produced exhaustive recommendations for preoperative testing based upon these four investigations and the patients' fitness and grade of surgery. Other bodies such as the UK Royal College of Radiologists have published their own guidelines on preoperative CXRs.

Your own institution may have in-house protocols for specific surgical specialities and procedures but fixed recommendations can never deal with every situation and particularly so with emergency surgery. Investigations must be matched to the patient's history, current physiological status and the scope of the proposed surgical procedure.

Note that:
1 Patients receiving digoxin or thiazide diuretic therapy must have their electrolytes checked – significant hyponatraemia and hypokalaemia are unacceptable prior to surgery.
2 Patients who have had recent major surgery may be anaemic.
3 The sickle-cell status should be checked in any patient originating from Afro-Caribbean, African and Mediterranean areas. The homozygous state is sickle-cell disease and these patients would have an established medical history. Of more practical importance is the heterozygous trait which is not infrequent. Hypoxia and hypotension can precipitate an ischaemic crisis in these patients.
4 Arterial blood gas analysis is usually necessary in patients with significant respiratory problems.

Blood transfusion

Blood is a valuable resource and your hospital should have an MSBOS (maximum surgical blood order schedule) protocol which attempts to match the surgical procedure and the number of units of concentrated red cells needed. As discussed above, such protocols cannot fully anticipate requirements in the emergency setting. If in doubt about the need for blood or the amount required then ask.

Be clear that a group and save (identifying the patients ABO blood group/Rhesus type and testing the sample for red cell antibodies) and an actual cross match (preparing units of compatible blood ready for that patient) are two distinct stages in the pathway to transfusion. A group and save should be requested for all patients undergoing emergency surgery.

Analysis of critical incidents during blood transfusion reveals the commonest problem occurs because the 'wrong unit of blood is given to the wrong patient'. It is essential to avoid mis-identification of samples. When withdrawing blood, take the sample tube and request forms to the patient's bedside. Ensure that sample tube and request form are completely and properly labelled (for the sample tube always do this by hand and preferably likewise for the form). The patient's full name and date of birth must be confirmed by checking their identity wristband.

Concurrent medication

Patients with chronic medical conditions are invariably receiving medication. Drugs can interact with anaesthesia and surgery in various ways. Your responsibility is to document the patient's medication on admission and record any declared allergies. In certain cases ensuring accurate information will require contact with the patient's general practitioner. With elective surgery it is a usual practice to initially prescribe the patient's normal regime and then make any subsequent adjustments or omissions according to perioperative needs. In emergency surgery the situation can be very different – you should be aware of the following:

1 Failure to absorb oral medication because of vomiting related to the surgical condition – this may have been happening for some time preadmission. This may increase the risks to patients with drug-dependent medical conditions.

2 Those drugs which should be maintained throughout the perioperative period with the normal dose and those which will require increased doses during any period of physiological or surgical stress – in particular steroids and insulin. These considerations may include the need for IV administration to achieve the therapeutic effect (see below).

3 The recognition of drugs whose action needs to be minimised or reversed during the perioperative period. This relates specifically to drugs given for anticoagulation and particularly to warfarin whose therapeutic effect (as measured by clotting studies) is often initially exacerbated during any acute illness.

Cardiovascular medication

There is no universal agreement as to the need to maintain antihypertensive drugs in the perioperative period but many clinicians will insist that strict control should be maintained. There is considerable evidence that beta-blockers can protect against cardiac ischaemia and for this reason some anaesthetists will occasionally prescribe them before operation.

The reduced plasma volume of the starved or hypovolaemic patient means that diuretics and/or ACE inhibitors/angiotensin receptor antagonists may be omitted before surgery. The anaesthetist will often direct such choices.

Control of angina in any acute medical situation is important and nitrates and calcium channel blockers should not be omitted. If the patient has a glyceryl trinitrate spray it should accompany them to theatre. Anti-arrhythmia treatment should **not** be withheld.

It may also be sensible for the patient to take any prescribed statins as there is increasing evidence that they have a cardioprotective effect.

The patient on long-term warfarin

Patients with valvular heart disease, atrial fibrillation or who have suffered a recent (within the last 6 months) thromboembolic event may take warfarin. A daily maintenance dose of 3–9 mg is adjusted by monitoring the International Normalised Ratio (INR). The patients' target INR will reflect their underlying condition and normally range between 2.0 and 3.5.

Warfarin is long acting and also interacts with many drugs; hence, the usual practice during the perioperative period is to change the warfarin to shorter acting alternatives. Prior to emergency surgery this is done in a controlled fashion often including substitution with heparin. In the emergency situation there is no time for such considerations and the problem may be exacerbated in an acutely ill patient by the INR being significantly elevated.

It may be necessary to:

1 Initially reverse the action of warfarin with IV vitamin K (1 mg).

2 Provide additional cover with fresh frozen plasma (initial dose, 10–15 mL/kg) and/or further doses of vitamin K.

Delaying surgery, where possible, for 12–24 hours will increase the effectiveness of these measures and allow the INR to be monitored but the management throughout the perioperative period will often require supervision by a haematologist. Beriplex® is another means of reversing warfarin anticoagulation – seek haematology advice.

Clopidogrel

This drug inhibits platelet aggregation and is in increasing use by physicians to manage various ischaemic vascular

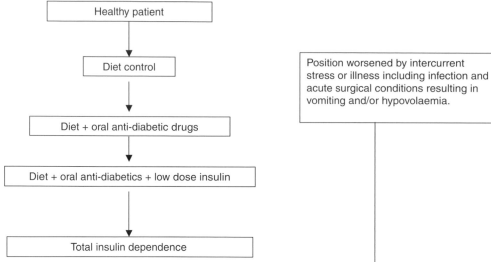

Figure 2.2 The surgical diabetic ladder.

conditions including thromboprophylaxis in coronary stents. Once discontinued, its anti-platelet effects continue for 24 hours. Surgery undertaken in the presence of clopidogrel can be associated with significant bleeding.

In the emergency situation the possibility of haemorrhage may be minimised by delaying surgery, if possible, for 24 hours. In elective surgery the British National Formulary (BNF) recommends discontinuing 7 days before hand if possible.

The complicating factor is often those patients with coronary stents – here the overall perioperative risks must be considered by the type of stent (drug eluting stents require longer treatment), the insertion – surgery interval and the stent location (proximal versus distal). These patients should be discussed with a cardiologist before surgery.

Respiratory medication
Patients should use their usual inhalers as normal to minimise the potential hazards of bronchospasm. If they are currently experiencing a worsening of their condition the same drugs (or alternative bronchodilator) may need to be prescribed in nebulised form as part of the preoperative preparation. Inhalers should also accompany the patient to theatre.

The diabetic patient
Diabetes mellitus results from a lack of insulin or from resistance to its action. In pathological terms diabetes is a vascular disease and this is reflected in many of its complications. Strict perioperative control of blood sugar reduces the risk of acute problems including infection.

Traditionally diabetic patients are classified as:
1 Insulin-dependent diabetes mellitus (IDDM) = type 1. These patients will take regular sub-cutaneous injections of insulin which will be prescribed in combinations of short- and medium/long-action preparations. The choice of insulin and the exact dosing regime will depend upon the patient.
2 Non-insulin-dependent diabetes mellitus (NIDDM) = type 2. These patients are managed by a combination of diet or diet and oral hypoglycaemics.

Diabetes and surgery
Any intercurrent illness will worsen diabetic control – the greater the physiological stress the larger the disturbance in sugar homeostasis (Figure 2.2). Surgery and anaesthesia cause a neuroendocrine stress response which further raises blood glucose.

In elective surgery the perioperative management of diabetes is dictated both by the nature of the surgery and by the patient's normal diabetic control including the period of preoperative starvation. Paradoxically, in emergency surgery the situation in some cases is simplified. This is because aside from the most trivial conditions, strict control of blood sugar in both type 1 and type 2 diabetics will invariably require an IV insulin infusion.

Sliding scale insulin
The principle here is that the patient is managed throughout the perioperative period by an IV infusion of 5% dextrose and short acting insulin until such time as their general medical condition permits them to return to their normal management. The infusions are started preoperatively and monitored by regular blood glucose measurements, aiming to maintain a blood glucose of 6–9 mmol/L. If the patient's blood glucose at the time of admission is in excess of 15 mmol/L then normal saline is initially substituted for 5% dextrose.

All hospitals should have protocols for initiating and managing sliding scale regimes including guidance on what actions to be taken in the event of hypoglycaemia or persistent hyperglycaemia, but you should note the following:

1 The infusion rates prescribed by the sliding scale protocol may need to be increased by up to 2–4 times in sick patients – this includes some steroid-dependent patients.

2 IV insulin decreases serum potassium which needs to be monitored. The sliding scale protocol should contain instructions for potassium supplementation. Be particularly aware of those patients who take diuretics.

Steroids

Any acute surgical condition and its associated physiological stress will increase the requirements of a steroid-dependent patient. When oral intake is not possible or uncertain the drug must be given intravenously. Any higher dosage must be maintained until the patient's recovery is established.

Guidance on suitable doses of perioperative corticosteroids can be found in the British National Formulary – in difficult cases the advice of a physician may be necessary.

Premedication and other drugs

The delivery of thyroxine (hypothyroidism), anti-epileptics and anti-Parkinson medication should also be consistent in the perioperative period.

If uncertain, always take advice from the anaesthetist as to which of the patient's usual medical therapy to stop or continue – otherwise, apart from analgesia do not prescribe any premedication unless instructed.

Analgesia

Pain is a symptom of many acute surgical conditions. Its treatment is important for humanitarian and physiological reasons. Various objective scales can be used to assess the degree of pain but in the final analysis pain is 'what the patient says it is'.

Modern treatment of pain emphasises the need to interrupt the pain mechanism at various anatomical levels between the site of 'injury' and its final perception in the cerebral cortex. Such an approach relies on combining different analgesic drugs and techniques of administration.

Analgesics can be given by a variety of routes but oral, intramuscular, rectal and sublingual are the standard routes of administration. The IV route is the most important analgesic strategy in the preoperative period as it is the most direct method of control, avoiding most of the disadvantages associated with the other routes of administration.

It is used in three ways:

1 By bolus injection of morphine or by a synthetic opiate: This is given in small divided doses until initial control of acute pain has been achieved. In the emergency setting this should be considered the gold standard of analgesia for general and vascular surgery.

2 By patient-controlled analgesia (PCA): This is an apparatus which affords continuation of the benefit achieved by bolus injection. The patient injects themselves directly into a vein from a reservoir of opiate. The drug cassette is programmed to deliver a fixed dose within a prescribed time so the patient cannot inject themselves indiscriminately. Such apparatus can be very useful if the patient's surgery is to be delayed. Morphine is the standard PCA opiate.

3 Bolus and fixed dosing of non-opiate analgesics are usually given orally and may also be given intravenously, e.g. paracetamol.

It is always necessary to prescribe an anti-emetic when opiates are used because of the possibility of nausea and vomiting.

The role of simple non-opiate analgesics is important but in the emergency setting their usefulness (paracetamol aside) can be limited. For instance, the otherwise excellent non-steroidal anti-inflammatory drugs (e.g. diclofenac and ibuprofen) are associated with gastrointestinal irritation and the possibility of exacerbating haemorrhage and renal dysfunction.

Fasting and IV fluids

In elective surgery the need for patients to be starved prior to general anaesthesia is a fundamental consideration in preoperative planning. In life- or limb-threatening injuries, this 'rule' is bypassed and it is the responsibility of the anaesthetist to manage the situation. In practice, many emergencies are in fact 'urgencies' and for various reasons such patients may experience variable delays before arriving in the operating theatre. For this reason, you must remain aware of the following considerations:

1 Fasting periods for elective surgery are historically based on studies of gastric emptying and pH. The accepted 'nil by mouth' period for elective patients has decreased – the accepted general guidelines are:

Food – 6 hours and clear fluids – 2 hours.

Clear fluids are non-particulate and include water, apple juice and tea without milk. 'Sips' of water should be allowed closer to the operation as may small quantities of water to take any essential medications with.

2 Patients without a surgical condition causing intestinal obstruction may still be at risk of aspiration of gastric contents. Obesity, hiatus hernia or diabetes can influence the mechanics of gastric emptying or promote oesophageal reflux and opiates given for pain relief will also slow gastric emptying.

3 Attempts to match a patient's period of starvation against the likely time of surgery are doomed to failure. When this is attempted, unforeseen events invariably result in patients coming to the operating theatre unnecessarily dehydrated. Surgical considerations aside it is good practice to establish a crystalloid infusion during the interim period.

Table 2.3 Composition of a 1L bag of common crystalloid solutions.

	0.9% saline (normal saline)	Hartmann's solution (lactated ringers)	0.18% saline + 4% dextrose (dextrose saline)	5% dextrose
Water (L)	l	1	1	1
Na$^+$ (mmol)	150	130	30	
Cl$^-$ (mmol)	150	109	30	
K$^+$ (mmol)		4		
Ca^{2+} (mmol)		1.5		
Lactate (mmol)		28		
Glucose (g)			40	50

Routine preoperative fluid requirements will usually be supplied with isotonic crystalloids which are aqueous solutions of electrolytes or other water-soluble molecules that are isotonic with plasma. The usual choices are 0.9% saline and lactated Ringer's (Hartmann's) solution (Table 2.3).

The choice of maintenance of IV fluid and the volume and rate of the replacement must be considered – careful correction of perioperative dehydration and electrolyte imbalance is not the same exercise as rapid volume restoration in resuscitation.

The formula will vary according to the surgical condition but the maintenance fluid prescription for adults should equal the:

normal daily requirement (1.5 mL/kg/hour) + extra insensible losses + electrolyte requirements.

Pay careful attention to patients taking diuretics. These drugs cause sodium and potassium loss in the urine which is easily worsened by using the incorrect fluid for replacement therapy – in particular, do not routinely prescribe 5% dextrose in large volumes.

In elderly patients respect both the body weight and rate of infusion as it is otherwise easy to precipitate acute heart failure. A controlled rate of blood transfusion preoperatively in an elderly patient also means that the practice of 'covering' the transfusion with diuretics is unnecessary.

Consent and identification for surgery

By definition obtaining informed consent for any operative procedure requires a wide knowledge of the surgery and should be the duty of the operating surgeon. However, listing the patient for surgery is likely to be your responsibility and you must be clear as to safe practice.

A properly constructed theatre listing requires that:
1 Printed operating schedules identify both the surgeon responsible for care and the surgeon(s) operating on the patient.

2 Every patient on the operating list should be named fully and identified with a unit number and date of birth.
3 Should two patients on the same list have the same name – this must be made explicit e.g. 'WARNING: TWO PATIENTS ON THE LIST WITH SAME SURNAME'.
4 The procedure the patient is consented for and that written on the operating list should be identical.
5 Operative descriptions should be comprehensive, unambiguous and devoid of abbreviations. In particular, Right and Left must be written as such – not R or L.
6 If a limb is involved it must be marked. In bilateral limb operations involving different procedures the limbs should be annotated.
7 You should not change a submitted list once operation has begun without first informing the operating surgeon, anaesthetist and the appropriate theatre team.

Summary

The extent to which any of the above points is necessary or fully completed prior to surgery will be dictated by the nature of the surgical problem.

Once the patient is undergoing surgery you should continue to follow through and communicate with your own surgical team and others in respect of outstanding results and postoperative care.

The essentials of preoperative preparation are:
1 Patient's history and physical examination documented.
2 Investigations taken and results where available recorded.
3 A 12-lead ECG.
4 Referral made to other specialties as required.
5 Postoperative placement considered – HDU/ITU.
6 Medication – oxygen and analgesia.
7 IV fluids/infusions – running as intended.
8 Catheterised?
9 Blood cross-matched OR group and save as required.
10 Patient consent and where relevant limbs marked and/or annotated.
11 Radiological imaging bundled with patient notes.

Further reading

Arozullah AM, Khuri SF, Henderson WG, Daley J, for Participants in the National Veterans Affairs Surgical Quality Improvement Program. Postoperative pneumonia risk index: multifactorial risk index for post op pneumonia. *Ann Intern Med* 2001;**135**:847–857.

Goldman L, Caldera DL, Nussbaum SR. Multifactorial index of cardiac risk in noncardiac surgical procedures. *N Engl J Med* 1977;**297**:845–850.

McAlister FA, Khan NA, Straus SE, et al. Accuracy of the preoperative assessment in predicting pulmonary risk after nonthoracic surgery. *Am J Repir Crit Care Med* 2003;**167**:741–744.

Smetana GW, Lawrence VA, Cornell JE. Preoperative pulmonary risk stratification for noncardiothoracic surgery: systematic review for the American College of Physicians. *Ann Intern Med* 2006;**144**:581–595.

Emergency Anaesthesia

Giles R. Nordmann

Department of Military Anaesthesia and Critical Care, Royal Centre for Defence Medicine, Birmingham, UK

Introduction

In elective surgery, patients are usually in optimal physical and mental health; any medical disorders are identified and treated; a definitive surgical diagnosis is made and an appropriate period of starvation has occurred.

In emergency surgery, however, one or more of these conditions may not be met. They may have an uncertain diagnosis in conjunction with uncontrolled coexisting medical disease with related cardiovascular, respiratory, renal and metabolic abnormalities in addition to the presence of:

- Haemorrhage
- Hypovolaemia
- Abnormal electrolytes
- Pain

The key factor in the practice of emergency anaesthesia is a thorough preoperative assessment and to be prepared for all potential complications including vomiting, dehydration, haemorrhage and atypical drug reactions in the face of electrolyte disorders.

Preoperative assessment

The success of minimising the risk to the patient from emergency surgery is a thorough preoperative assessment of the patient.

History and examination

A full medical and drug history is taken with emphasis on assessing the patient's cardiorespiratory reserve and in particular the existence of angina, orthopnoea, dyspnoea and a productive cough. The presence of these in the patient should elicit further detailed enquiry into, and examination of, their cardiovascular and respiratory systems and with the

Emergency Surgery, 1st edition. Edited by Adam Brooks, Peter F. Mahoney, Bryan A. Cotton and Nigel Tai. © 2010 Blackwell Publishing.

assistance of pertinent investigations their premorbid physiological reserve should be assessed.

Assessment of airway

It is important to take an anaesthetic history and evaluate the patient's airway particularly if a rapid sequence induction (RSI) is to be carried out. A difficult view at laryngoscopy is suggested by the presence of limited mouth opening, prominent incisors and poor atlanto-occipital joint movement; however, there is no specific test for estimating the ease of intubation after induction of anaesthesia. As part of the examination, two airway assessment tests (shown in Box 3.1) undertaken in conjunction with each other predict 80% of difficult intubation scenarios (see Figure 3.1).

Hypovolaemia

Diminution of the sympathetic nervous system occurs with general or regional anaesthesia. The resultant loss in vascular tone of both arteriolar and venous systems can lead to circulatory collapse and cardiac arrest on induction of anaesthesia when undertaken in the presence of significant unrecognised hypovolaemia. If the surgical condition leads to significant fluid loss or haemorrhage, the patient requires an assessment of their losses and deficits that need to be addressed.

Blood loss

Clinical examination in conjunction with history and measured losses will assist the assessment of the patient's circulatory status. Throughout the spectrum of the response to haemorrhage, heart rate, arterial pulse pressure and central venous pressure are useful indicators. Assessment of cardiac output and tissue flow, however, is more difficult.

Although it is relatively easy to recognise the effects of profound shock, the early manifestations (tachycardia and peripheral vasoconstriction) are more difficult to recognise. End-organ perfusion can assist in this assessment process and the clinical evaluation of urine output and peripheral circulation are important.

The classic division of grade of shock is further polluted by the differing physiological reactions of different age groups

Box 3.1 Difficult laryngoscopy view prediction tests

- Mallampati scoring
  - Assessment of visibility of soft palate and uvula on mouth opening with tongue protruded
  - Scored 1 to 4
  - The significant scores are that of 3 or 4 and mean only the soft and hard palate are visible
- Thyromental distance
  - Measurement of length between superior notch of the thyroid cartilage and the mental protuberance of the mandible
  - The threshold is 6.5 cm
  - A distance less than this is significant
- A poor view at direct laryngoscopy is predicted with 80% accuracy if there is a Mallampati score of 3 or more in addition to a thyromental distance of less than 6.5 cm

to haemorrhage. Very young children have an undeveloped sympathetic nervous system rendering them unable to influence blood pressure and flow significantly. In addition to a fixed stroke volume, tachycardia is their only response. Young fit adults can mount such a significant compensatory

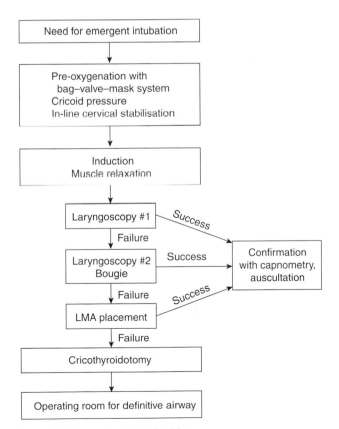

Figure 3.1 Emergency airway algorithm.

response that blood pressure may only be affected after there is a loss of a third of the patient's blood volume. In contrast, elderly patients have a limited cardiac reserve and with a relatively fixed vascular tree, signs of severe shock can become evident after a loss of only 10% of blood volume.

Normally clinical signs occur after 20% blood loss (1000 mL in an adult) and the classical signs of tachycardia, hypotension, oliguria and peripheral vasoconstriction occur after 30% blood loss. A 2 L blood loss will lead to cerebral manifestations, agitation and restlessness leading to loss of consciousness.

Massive blood loss particularly in a trauma situation can be exacerbated by the presence of hypothermia and acidosis, both of which lead to a significant coagulopathy. This is worsened by further dilution of coagulation factors from crystalloid/colloid fluid resuscitation or blood transfusion without the use of coagulation products.

Extracellular fluid loss

Estimation of the quantity of fluid loss from the extracellular space is difficult and there may be a significant deficit before there are any signs or symptoms elicited. A high degree of suspicion should be maintained in the patient with any emergent surgical condition and this would be supported by a number of factors:

- Surgical condition, e.g. bowel obstruction
- Duration of starvation, i.e. diminished fluid intake
- Evidence of further fluid loss, e.g. diarrhoea or vomiting

A history and examination can provide further evidence and the commonest symptoms and signs are detailed in Box 3.2. Of note is the fact that almost 3 L of fluid needs to be lost before clinical signs become apparent.

Orthostatic hypotension is a potent indicator of incomplete resuscitation and particularly important for induction of anaesthesia in this state without resuscitation will lead to significant hypotension.

In addition to haemoconcentration (increased haemoglobin concentration and packed cell volume), other laboratory results will help confirm the diagnosis of extracellular fluid loss. With worsening dehydration, diminished renal blood flow will lead to a rise in blood urea as less is cleared and this would be out of proportion to any elevation in creatinine.

Electrolyte disturbance

Caused by both concurrent medications and co-morbidities, and amplified by fluid loss from the surgical condition the presence of electrolyte disturbances are common. Potassium and magnesium deficiencies are the most prevalent and can have significant consequences as shown in Box 3.3. In addition, abnormalities of acid–base balance can be caused directly by the surgical condition (metabolic acidosis secondary to fluid loss or bowel ischaemia) and indirectly (abdominal pain decreasing respiratory effort and ability to

---

Box 3.2 Signs/symptoms of extracellular fluid loss

- Mild 3000 mL loss
  - Thirst
  - Reduced skin elasticity
  - Dry tongue
- Mild 4000 mL loss
  - Nausea
  - Apathy
  - Oliguria
  - Orthostatic hypotension
  - Haemoconcentration
  - Low CVP
- Moderate 5000 mL loss
  - Hypotension
  - Diminished pulse
  - Cool peripheries
- Severe 7000 mL loss
  - Coma
  - Shock
  - Death

---

compensate for metabolic acidosis). Significant electrolyte abnormalities should trigger an early move to initiate resuscitation in a critical care environment.

Resuscitation

Once the extent of blood loss or fluid loss has been estimated, it is preferable for correction and resuscitation to occur prior to surgery. An isotonic solution such as Hartmann's solution (compound sodium lactate) will equilibrate to remain predominantly in the extracellular space and is the fluid of choice for replacing fluid loss here. Anaemia or blood loss is treated preferably by blood transfusion, if nec-

---

Box 3.3 Signs/symptoms of hypokalaemia

- Muscle weakness/hypotonia
- Cramps
- Tetany
- Cardiac arrhythmias
- ECG
  - Small/inverted T waves
  - Prominent U waves
  - Prolonged P-R interval
  - Depressed ST segment

---

essary preoperative optimisation should be undertaken in a critical care scenario.

Timing of surgery

On the basis of a thorough preoperative assessment and with the results of relevant investigations, a decision can be made about the appropriate time to operate in view of the extent of resuscitation required. There are a few life-threatening conditions that need immediate surgery. The vast majority of patients benefit from correction of both hypovolaemia and electrolyte abnormalities and the stabilisation of medical problems. The optimal time to operate is when all fluid deficits have been corrected, but if urgent requirements for surgery exist a compromise is necessary.

Anaesthetic conduct

Aspiration

In emergency surgery, any fasting time regimes are unreliable and all emergent patients should be treated as having a full stomach. As such they are at risk of vomiting, regurgitation and aspiration, the commonest hazards of emergency anaesthesia.

Vomiting occurs in lighter planes of anaesthesia at induction or emergence. It is an active process and causes spasm of the vocal cords (laryngospasm) preventing material entering the larynx. This safety reflex allows the anaesthetist's time to clear the pharynx of vomitus before respiration resumes. In contrast, regurgitation is a passive and 'silent' (the anaesthetist is unaware) process that can occur at any time but is more usual during deeper planes of anaesthesia.

If aspiration occurs the respiratory sequelae that result can range from minor pulmonary impairment to acute respiratory distress syndrome (ARDS). Three different mechanisms are involved: physical airway obstruction from particulates, a chemical pneumonitis from the acidic material and bacterial contamination. Treatment includes suctioning the trachea with or without the need for bronchoscopy, oxygen and continued ventilation to treat hypoxia with the possible addition of antibiotics. Postoperative admission to critical care with continued ventilation and daily physiotherapy is not unusual particularly in the face of ARDS.

Elective surgery has specified starvation times of 6 hours for solids to minimise the chances of such sequelae. In emergency surgery, however, various mechanisms affect the normal gastrointestinal physiology and validity of normal starvation times (Box 3.4).

In patients with an acute abdomen or trauma it is prudent to assume that they have a full stomach. A 6-hour fasting is unreliable and commonly inadequate as it is not uncommon in these situations to encounter vomiting 24 hours after the

---

Box 3.4 Influences on starvation times

- Timing of surgery cannot be delayed
- Lower oesophageal sphincter tone diminished by drugs (e.g. opioids and alcohol)
- Gastric emptying delayed by:
  - Abdominal pathology (e.g. trauma, ileus, obstruction and peritonitis)
  - Drugs (e.g. opioids, anticholinergics and alcohol)
  - Fear, anxiety and pain
  - Pregnancy

Box 3.5 RSI basic requirements

- At least one skilled assistant
- Tipping trolley
- Suction apparatus working, left on and within easy reach of the anaesthetist – commonly positioned under the patient's pillow
- Patient in correct position – supine with head in the classic 'sniffing position'
- All drugs ready and labelled
- IV fluids connected and infusing
- Range of sizes of endotracheal tubes available
- Spare laryngoscope and laryngoscope blades
- Ancillary intubation aids including:
  - Gum elastic bougie
  - Stilletes
  - Difficult intubation laryngoscopes
  - Laryngeal mask airway

---

last ingestion of food. In emergency anaesthesia the airway must be secured, intubating the trachea as rapidly as possible after induction of anaesthesia. Although various predominantly pharmacological methods can be used to aid gastric emptying (nasogastric tube and metoclopramide) and neutralise stomach acidity (ranitidine and sodium citrate), these are not infallible.

The only reliable method to prevent aspiration is to use the correct anaesthetic technique, the RSI.

Anaesthetic choice

Not all emergency surgery needs a general anaesthetic. In many scenarios an alternative may be beneficial to both the patients' surgical condition and their medical co-morbidities.

Regional anaesthesia, in particular, is useful for any surgery on the extremities. It will provide anaesthesia, analgesia, muscle relaxation and immobility. In addition, it can have minimal impact on the cardiovascular and respiratory systems; a potential benefit in a patient who has significant cardiorespiratory co-morbidities and diminished physiological reserve.

Central neuraxial blockade (spinal or epidural) can also be beneficial for lower extremity anaesthesia; however, these must be undertaken with great care in cases of significant hypovolaemia and haemorrhage as they can cause large decreases in arterial pressure. In these situations they are not safer than general anaesthesia and in patients with trauma or intra-abdominal pathology they are more dangerous particularly in inexperienced hands.

Induction of anaesthesia

Rapid sequence induction

If general anaesthesia is to be utilised, the decision to undertake an RSI is a balance between the risk of losing control of the airway and the risk of aspiration. It disregards one of the basic rules of anaesthesia – muscle relaxants are not normally used unless control of the airway is certain. It is for this reason that the airway is assessed to ascertain whether intubation will be difficult (Box 3.1). The anaesthetist should also have a plan if intubation is not possible. If the airway is predicted to be difficult then an alternative plan can be used (see sections 'inhalational induction' or 'fibreoptic intubation').

The basic requirements for RSI are shown in Box 3.5. For RSI to be carried out successfully and safely these requirements must be present. The RSI can be divided into three phases.

Pre-oxygenation

With the patient adequately monitored (as per the guidelines of the Association of Anaesthetists of Great Britain and Ireland), he or she should breathe 100% oxygen for at least 3 minutes from a suitable breathing circuit and a well-fitting mask.

Air contains 78% nitrogen, so when the patient breathes oxygen only, the lungs will denitrogenate and contain only oxygen and carbon dioxide. This will provide a larger respiratory reservoir of oxygen to utilise before hypoxia occurs.

Cricoid pressure

Also known as Sellick's manoeuvre, this is the process of a skilled assistant pushing down on the cricoid cartilage with firm pressure from the thumb and forefinger on induction of anaesthesia. This pressure is maintained until the anaesthetist tells the assistant to stop. It is imperative that the cricoid cartilage is identified before anaesthesia is induced.

It is important that the identification is correct as pressure on the thyroid cartilage can have a detrimental effect on the view at laryngoscopy making intubation difficult. The pressure used is similar to that which would cause mild pain when exerted on the nasal bridge. The object of Sellick's manoeuvre is to compress the oesophagus between the cricoid cartilage and the vertebral column. Because the cricoid cartilage is a complete ring the tracheal lumen is not distorted and compression of the oesophagus prevents any regurgitated material from the stomach entering the pharynx.

Intubation

With the skilled assistant in position an anaesthetic dose of sodium thiopentone is given intravenously. Without waiting to assess the effect of the induction agent a paralysing dose of suxamethonium is given immediately. When the jaw is judged to be relaxed, direct laryngoscopy is performed and the trachea is intubated. Cricoid pressure is maintained until the endotracheal tube cuff is inflated and its position is ascertained by auscultation of the lungs and there is evidence of the presence of end-tidal carbon dioxide.

One of the major disadvantages of an RSI is the potential haemodynamic instability. Hypotension and circulatory collapse (including electromechanical dissociation arrest) can occur if the induction agent dose is too excessive particularly in the presence of hypovolaemia and haemorrhage. If the dose is inadequate, hypertension and tachycardia (and other arrhythmias) can occur. Unfortunately, it is difficult to select the correct dose, whereas a dose of 4 mg kg^{-1} of thiopentone is adequate for a healthy young adult, 2 mg kg^{-1} may be excessive for an elderly, frail patient. The bleeding hypovolaemic patient needing emergency surgery as part of their resuscitation will need even less. The other main disadvantage is the uncertainty of ease of intubation and alternative methods of induction are discussed below.

Alternative or additional drugs can be used; however, the decision to use a different combination of drugs lies with the anaesthetist and remains a careful risk benefit balance. By far the simplest and safest drugs to use are those discussed above; however, in certain situations alternatives are viable and will depend on the experience of the anaesthetist present.

Both induction agent and neuromuscular blocking drug must act rapidly and have a short duration of action. A rapid onset of action will allow quick endotracheal intubation and a short duration of action will allow the return of spontaneous respiration in the situation of failed intubation. For neuromuscular blockade suxamethonium is an effective drug but it has many side effects (Box 3.6).

Rocuronium, a non-depolarising muscle relaxant that has appreciably less side effects than suxamathonium, has a rapid onset if given in the right dose but its disadvantage is its prolonged duration of action. Promising recent studies have shown that it can be reversed with a selective relaxant

---

Box 3.6 Side effects of suxamethonium

- Anaphylaxis – suxamethonium is the most common muscle relaxant to cause anaphylaxis
- Malignant hyperthermia – a rare condition with 5% mortality
- Prolonged block – also termed suxamethonium apnoea, necessitating prolonged ventilation in critical care
- Hyperkalaemia – large enough to provoke cardiac arrest in certain conditions; burns, paraplegia, myopathies
- Arrhythmias – bradycardias and ventricular arrhythmias
- Muscle pains – particularly in young adults
- Raised intraocular pressure
- Raised intragastric pressure

---

binding agent called sugammadex within an acceptable time period.

Different induction agents are used in emergent situations. There are various alternatives used that have an improved cardiovascular stability (e.g. ketamine, opioid/benzodiazepine combination) but there are potential disadvantages to their use, in particular prolonged induction time and prolonged duration of action.

Complimentary drugs can also be utilised. In the presence of significant hypovolaemia or haemorrhage it is not unusual to need a vasoconstrictor (ephedrine, metaraminol and adrenaline) to diminish the vasodilatory properties of the induction agent. In situations where a further increase in blood pressure or heart rate would be detrimental (uncontrolled hypertension and pre-eclampsia), a number of agents have been shown to have benefit, most of which have a short duration of action: opioids (alfentanil and remifentanil), beta-blockers (esmolol) and magnesium.

Inhalational induction

If it is not possible to predict whether intubation is going to be difficult, an inhalational induction can be used with the volatile agent sevoflurane and oxygen. The key part of the process is to keep the patient breathing spontaneously. Induction of anaesthesia takes longer and in the emergency scenario cricoid pressure is still required in the presence of a potentially full stomach. When a deep plane of anaesthesia is achieved laryngoscopy is performed with a subsequent attempt at intubation whilst the patient is breathing spontaneously. There is a significant risk of laryngospasm and apnoea throughout this process and it is important to ensure that laryngoscopy is only undertaken in a deep plane of anaesthesia. Some practitioners spray local anaesthetic on the vocal cords before intubation is attempted.

Fibreoptic intubation

Nasal intubation with the use of a fibreoptic intubating laryngoscope in the awake patient can secure the airway in controlled circumstances minimising the risk of loss of the airway. The procedure takes time as full anaesthesia of the airway is required beforehand. It is also labour-intensive as two skilled anaesthetists are preferable.

Maintenance of anaesthesia

The maintenance of a balanced anaesthetic technique will be similar to that of an elective patient with a number of additions. A balanced technique will include:
- Anaesthesia – loss of awareness
- Analgesia – in order to attenuate the reflexes of the autonomic system to a painful stimulus
- Muscle relaxation

Anaesthesia is sustained with either intravenous or inhalational means. With both, it is not uncommon to use a smaller dose than usual if there is ongoing haemorrhage or the patient is inadequately resuscitated.

Analgesia can be assisted by the use of nitrous oxide (50–66%) in addition to an intravenous opioid before incision. Further analgesia is titrated throughout depending on the condition of the patient and the extent of surgery. A combined regional technique, peripheral (nerve plexus block) or central (epidural or spinal) will assist perioperative analgesia. As a rule in the emergent situation less drugs are needed and it is prudent to start with half the dose normally given to an elective patient.

Muscle relaxation is continued using a non-depolarising muscle relaxant once the effects of suxamethonium wear off. Pancuronium increases heart rate and blood pressure and can be of use in the face of hypovolaemia; atracurium has minimal cardiovascular effects but is metabolised easily and useful if there is renal impairment.

Summary

In emergency anaesthesia the key factors are:
- A thorough preoperative assessment to assess the effects of the emergent surgical condition and the patients' existing medical co-morbidities.
- Adequate resuscitation to compensate for blood loss and extracellular fluid loss in addition to optimisation of concurrent medical problems.
- Devising an appropriate anaesthetic technique that deals with the surgical condition of the patient, their medical co-morbidities and the needs of the surgeon. This will almost always involve the need for an RSI.

Further reading

Flockton EA, Mastronardi P, Hunter JM, et al. Reversal of rocuronium-induced neuromuscular block with suggamadex is faster than reversal of cisatracurium-induced block with neostigmine. *BJA* 2008;**100**(5):622–630.

Mallampati SR, Gatt SP, Gugino LD, Desai SP, Waraksa B, Freidberger DA. Clinical sign to predict difficult tracheal intubation: a prospective study. *Can Anaesth Soc J* 1985;**32**:429–434.

Sellick BA. Cricoid pressure to control regurgitation of stomach contents during induction of anaesthesia. *The Lancet* 1961;**2**:404–406.

The Association of Anaesthetists of Great Britain and Ireland. *Recommendations for Standards of Monitoring During Anaesthesia and Recovery*, 4th edn. The Association of Anaesthetists of Great Britain and Ireland, London, 2007.

4 Analgesia

Jeff L. Tong

Department of Military Anaesthesia and Critical Care, Royal Centre for Defence Medicine, Birmingham, UK

Introduction

Pain may be defined as an unpleasant sensory and emotional experience associated with actual or potential tissue damage. However, an individual's perception of what is painful may be influenced by differences in age, gender, culture, previous pain experiences, beliefs, mood and ability to cope.

Acute pain commonly occurs following the stimulation of nociceptors (visceral or somatic) by noxious stimuli and transmission of an impulse along intact neurons to the central nervous system (CNS). This is classified as nociceptive pain, which is common following trauma and responds to analgesics. In the presence of nerve damage, neuropathic pain may be present, which has different characteristics and responds poorly to traditional analgesics.

Acute nociceptive pain can be classified as mild, moderate or severe and the most appropriate choice of analgesia is determined by the severity of the pain. This may be established using one of the numerous pain assessment tools which determine an appropriate level of entry onto the analgesia ladder. Strong opiate analgesics are widely used to treat severe pain, e.g. morphine; and weak analgesics or non-steroidal anti-inflammatory drugs (NSAIDs) are used in mild-to-moderate pain, e.g. codeine and diclofenac.

In addition to the stimulation of nociceptors the perception of pain is influenced by strong psychological and emotional factors. Anxiety and fear are common following a sudden injury, which explains why reassurance and comfort may contribute to the analgesic and anxiolytic effect. Non-pharmacological strategies can also provide transient pain relief, so distraction techniques may be a useful measure.

In the emergency surgical patient, it is important to establish the likely cause of the pain and how it may be relieved, e.g. the management of distension pain (bowel or bladder) is different from pain due to ischaemic limbs, bowel or the myocardium (angina).

For a particular cause of nociceptive pain, a single analgesic option is unlikely to meet the needs of all patients or all conditions, and adopting a multi-modal approach by combining different analgesics, may provide superior analgesia.

Why is analgesia needed?

Following tissue injury, tachypnoea, tachycardia and hypertension commonly occur, due to autonomic stimulation and endogenous catecholamine secretion, initiating the 'flight or fight' response. In the presence of coexisting cardiac disease, this response may compromise myocardial perfusion, resulting in myocardial ischaemia. In the presence of non-compressible haemorrhage, the cardiovascular response to pain can perpetuate intravascular volume depletion, which decreases oxygen-carrying capacity. It is therefore, therapeutically beneficial to administer supplementary oxygen to all patients in pain. In general terms, administering adequate analgesia should cause the respiratory rate, heart rate and arterial blood pressure to decrease to within a physiologically acceptable range.

Wound pain is worse on movement and is usually maximal in the first 72 hours. Analgesia is important as it allows the patient to move, which reduces the risk of venous thromboembolism, and cough which reduces the risk of sputum retention and respiratory infection. Inadequate analgesia following a laparotomy may result in significant morbidity due to hypoventilation and pulmonary atelectasis, leading to inefficient alveolar gas exchange and hypoxaemia.

Assessment of pain

Poor provision of analgesia frequently occurs because the needs of the patients are often underestimated. A variety of tools are available to assist in the rapid objective assessment of the severity of pain both before and after analgesia.

Based on the patient's age and communicative ability, a pain score may be established using visual analogue,

Emergency Surgery, 1st edition. Edited by Adam Brooks, Peter F. Mahoney, Bryan A. Cotton and Nigel Tai. © 2010 Blackwell Publishing.

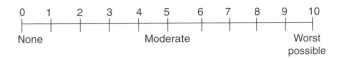

Figure 4.1 Numeric pain intensity scale.

numerical or facial pain scales (Figures 4.1 and 4.2). High scores are associated with more severe pain and vice versa. However, patients who state that their pain is 'eleven out of ten' indicate their anxiety.

These pain assessment tools allow appropriate analgesia to be selected: weak opioid analgesics are used in mild-to-moderate pain and strong opioid analgesics are used to treat severe pain. This is the fundamental principle of the analgesic ladder.

Sedation and a decrease in the Glasgow Coma Score (GCS) may be observed as the dose of opiates increases, consequently obtaining critical information from the patient should be performed promptly.

Whilst concerns exist over the accuracy of clinical examination in patients who have been given strong analgesia, e.g. clearing the cervical spine, intravenous (IV) morphine should not be delayed.

Dosage

When calculating the dose of a specific drug, it is important to know the metric body weight (kg) of the patient. In children, from the age of 1 year until they reach puberty, a formula (based on their age in years) may be used to calculate their estimated body weight in kilogram, e.g. a 4-year old should weigh 16 kg (Figure 4.3).

Route and frequency

IV analgesia is the preferred route of administration in the emergency surgical patient. This route allows rapid administration, onset of action and the drug may be titrated to effect, thus side effects are minimised. Regular small IV doses are preferred followed by a period of assessment (titrate to effect), with further small doses administered as necessary. In the absence of IV access, the intraosseous route provides an effective alternative.

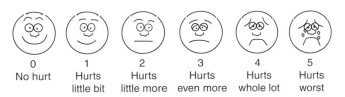

Figure 4.2 Wong–Baker FACES pain scale (with permission).

$$(\text{Age} + 4) \times 2 = \text{Body weight}$$

Figure 4.3 Formula for calculating body weight in children.

Absorption from the gastrointestinal tract or following intramuscular (IM) injection is unpredictable, inconsistent and may be delayed. Whilst inhaled analgesia is popular in the pre-hospital environment, it has a limited role within hospitals. If analgesia is prescribed 'p.r.n.' (as required) then the patient should be informed of this so that he or she can ask for it when required.

Patient-controlled analgesia

A patient-controlled analgesia (PCA) system delivers intermittent IV boluses of opioid that are demand activated by the patient (Figure 4.4). For small children and infants a nurse-controlled analgesia (NCA) system is used, and when analgesia is required the nurse activates the system.

Overdosage is avoided by limiting the dose of the bolus and the total dose administered within a period of time. A lockout interval is also set with the option of a background infusion (Table 4.1). PCA may also be used in conjunction with epidural analgesia (opioid free).

The PCA should be delivered through a dedicated IV line. When attached via a three-way tap to a fluid infusion, a one way valve should be incorporated into the system to prevent backflow into the tubing and the delivery of a large bolus. The management of opioid-induced respiratory depression is shown in Figure 4.5.

PCA has been shown to provide consistent plasma drug levels when compared with intramuscular techniques and with fewer side effects. It is mostly used for the control of postoperative pain. Respiratory depression, over sedation and hypotension are not usually a problem if PCA is used correctly and may be due to some other pathological process.

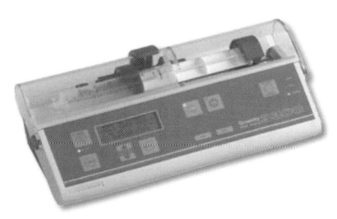

Figure 4.4 The Graseby 3300 PCA pump (with permission).

Table 4.1 A standard morphine PCA prescription.

Drug concentration	1 mg/mL
Bolus dose	1 mg
Bolus duration	Stat
Lockout period	5 minutes
Maximum per hour	12 mg
Background infusion	Nil

Intra-abdominal bleeding, development of septicaemia, myocardial insufficiency and hypoxaemia are all serious complications which may occur in any surgical patient. It is important to exclude these complications in any patient on PCA who becomes excessively drowsy with or without hypotension or respiratory depression.

Narcotic analgesia

Opioid analgesics are widely used in the treatment of dull, poorly localised (visceral) pain. They share many side effects, which commonly include nausea, vomiting, drowsiness and constipation. Higher doses produce cardiovascular and respiratory depression.

Morphine is the most frequently administered analgesic for severe pain and is the standard against which other opioid analgesics are compared. Morphine may cause histamine release with vasodilatation, bronchospasm and a pruritic cutaneous rash. The reaction may be limited or it may proceed to a full immunological reaction (anaphylaxis).

Diamorphine (diacetylmorphine) is twice as potent as morphine and it causes more euphoria but less hypotension and nausea. It is also known as 'heroin' and is unavailable in the United States.

Pethidine is similar to morphine but due to being more lipid-soluble it has a more rapid onset of action. Analgesia is

short-lasting which limits its use. It has weak atropine-like activity causing pupillary dilatation, tachycardia and may cause convulsions.

Codeine (methylmorphine) is a weak opiate that has one-twelfth the analgesic potency of morphine. It has a side effect profile which restricts its dosage to levels that produces less analgesia than morphine. It is effective for the relief of mild-to-moderate pain and is commonly prescribed following head injury. Dihydrocodeine is an analgesic with similar efficacy to codeine.

Fentanyl is a commonly used opioid for intraoperative IV analgesia. It may be administered via numerous routes including neuraxial, transdermal and oromucosal, e.g. adhesive patches, lozenges, lollipops and nasal sprays. Large doses may cause muscle rigidity, especially of the chest wall, which can require assisted ventilation and the use of muscle relaxants.

Tramadol provides analgesia through traditional binding of opioid receptors and by enhancing serotonergic and adrenergic pathways. It is effective against moderate pain and causes less respiratory depression.

Ketamine

This is an NMDA receptor antagonist, which can provide dose-dependent, rapid and effective analgesia and sedation following IV or IM administration. It can be used to induce general anaesthesia (GA) and is considered the drug of choice in cardiovascularly unstable or hypovolaemic patients. It may cause an increase in arterial blood pressure and so should be used with caution in head injuries. When used in sub-anaesthetic doses, spontaneously breathing patients frequently maintain a patent airway, though increased salivation is common. Ketamine is a phencyclidine derivative and its use has been associated with hallucinations or nightmares, the effect of which may be diminished if it is used in conjunction with a benzodiazepine.

Non-narcotic analgesia

Somatic pain is sharply defined and may be relieved by a weak opioid analgesic or NSAIDs. Paracetamol and diclofenac are both available for IV administration and may provide effective relief as single agents or in combination with another class of analgesic.

Anti-emetics

The aim of administering an anti-emetic should be the prevention of nausea and vomiting, which is the commonest side effect of opiates. They should be given early as this side effect is found, by many patients, to be just as unpleasant

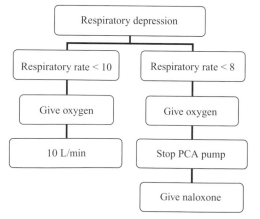

Figure 4.5 Management of opioid-induced respiratory depression.

Table 4.2 Anti-emetic doses and side effects.

Drug	Dose	Notes
Cyclizine	50 mg	Tachycardia is common
		Pain on injection
Ondansetron	4 mg	May prolong QT interval
Prochlorperazine	12.5 mg	Only IM
		Dystonic reactions
Metoclopramide	10 mg	Prokinetic effect
		Dystonic reaction

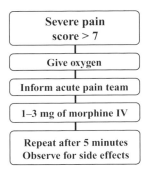

Figure 4.6 Management of severe acute pain.

as pain. The prevention of nausea and vomiting may be achieved using several classes of drug, which antagonise different receptor types at the chemoreceptor trigger zone (CTZ) and vomiting centre. The choice of drug is determined by the aetiology of the vomiting and its side effect profile (Table 4.2). Unpredictable absorption from the gastrointestinal tract and delayed onset restricts the oral route of administration, so the route of choice for anti-emetics is IV.

Cyclizine is an antihistamine that is often administered with IV morphine. Tachycardia is a common anti-cholinergic side effect of cyclizine and may last several minutes. Slow IV administration causes less cardiovascular disturbance and it should be diluted to minimise the risk of causing pain on injection; however, mild sedation has been described.

Ondansetron is a 5HT-3 receptor antagonist which blocks this receptor in the CNS and gastrointestinal tract. It is relatively free from adverse side effects though it has been known to prolong the QT interval.

Prochlorperazine acts centrally by blocking dopamine receptors at the CTZ. It cannot be given intravenously. All dopamine antagonists can induce acute dystonic reactions (skeletal and facial muscle spasms) and oculogyric crises.

Metoclopramide is a dopamine antagonist which acts directly on the gastrointestinal tract. It has a prokinetic effect on peristalsis and is contraindicated in intestinal perforation, haemorrhage and obstruction. As an anti-emetic it has limited efficacy.

Managing severe pain

Medical staff should be able to deal with the initial management of inadequate analgesia and to diagnose and respond to any complications that may occur. In the emergency surgical patient this can occur frequently in the perioperative period and should be managed by careful IV titration of dilute opiate, e.g. morphine diluted to a 1 mg/mL solution. IV boluses of 1–3 mg of morphine may be repeated at 5-minute intervals until analgesia is achieved (Figure 4.6). The time interval is important as this is the latency of onset of morphine administered intravenously. During this titration period, the patient should be observed for side effects, particularly respiratory depression or excessive sedation. If

analgesia is still inadequate or becomes inadequate within 2 hours after the initial morphine titration, further IV morphine should be titrated as before, until effective analgesia is established. The acute pain team should be informed, who may suggest an additional analgesic prescription or if appropriate, alter the PCA pump settings. Whilst adequate pain relief may take longer to achieve using this method, control is maintained and the risk of administering excessive doses is reduced.

Analgesia or anaesthesia

Occasionally, patients may be combative or confused and there is a tendency to administer IV sedation to these patients, e.g. midazolam. Pain and hypoxaemia are common causes of confusion and should be promptly treated. Anxiolysis and sedation are common side effects of strong opiate analgesia, but benzodiazepines have no analgesic properties.

Increasing doses of IV morphine will cause the level of consciousness to fall and when the GCS is less than 8, aspiration of gastric contents may occur unless the airway is appropriately protected. Since all emergency surgery patients should be considered to have a full stomach, achieving adequate analgesia in a polytrauma patient may compromise their ability to protect their own airway. In some situations GA may be induced and maintained within the emergency department or in the pre-hospital environment prior to being transferred for surgery. Effective analgesia can then be administered following tracheal intubation and airway protection.

Painful procedures, e.g. reducing fractures or dislocated joints, can be performed more efficiently with shorter recovery times following a GA, than after large doses of IV midazolam and morphine.

Nitrous oxide has analgesic properties and is used as an anaesthetic carrier gas and is a component of Entonox (50% oxygen and 50% nitrous oxide). However, nitrous oxide diffuses into air-filled cavities causing the air space to expand and its use is not recommended in injuries to the head, eye, lungs or bowel. Supplementary oxygen should be given to patients for 20 minutes after using nitrous oxide to reduce the risk of diffusion hypoxia.

Naloxone is a specific antagonist at opioid receptors, which can reverse the respiratory depression, sedative effect and analgesia produced by morphine-like drugs. It should be administered intravenously for rapid response, but has a short half-life and a repeat dose may be required. Diluting 400 mcg (1 mL) of naloxone in 10 mL of saline produces an easy to administer concentration of 40 mcg/mL. At 1-minute intervals 1 mL IV bolus doses should be given until the respiratory rate exceeds 10 per minute. A whole pre-filled syringe of undiluted naloxone is rarely required, except in dire circumstances.

Local anaesthetics

Local anaesthetic (LA) drugs can provide effective pain relief by blocking membrane depolarisation, which reversibly blocks conduction along neurons. They can be administer by various routes, e.g. topical, local infiltration, peripheral nerve block, intravenous regional anaesthesia (Bier's block), plexus block, subarachnoid block (spinal) and extradural block (epidural). The effective use of LAs reduces the need for additional forms of analgesia and they are said to have an opioid sparing effect.

Following superficial surgery or when skin incisions are small, infiltrating the wound with local anaesthetic at the time of surgery or performing a field block may reduce postoperative pain.

Prolonged analgesia may be achieved with regional nerve blocks, e.g. femoral nerve or digital nerve blocks, and using longer-acting LA agents such as bupivacaine may provide effective analgesia for many hours.

Local anaesthetics generally cause vasodilatation, so the addition of a low-dose vasoconstrictor, such as adrenaline (1 in 200,000), reduces local blood flow, slows the rate of absorption and prolongs the duration of local anaesthetic effect. Local anaesthetic solutions containing a vasoconstrictor should not be injected into digits or appendages (ring block/dorsal nerve block), as this may produce ischaemic necrosis. Inadvertent intravenous and intra-arterial administration should similarly be avoided.

In addition to diffusing into nerves at the injection site, the drug also enters capillaries and is removed by the circulation. The tissue concentration of drug will eventually fall below that in the nerves and the drug will diffuse out, thus restoring normal function.

Although uptake into the circulation is important in terminating the action of local anaesthetics, it is also responsible for producing toxicity. Maximum plasma concentrations of local anaesthetic usually develop within 30 minutes of administration, so careful surveillance for signs of toxicity is necessary during this period.

Table 4.3 Standard doses of local anaesthetic agents (4-hour period).

	Dose*	Notes
Lidocaine	3–4 mg/kg	Double the dose when with adrenaline
Bupivacaine	2 mg/kg	Malignant dysrhythmia
Ropivacaine	2 mg/kg	
Prilocaine	7 mg/kg	Methaemoglobinaemia may occur

* 1 mL of a 1% solution contains 10 mg

Following single injections of LA, the block duration is dependent on the half-life of the agent used. Whilst it is not technically difficult to perform a peripheral nerve block, a degree of anatomical knowledge and repetitive practice is required for consistent results. Continuous catheter-based peripheral nerve blocks or epidural anaesthesia techniques are used to prolong the duration of the block, by infusing LA down an appropriately placed catheter. They are increasing in popularity and may provide superior pain control to opioid-based analgesia without their side effects.

When calculating the safe dose of local anaesthetic which can be administered over a 4-hour period, the patient's body weight (kg) is required (Table 4.3). The concentration of local anaesthetic solutions is commonly presented as a percentage, which can easily be converted into mg/mL by recalling that '1 mL of a 1% solution contains 10 mg'. Practically, a 100 kg patient could safely be given 40 mL of 0.5% bupivacaine, or 80 mL of 0.25% ropivacaine. Doses should be adjusted according to any coexisting diseases and the nature of the surgical procedure.

Lidocaine is the most widely used agent. It acts more rapidly than most other local anaesthetics and has a duration of action of about 90 minutes. When the solution contains adrenaline, up to twice the 'plain' dose of lidocaine may be safely administered.

Bupivacaine has a slow onset time, but it has the longest duration of action. Bupivacaine exists as a racemic mixture of isomers and is associated with severe cardiotoxicity following inadvertent intravascular injection or when its concentration in the plasma reaches toxic levels. Dysrhythmias which are resistant to treatment and cardiac arrest may follow. **Levobupivacaine** (L-bupivacaine) represents a purified local anaesthetic solution containing only the L-isomer of bupivacaine. It has similar properties to bupivacaine but has a pharmacological profile that is associated with fewer adverse effects. The addition of adrenaline to bupivacaine solutions does not allow greater than 2 mg/kg to be given over a 4-hour period.

Ropivacaine is similar to bupivacaine but is less potent and cardiotoxic.

Prilocaine is similar to lidocaine but is less toxic in equipotent doses. High doses can cause methaemoglobinaemia, which may require IV treatment with 1%

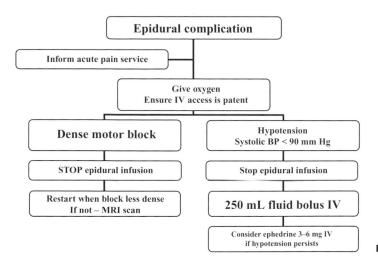

Figure 4.7 Management of epidural complications.

methylene blue (1 mg/kg). The addition of adrenaline to prilocaine solutions does not allow greater doses to be given over a 4-hour period.

Epidurals

Epidurals are frequently used to provide analgesia following thoracotomy, laparotomy and lower limb procedures. Weak concentrations of LA are used with the aim of producing a sensory block in the dermatomes at the surgical site. The ideal height of anaesthesia provided by an epidural is the dermatome above the highest point of the surgical incision. Patients should normally have a low pain score when the epidural is functioning correctly, so the acute pain team should be informed of any patient with a pain score >5.

Opiates may also be added to the LA solution, which can improve the quality of the analgesia. However, no other opioids or sedative drugs should be administered to patients receiving an epidural infusion containing opiates.

Complications

The presence of a dense motor block may be a neurological emergency and the acute pain service must be informed immediately. If persistent, the epidural should be stopped but if the block is not resolving within 3–4 hours after stopping the epidural, the patient may need an urgent MRI scan to exclude a treatable lesion, e.g. haematoma. Once the motor block has started to resolve, the epidural may be restarted. The patient may require alternative analgesia while the epidural is stopped.

A sympathetic block routinely occurs when LAs are injected into the epidural (extradural) space, which may cause the arterial blood pressure to fall. Usually this responds to a bolus of IV fluids, but when the height of the block reaches the mid-thoracic dermatomes, hypotension and bradycardia may occur. Supplementary oxygen and further IV fluids are indicted and the epidural infusion should be stopped and the acute pain service must be informed. Intravenous ephedrine

given in 3–6 mg boluses every 2 minutes may be required if the systolic blood pressure is below 90 mm Hg (Figure 4.7).

The acute pain team should also be informed if the epidural catheter is exposed or the filter becomes disconnected; the epidural site looks red, swollen or is painful.

Neuropathic pain

Neuropathic pain is defined as 'pains resulting from disease or damage of the peripheral or central nervous systems, and from dysfunction of the nervous system'. Inflammatory mediators cause peripheral sensitisation of nociceptors making them more sensitive to stimulation (Table 4.4). This process can be primary (at the site) or secondary (at a remote site) leading to 'wind up' of spinal cord activity which may result in a continuation of the pain. If untreated 'central sensitisation' may occur, resulting in lasting perceptions of pain that continue after tissue repair is complete.

Table 4.4 Chemicals that can facilitate or mediate the inflammatory process.

Bradykinin
Prostaglandins
Leukotrienes
Serotonin
Histamine
Substance P
Thromboxanes
Platelet activating factor
Adenosine and ATP
Protons and free radicals
Cytokines
Interleukins
Tumour necrosis factor
Neurotropins (nerve growth factor)

The pain which may be burning, tingling, shooting or scalding, occurs in areas of sensory deficit and can be evoked by non-noxious stimuli. Symptoms include allodynia, hyperalgesia, hyperpathia and signs of sympathetic dysfunction are common.

The neurobiological changes that characterise neuropathic pain may occur within hours of an acute injury and the response to opioid analgesia is frequently poor. Within this group, tramadol and oxycodone are the most effective. In the face of increasing opioid requirements with partial or no effect, the use of regional anaesthesia and the addition of non-narcotic analgesia may be of benefit.

Summary

- Obtain *ample* information early.
- Give oxygen to patients in pain.
- Provide analgesia rather than sedation.
- IV morphine should be titrated to effect.
- Anti-emetics should be given with opiates.
- Do not give IM opioids to patients on PCA.
- Do not give opioids to patients receiving epidural infusions containing opioids.

2   Abdomen

5 Acute Appendicitis

Tom Palser[1], David J. Humes[2] & Adam Brooks[2]
[1]Royal College of Surgeons of England, London, UK
[2]Queen's Medical Centre, Department of Surgery, Nottingham, UK

Introduction

Appendicectomy is the most common emergency surgical operation, with more than 40,000 performed each year in England alone. The chance of a person developing appendicitis over the course of his or her lifetime is ~7%. Many other patients are admitted with suspected appendicitis but either resolve before surgery or are diagnosed with other pathologies. Although generally considered a 'benign' disease, complication rates following appendicitis are high (up to 30% in some series). Some patients, particularly the elderly or those who present late, can be extremely septic and require critical care support. Careful assessment and treatment of the patient with suspected appendicitis is therefore essential.

Clinical presentation

The main features of acute appendicitis are abdominal pain and symptoms of systemic illness such as fever, loss of appetite and malaise. Classically the pain is initially colicky or aching in nature and located in the centre of the abdomen. As the disease progresses it becomes sharper and localised in the right iliac fossa. However, due to the varying position of the appendix, many patients present with a different pattern of pain. A systematic review of the value of clinical symptoms, examination findings and laboratory investigations showed that the features in the history that are most predictive of appendicitis are:
- A relatively short history
- Fever
- Pain migration
  Other important symptoms include:
- Malaise
- Loss of appetite

- Nausea or vomiting
- Diarrhoea (if the appendix tip lies against the bowel)

Typical presentations include the child who is generally irritable and off his food and the confused, shocked, elderly patient. Although pain is the usual presenting feature it is not absolutely universal, especially in the extremes of age.

It is also essential to ask about symptoms related to other potential diagnoses. If the patient is female, a full gynaecological history (especially the date of the last menstrual period) should be taken. In older patients, it is important to consider the possibility of malignancy, so questions about their recent weight, appetite, bowel habit and any rectal bleeding should be asked. Diabetic ketoacidosis, acute pancreatitis and a perforated peptic ulcer can all mimic acute appendicitis in their early stages so these too should be considered. The differential diagnosis of suspected appendicitis is shown in Box 5.1. Those that can cause the patient to deteriorate rapidly are highlighted in bold.

On examination, the patient may be septic and shocked, especially if they are presented late, are elderly or immunocompromised. The patient is often febrile, flushed and lying still. They may have their right hip flexed and complain of pain on passive hip extension (the psoas stretch sign – caused by irritation of psoas major by a retrocaecal or retrocolic appendix).

If the appendix is perforated, there may be generalised peritonitis and abdominal rigidity. More commonly there is tenderness and guarding in the right iliac fossa, although the location may vary depending on the position of the appendix tip. For example, it is not uncommon for the point of maximal tenderness to be more suprapubic than lateral. The systematic review by Andersson identified the following examination features as having the highest specificity and sensitivity for acute appendicitis:
- Temperature >37.7°C
- Localised (rather than diffuse) tenderness
- Indirect tenderness (where the pain is worst at the point of maximal tenderness when the patient is palpated in the left iliac fossa, also known as Rovsing's sign)
- Rebound or percussion tenderness
- Guarding

Emergency Surgery, 1st edition. Edited by Adam Brooks, Peter F. Mahoney, Bryan A. Cotton and Nigel Tai. © 2010 Blackwell Publishing.

Box 5.1 Differential diagnosis of acute appendicitis

Surgical
- **Perforated colonic tumour**
- **Pancreatitis**
- **Perforated peptic ulcer**
- **Intestinal obstruction**
- Mesenteric adenitis
- Diverticulitis
- Acute cholecystitis
- Rectus sheath haematoma

Gynaecological
- **Ectopic pregnancy**
- Ruptured ovarian follicle
- Salpingitis/pelvic inflammatory disease
- Torted ovarian cyst
- Mittelschmerz

Urological
- Ureteric colic
- Pyelonephritis
- Urinary tract Infection

Medical
- **Diabetic ketoacidosis**
- Gastroenteritis
- Terminal ileitis
- Pneumonia

Tenderness on rectal examination may be present but its specificity is low (likelihood ratio is 1.03 in Andersson's review), so its utility is debated.

Investigations

Despite advances in imaging technology, the diagnosis of acute appendicitis remains essentially a clinical one. Certain laboratory investigations may help make the diagnosis while others are important in excluding other potential differential diagnoses and preparing the patient for possible surgery. Andersson's systematic review identified a raised white cell count, C-reactive protein and a neutrophilia as being most predictive for appendicitis. An amylase and a blood glucose should be checked to investigate for pancreatitis and diabetic ketoacidosis and as with all surgical patients, a full blood count, urea and electrolytes and clotting profile should also be taken.

All women of childbearing age presenting with abdominal pain are assumed to have a ruptured ectopic pregnancy until proven otherwise, so a urine sample should always be tested for B-HCG as soon as possible. The presence of white cells and protein in the urine may well be due to bladder irritation caused by an inflamed retrocaecal or pelvic appendix, so it should not be assumed that they indicate a urinary tract infection.

The use of further imaging should be guided by the clinical picture. A meta-analysis by Terawasa et al. showed that ultrasound has a sensitivity of 86% and a specificity of 81% for diagnosing appendicitis. It has several advantages it is non-invasive, carries no radiation risk and is cheap and often easily available. However, it is operator-dependent and, as shown above, can neither exclude nor confidently predict acute appendicitis. It is most useful in helping to exclude gynaecological pathology in stable female patients rather than in diagnosing appendicitis itself. The same review showed that computed tomography (CT) scanning has a sensitivity of 94% and specificity of 95%. CT has the added benefit of more accurately imaging the rest of the abdomen so is very useful if the diagnosis is unclear. This is particularly true in older patients where perforated tumours and diverticulitis are more common. Although the sensitivity is relatively high, 1 in 20 patients with a negative CT will still have appendicitis. Magnetic resonance imaging (MRI) confers no added benefit over CT but may be useful in patients in whom CT is contraindicated (in particular pregnant patients).

In summary, therefore, laboratory and radiological investigations may help confirm the diagnosis of appendicitis but are most useful in excluding other causes. Urinalysis should always be performed in women of childbearing age to exclude an ectopic pregnancy and ultrasound should be considered in stable female patients to help exclude gynaecological pathology. CT should be considered in patients with suspected appendicitis in whom the diagnosis is unclear and cannot be confirmed by clinical and laboratory findings. In most patients, the diagnosis and decision to operate remains a clinical one. Box 5.2 shows a suggested management algorithm.

Initial management

Although many patients with suspected acute appendicitis are relatively stable, some present with overt sepsis. In 2005, 118 patients in England and Wales died of acute appendicitis, so the need for careful monitoring and rapid resuscitation is essential. The principles of resuscitation are the same as for other causes of the acute abdomen.

The hypothesis that analgesia may mask the pain and result in an incorrect diagnosis has no evidence base, so all patients should be given appropriate analgesia, prescribed intravenous fluids and thromboprophylaxis. The patient

Box 5.2 Proposed management algorithm for acute appendicitis

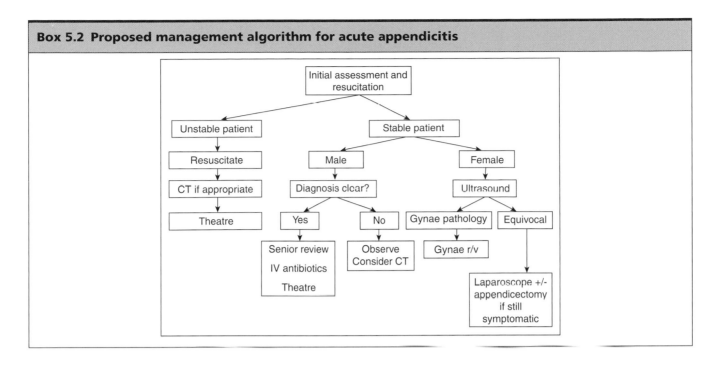

should be nil by mouth until reviewed by a senior, unless they are stable in which case they may be allowed to drink water overnight.

Once the decision to operate has been taken, broad-spectrum antibiotics should be started. A Cochrane review showed that perioperative antibiotics decrease the wound infection and intra-abdominal abscess rate, but there was no consensus on the regimen that should be given. Many surgeons give three doses if the appendix is not obviously inflamed at operation, but give a full 5-day course if it is. Antibiotics should not be started until the decision to operate has been made by a senior as they may potentially mask the examination signs, but there is little evidence that they are a feasible alternative treatment in themselves.

Operative management

Several controversies exist in the operative management of appendicitis, principally the timing of the operation, the choice of an open or laparosopic approach and whether to remove a macroscopically normal appendix. When consenting the patient ensure the risks of infection, bleeding, intra-abdominal abscess, the need for conversion (if appropriate) and the (rare) potential need for laparotomy and/or bowel resection and/or stoma formation are discussed.

Timing of operation

Once a diagnosis of acute appendicitis is made surgery should be undertaken within 24 hours to prevent an increase in morbidity and mortality which results from perforation. A recent retrospective study found no difference in the complication rate when appendicectomy was performed

up to 24 hours after symptom onset compared to when it was performed up to 12 hours. A further study showed that after the first 36 hours after the onset of symptoms, the risk of perforation is 16–36% and increases by approximately 5% per 12-hour period.

Choice of operation

Currently, the main area of debate in the management of appendicitis is whether the open or laparoscopic approach should be used. Some studies have claimed that laparoscopic appendicectomy is superior to the open approach in terms of less postoperative pain, fewer postoperative complications, a faster recovery time and a better cosmetic result. In addition where the diagnosis is equivocal, particularly in female patients in whom the differential diagnosis is much broader, it offers the advantage of being able to perform a diagnostic laparoscopy without the disadvantages of the open operation.

There have been two recent systematic reviews, one of which concluded that laparoscopic appendicectomy was associated with a decreased wound infection rate, a decreased hospital stay and a faster return to work, but a higher rate of intra-abdominal abscesses. The other felt that based on the available evidence 'a conclusive decision is not yet practicable'.

If the open approach is chosen, both the oblique grid-iron incision and the transverse Lanz incision are equally effective. If the diagnosis is in doubt or the patient is grossly peritonitic, a lower midline approach should be considered because of the improved access it gives. Surgical drains should not be placed except in the case of gross peritoneal contamination, as there is no evidence of benefit and they have been associated with an increased risk of faecal fistula. If there is gross peritoneal contamination ensure that a thorough washout is performed and consider closing the skin with clips rather than a subcuticular stitch to aid treatment of a potential wound infection.

Macroscopically normal appendix

It is universally accepted that when an open approach is used, the appendix should always be removed to prevent diagnostic confusion in the future. Current practice in most surgical units is to leave a macroscopically normal appendix at laparoscopy. Evidence either way is poor but a retrospective study by Chiarugi et al. found that 58% of macroscopically normal appendices showed microscopic evidence of inflammation. Another study showed that 4–13% of patients who underwent diagnostic laparoscopy but in whom the appendix was left eventually underwent appendicectomy for recurrent abdominal pain. The same study showed that there was no significant difference in morbidity rates whether appendicectomy was performed or not. These studies indicate that when laparoscopy is performed for suspected appendicitis, the appendix should be removed whatever its macroscopic appearances. However, the evidence either way is not strong and currently there are no randomised controlled trials to support either strategy.

Complications

Although historically considered a benign disease, a recent study showed that up to 30% of patients undergoing appendicectomy suffer a postoperative complication and ~5% will require a further procedure. Particular complications to consider are wound infection and intra-abdominal abscesses. The latter may present any time up to 2 weeks after surgery. Although classically accompanied by a swinging pyrexia, it should be considered in any post-appendicectomy patient returning with continued lower abdominal pain. The diagnosis can be confirmed by an ultrasound or CT scan. Most can be treated radiologically, but a small proportion will need further surgery to drain.

Special situations

Pregnancy

Appendicitis is the most common non-obstetric surgical complication during pregnancy and is associated with a high rate of perforation (up to 43% in some studies). This is thought to be due to delayed diagnosis and a reluctance to operate on pregnant patients. However, whereas uncomplicated appendicitis is associated with a foetal loss rate of ~3–5%, in perforated appendicitis this rises to between 20

and 35% and is associated with a maternal mortality of ~4%. No increased risk of major birth defects has been found but pre-term delivery has been reported to be as high as 20%. It is therefore essential to consider and exclude the diagnosis early in any pregnant woman presenting with abdominal pain and/or systemic illness.

As the uterus grows, the appendix moves progressively superolaterally so that by late pregnancy it may be as high as the right upper quadrant and mimic gall bladder pain. In addition as the uterus grows, the two layers of peritoneum become separated which decreases the somatic sensation of pain and decreases the ability to localise pain on examination. The classic features of sharp pain with localised guarding may therefore not be present. The imaging modality of choice remains ultrasound, but if the diagnosis remains unclear an urgent MRI should be performed. CT should be avoided if possible because of the ionising radiation.

Due to the risks of foetal and maternal mortality from perforation, once the diagnosis is made surgery should be undertaken without further delay, even in the middle of the night. Before 20 weeks' gestation a laparoscopic approach is reasonable, but after this approach a standard open approach should be used. The review by Dietrich et al. gives more details about surgical diseases during pregnancy.

Appendix mass/abscess

Occasionally, a localised perforation can become walled off and present late with a tender mass in the right iliac fossa. This varies in severity from a simple inflammatory mass to a large pus-filled abscess causing severe systemic illness. The patient may give a history indicative of recent appendicitis and systemic symptoms of fever, anorexia and nausea are common. An ultrasound or CT should be performed to investigate the mass further. There is currently no consensus on how these masses should be managed. If the patient is systemically unwell, many would advocate radiological drainage but in milder cases, systemic antibiotics followed by interval appendicectomy may be sufficient.

Summary

Surgery for suspected appendicitis remains the commonest general surgical operation performed in the UK. Although often considered a benign disease it still results in significant morbidity and even mortality, especially in elderly patients. The most important features to note in the history are fever and the character of the pain and on examination the most specific features are pyrexia, localised tenderness and guarding. Investigations may not be needed but ultrasound or CT scan should be used in the first instance if necessary. Once the patient has been resuscitated, the diagnosis has been made and the decision to operate has been taken, antibiotics should be started and surgery should be performed without undue delay.

Further reading

Andersen BR, Kallehave FL, Andersen HK. Antibiotics versus placebo for prevention of postoperative infection after appendicectomy. *Cochrane Database Syst Rev* 2005;CD001439.

Andersson REB. Meta-analysis of the clinical and laboratory diagnosis of appendicitis. *Br J Surg* 2004;**91**:28–37.

Dietrich CS, Hill CC, Hueman M. Surgical diseases presenting in pregnancy. *Surg Clin N Am* 2008;**88**:403–419.

Humes DJ, Simpson J. Acute appendicitis. *BMJ* 2006;**333**:520–534.

Kapischke M, Caliebe A, Tepel J, et al. Open versus laparoscopic appendicectomy. A critical review. *Surg Endosc* 2006;**20**:1060–1068.

Sauerland S, Lefering R, Neugebauer E. Laparoscopic versus open surgery for suspected appendicitis. *Cochrane Database Syst Rev* 2004;CD001546.

Terawasa T, Blackmore CC, Bent S, et al. Systematic review: computed tomography and ultrasonography to detect acute appendicitis in adults and adolescents. *Ann Intern Med* 2004;**141**:537–546.

Colonic Diverticulosis

David Luke & Douglas M. Bowley

Department of Colorectal Surgery, Heart of England NHS Foundation Trust, Birmingham, UK

Introduction

In a busy District General Hospital, in the UK, it would be unusual for a 24-hour acute take not to include a patient with symptoms arising from suspected or proven colonic diverticulosis. This is a reflection of the incidence of diverticulosis in the developed world. In contrast, diverticulosis is rare in less developed parts of the world such as rural Africa and Asia. In the developed world, by the age of 50 years, approximately half of all individuals will have colonic diverticulosis and this proportion increases to 70% by the age of 80 years. The majority of those with diverticulosis (approximately 75%) are asymptomatic.

The symptomatic presentation of diverticular disease varies with some patients presenting with pain only, secondary to colonic spasm. Alternatively, the presentation can be that of diverticulitis and its complications, or diverticular haemorrhage. Of the 25% of those with symptomatic diverticulosis, three quarters will have at least one presentation of diverticulitis. There is recent evidence to suggest that colonic diverticulosis is affecting younger patients (in their 30s and 40s) and that the condition is linked to obesity. Diverticulitis appears to be more virulent in young patients, with up to 80% needing urgent surgery during their initial attack, with a high risk of recurrences or complications.

Pathophysiology and aetiology

Diverticulum literally means a 'blind alley'; it is derived from the Latin verb *devertere* 'to turn aside'. A diverticulum is an abnormal sac or pouch formed at a weak point in the intestinal wall. These diverticula are more common in the colon than the small intestine and throughout the colon the most common place for them to be found is the sigmoid colon. Diverticula can vary in size but the majority are small, between 0.5 and 1.0 cm in diameter. They can also vary in number in different individuals from a 'few' to a 'few hundred'. Diverticulitis is defined as inflammation of one or more of these diverticula.

Diverticula form at the site of potential weak spots when there is a sustained increase in intraluminal pressure in the bowel. The weakest points in the bowel wall are those places where the 'vasa recta' nutrient arteries enter. With higher pressures inside the bowel, small herniations are created through these areas of weakness. Diverticula are only lined by mucosa with no muscular coating which is an important underlying reason for the complications of diverticulosis and diverticulitis described later in the chapter. The commonest explanation for sustained increases in intraluminal pressure within the bowel is the stereotypical 'western' low-fibre diet; resulting in smaller, compact stools, in turn resulting in colonic spasm. Chronic constipation is intrinsically linked with this theory. Diverticulitis is certainly much more common in Western countries such as the UK, USA and Canada where a low-fibre diet is more common. Diverticulitis also appears to be linked with a high meat intake and in support of this theory vegetarians appear to be protected to some extent.

Alterations in gut motility have also been linked with diverticula formation and hence diverticulitis. Manometric studies have been carried out which have shown higher resting, postprandial and neostigmine-induced intraluminal pressures in patients with diverticulosis compared to controls. Following such a study, a theory of segmentation has been proposed whereby a series of 'little bladders' are formed in the colon due to intramural muscle contraction. It is thought that these 'little bladders' result in slower intestinal transit and higher intraluminal pressures, increasing the chances of diverticular formation.

Histological analysis of colonic specimens from patients with diverticulosis demonstrates higher than normal elastin deposition in the muscle wall. This results in shortening of the taenia and bunching of the circular muscle leading to an increased risk of diverticula formation. Patients with connective tissue disorders such as Marfan and Ehlers-Danlos syndromes have a higher incidence of early diverticula

Emergency Surgery, 1st edition. Edited by Adam Brooks, Peter F. Mahoney, Bryan A. Cotton and Nigel Tai. © 2010 Blackwell Publishing.

formation. This supports the theory that intestinal wall connective tissue abnormalities can make individuals more likely to develop diverticula.

Clinical presentation

Patients can present with:

Uncomplicated diverticular disease (diverticulosis)
Diverticulitis
Diverticular abscess
Diverticular fistula (colovaginal, colovesical and colocutaneous)
Diverticular haemorrhage
Diverticular colitis

Diverticulosis

The majority of patients with diverticulosis remain asymptomatic and it is often the case that the diagnosis of diverticulosis is made incidentally during investigation of or screening for some other pathology. Diverticula can be seen at sigmoidoscopy or colonoscopy when it is done either to investigate bowel symptoms or as part of a screening programme. Generally these patients, in whom diverticulosis is picked up incidentally, require no treatment and no surgical follow-up. There is some evidence that advice to maintain a high-fibre diet, preferably with fruit and vegetables as the source of fibre, helps to prevent complications of diverticulosis arising. Patients presenting with uncomplicated diverticulosis can present with a number of non-specific symptoms. Generally they present with vague lower abdominal pain, often colicky in nature. This can be localised to the left iliac fossa; however, equally can localise across the whole of the lower abdomen. This pain can be accompanied by the sensation of feeling bloated or constipated. It can be difficult to attribute specific symptoms to uncomplicated diverticulosis. Patients can present with vague abdominal symptoms and investigations may find diverticula in the colon; however, a definite link between the symptoms and the presence of these diverticula can be difficult to prove. Some clinicians recommend the use of antispasmodic agents to reduce symptoms; however, there is no strong research-based evidence which supports this.

Diverticulitis

The commonest complication of diverticular disease is acute diverticulitis and inflammation of one or more diverticula. The presentation can vary depending on the site of the diverticula, the severity of the inflammation and whether or not the inflammatory process has become complicated. The commonest presentation is of localised left-sided lower abdominal pain, often associated with nausea, or altered bowel habit, either diarrhoea or constipation. Patients often present with the classic triad of left lower quadrant pain, fever and leucocytosis.

In Western populations, the affected diverticula tend to be in the sigmoid colon; however, all parts of the colon may be affected and indeed, in some populations, particularly people of Asian descent, right colonic diverticula are more often involved in active disease. As a result of this an individual with diverticulitis may present with right-sided abdominal pain. An alternative cause of symptoms and signs of diverticulitis occurring away from the left iliac fossa is if the patient has a long, redundant sigmoid colon; in this instance, the affected segment of bowel may lie centrally or on the right side of the abdomen, making diagnosis more difficult.

Pathogenesis of diverticulitis

The pathogenesis of diverticulitis is thought to be similar to that of appendicitis. The necks of the diverticula can become obstructed with faecal material; this can cause localised inflammation in the bowel mucosa leading to ischaemia, bacterial translocation and trans-mural inflammation. This can eventually lead to micro-perforations and complicated diverticulitis. Perforations secondary to diverticulitis can present in many ways depending on the extent of the perforation. Small localised perforations may cause localised abscesses and focal pain. More extensive perforations can result in more of the colon being affected and can result in an inflammatory mass (or phlegmon) affecting a large portion of colon and causing more significant symptoms. Large perforations can result in faecal contamination which can present with peritonitis, or sepsis and can be life-threatening.

Diagnosis of diverticulitis

The diagnosis of diverticulitis is initially made on the basis of history and clinical examination. Laboratory investigations, imaging modalities and (occasionally) endoscopic investigations are then used to support and confirm the diagnosis.

The clinical presentation of diverticulitis depends on the location and extent of the disease and the presence or absence of complications. The most common presentation is of left lower quadrant pain and this occurs in 70% of patients. The pain can be associated with a myriad of symptoms, including nausea, vomiting, bloating, constipation, diarrhoea, flatulence and fever. The location of the pain may vary with right-sided diverticulitis mimicking appendicitis or cholecystitis. Perforation and abscess formation may present with minimal symptoms if the perforation is contained in the retroperitoneum, or the patient may present with the non-specific symptom of spiking fevers of unknown origin. Perforation with intra-abdominal contamination can present with a generalised peritonitis over a short period of time. It is important to recognise that elderly patients or those on long-term steroid treatment may present with minimal symptoms and signs which can make prompt diagnosis difficult.

Clinical examination of the patient with diverticulitis most classically reveals left lower quadrant tenderness, with or without localised guarding of the abdominal muscles. Again the position of this tenderness may vary depending on the location of the affected bowel. More complicated diverticulitis may present with a tender mass in the left lower quadrant and a mass may also be palpable on pelvic or rectal examination. If there is perforation and faecal contamination then the patient will present with an acute abdomen and generalised peritonitis. Colovesical fistula formation may result in urinary symptoms such as suprapubic pain, flank pain, cystitis-type symptoms or faecaluria. Colovaginal fistula formation in women can present with a purulent or offensive vaginal discharge. Fistulas can also develop into the abdominal wall, resulting in signs of soft tissue infection and at its worst necrotising fasciitis.

Laboratory tests

On presentation the patient with possible diverticulitis should be investigated with a range of laboratory tests; full blood count may reveal a leucocytosis with a neutrophilia although this is not always the case. Haemoglobin may be reduced due to bleeding per rectum. There may be an electrolyte disturbance if the patient presents with vomiting or diarrhoea. Inflammatory markers such as CRP (C-reactive protein) may be elevated. Urinalysis and mid-stream specimen of urine are important in determining whether there is any possible fistulation with the urinary tract and a pregnancy test should be done on any female of childbearing age.

Imaging

Plain abdominal films can be used to show evidence of bowel obstruction or ileus which can be helpful in assessment of the patient. Erect chest radiograph can potentially show free gas under the diaphragm which would suggest perforation.

Contrast studies of the large bowel are not appropriate to be done during an acute presentation, however, may be appropriate in assessing the extent of diverticular disease in its quiescent phase.

Computed tomography (CT) scan of the abdomen is considered the gold standard imaging modality to confirm the diagnosis and assess the extent and severity of diverticulitis. In a patient thought to have acute diverticulitis a CT scan is safer than contrast studies and can also give information about the extraluminal anatomy which can help in the demonstration of complications and help with staging of the disease. Obvious colonic diverticulosis, pericolic fat stranding, bowel wall thickening, inflammatory masses or phlegmons, and abscesses can all be demonstrated on CT scan. CT scans can also help in the assessment of possible fistulas and it can be used to guide percutaneous drainage of diverticular abscesses.

Endoscopic examination of the colon should also be avoided during a suspected acute episode of diverticulitis as

Table 6.1 Modified Hinchey's classification of acute diverticulitis.

Stage	Characteristic symptoms
0	Mild clinical diverticulitis
Ia	Confined pericolic inflammation, no abscess
Ib	Confined pericolic abscess (abscess or phlegmon may be palpable, fever, severe and localised abdominal pain)
II	Pelvic, retroperitoneal or distant intraperitoneal abscess (abscess or phlegmon may be palpable, fever and systemic toxicity)
III	Generalised purulent peritonitis, no communication with bowel lumen
IV	Faeculent peritonitis, open communication with bowel lumen

the complication rate of such a procedure is high. It is useful in assessing the degree of colonic involvement of diverticulosis and to rule out other pathologies, such as malignancy, which may mimic diverticulosis. Endoscopic examination should be delayed until the acute episode has been adequately treated.

Staging of diverticulitis

Colonic diverticulosis can be considered as a spectrum of disorders with asymptomatic diverticulosis at one end of the spectrum and complicated diverticulitis at the other end. Acute diverticulitis can be staged using clinical findings, imaging appearance or based on the presence or absence of complications.

Hinchey's classification is simple, widely used, and can be used to plan appropriate surgical management (Table 6.1). As CT is now the accepted investigative modality, CT criteria are increasingly being used to ensure that patients with different severity of diverticulitis are managed appropriately (Table 6.2). Those with mild disease are better treated conservatively whereas those with severe disease are better treated invasively, either by percutaneous drainage or by surgical intervention (Figure 6.1).

Management of diverticulitis

Many mild attacks of diverticulitis are managed quite successfully in the primary care setting with rest, analgesia, antispasmodics and, sometimes, oral antibiotics. In the more

Table 6.2 Ambrosetti's CT staging of diverticulitis.

Mild diverticulitis	Severe diverticulitis
Localised sigmoid wall thickening (<5 mm) Inflammation of pericolic fat	Abscess Extraluminal air Extraluminal contrast

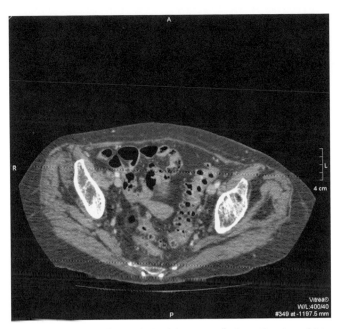

Figure 6.1 Colonic diverticulosis without complications. Courtesy of Dr Ben Miller, Consultant Radiologist, Heart of England NHS Foundation Trust, Birmingham.

acute setting, the patients with symptoms and signs of acute diverticulitis are generally admitted for inpatient treatment. Antibiotics should be started as soon as the diagnosis is made. Intravenous antibiotics are recommended, especially if the patient is systemically unwell. The antibiotic regime should target colonic anaerobic and gram-negative bacteria. Some form of bowel rest is usually instituted, with a clear fluid diet at first, depending on the severity of the presentation. If the patient is not taking adequate fluids orally or is felt to be dehydrated intravenous fluids should be administered. In patients who are going to respond to conservative management an improvement is generally seen within the first 2–3 days. The decision to investigate with imaging can be delayed if the patient does improve and can be performed as an outpatient once the patient has completed a course of antibiotics. Oral intake is gradually increased through clear fluids, free fluids to soft diet and eventually full diet at variable pace depending on the patient's clinical condition.

The majority of patients admitted with acute diverticulitis will settle with conservative treatment; however, between 15 and 30% of these patients will require surgical intervention. The most striking of these are the patients who present with generalised peritonitis secondary to diverticulitis and associated perforation. These patients generally present with clear symptoms and signs and require urgent surgical intervention. Mortality in these patients is high (up to 35% in some series) and morbidity is significant, particularly wound complications such as dehiscence, wound infection, and there is a high risk of incisional hernia formation.

The commonest surgical intervention during an acute episode of diverticulitis is a Hartmann's procedure (sigmoid colectomy and end colostomy formation). This is a safe operation and avoids the formation of an anastomosis in a contaminated environment. Often, Hartmann's procedure is the first of a two-stage operation, the second stage being the reversal of Hartmann's which is generally carried out at least 3 months after the initial procedure. The reversal of Hartmann's can be a technically difficult and challenging procedure and many elderly patients never have their stoma reversed.

A safe alternative can be a slightly different two-stage procedure. The first stage is a sigmoid resection with primary anastomosis and proximal defunctioning stoma – usually a loop ileostomy. The second stage is the closure of stoma which is technically less difficult than a reversal of Hartmann's. This two-stage procedure is used when the surgeon wishes to undertake a primary anastomosis but 'protect' the healing colonic suture line.

However, with increasing utilisation of laparoscopic surgery in the elective colorectal arena, surgeons are increasingly using a minimally invasive approach to the patient with diverticulitis who has failed conservative or percutaneous attempts at management. In patients with complicated acute diverticulitis and peritonitis without gross faecal contamination, laparoscopic peritoneal lavage, inspection of the colon and intraoperative drain placement of the peritoneal cavity appear to alleviate morbidity and improve the outcome. In one recent, multi-centre study of 100 patients with perforated diverticulitis, only eight patients with grade 4 diverticulitis required conversion to an open Hartmann's procedure. The remaining 92 patients were managed by laparoscopic lavage, with morbidity and mortality rates of 4 and 3% respectively. Two patients required postoperative intervention for a pelvic abscess and only two patients represented with diverticulitis at a median follow-up of 36 (range 12–84) months.

In patients who respond to conservative management there is debate about elective surgical intervention. The conventional wisdom has been that elective surgical intervention is warranted after two recurrent attacks of diverticulitis in order to prevent further attacks and more importantly the complications of an attack of diverticulitis. It has been suggested that recurrent attacks are less responsive to medical treatment and have a higher mortality rate thus justifying the aggressive surgical management. After one episode of diverticulitis one third of patients have a recurrence and one third of these go on to have a third recurrence. The incidence of perforation appears to be most likely during the first episode. Given these facts and the high complication rate after elective 'diverticular' surgery as well as the high rate of ongoing symptoms after elective resections for diverticulosis the decision to carry out elective resections must be carefully discussed with the patient. In some recent studies, only half of patients with severe, perforated diverticular disease who did not receive surgery on their index admission required elective colonic resection.

Those patients who go forward for elective colonic resection are increasingly likely to have laparoscopic-assisted sigmoid colectomy. This confers the benefits of reduced post-operative pain, decreased ileus and reduced length of stay and now represents the procedure of choice for elective resection for sigmoid diverticulitis. Conversion to open surgery appears to be associated with complicated diverticulitis involving abscess or fistulae but as experience with laparoscopic colorectal surgery increases, the conversion rate falls.

Diverticular abscess

Abscess formation results from perforated diverticulitis. After an initial perforation an inflammatory mass or phlegmon forms. A phlegmon is a spreading diffuse inflammatory process with the formation of suppurative/purulent exudate or pus. Further spread of the inflammatory process can lead to a larger abscess which can be local to the colon or indeed distant to it. Patients with a diverticular abscess present with pain, intermittent fever, altered bowel habit and a palpable mass on clinical examination. The diagnosis is best confirmed on CT scan and repeated CT is useful to assess the effect of treatment on the abscess. Treatment for diverticulitis complicated by abscess formation is variable. Small abscesses may be treated by the same conservative management as for otherwise uncomplicated diverticulitis; bowel rest, intravenous hydration and antibiotics are used successfully in some instances. The second alternative is to drain the abscess percutaneously. This can be done with the aid of an experienced interventional radiology service; usually using CT to guide drainage. Diverticular abscesses may need repeated drainage to achieve resolution and colocutaneous fistula may occur in up to 40% of diverticular abscesses drained percutaneously. The advantage is that percutaneous drainage is relatively non-invasive, and rapid control of the patient's condition can be achieved without the complications of a major laparotomy. The emergence of percutaneous drainage as a viable treatment option also removes the requirement to carry out an open two-stage procedure. Instead percutaneous drainage can be carried out followed by a delayed single-stage procedure – if indeed a further procedure is needed at all (Figure 6.2).

Diverticular fistula

The most common fistula associated with diverticular disease is colovesicular. Such fistulas are commoner in men, attributable to protection of the bladder by the uterus. Approximately, half of women with colovesical fistulas have had a hysterectomy. The presenting features are typically passage of gas or faecal debris in the urinary stream. The patients require investigation to establish the cause of the fistula (usually to exclude malignancy) including cystoscopy,

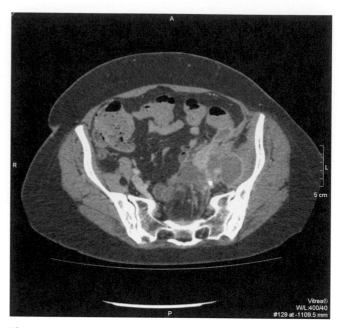

Figure 6.2 Colonic diverticulitis with pelvic abscess. Courtesy of Dr Ben Miller, Consultant Radiologist, Heart of England NHS Foundation Trust, Birmingham.

flexible sigmoidoscopy and cross-sectional imaging (usually by CT virtual colonoscopy) to define the fistula tracts. Single-stage operative resection with fistula closure can be undertaken in many patients; occasionally, high-risk elderly patients with minimally symptomatic fistulas can be treated by stool softeners and long-term prophylactic antibiotics. Colovaginal fistulas are the next most frequent diverticula-associated fistula, representing about 25% of all cases. Passage of stool or flatus via the vagina is pathognomonic. The treatment for this is surgical resection of the diseased colon. Coloenteric, colouterine, coloureteral and colocutaneous fistulas also arise, but are much less common.

Diverticular haemorrhage

Colonic diverticulosis is the cause of major lower gastrointestinal (GI) bleeding in approximately 40% of instances. Severe haemorrhage can arise in 3–5% of patients with diverticulosis. Despite the fact that most diverticula are in the left colon in Western populations, the site of bleeding may more often be located in the proximal colon. Lower GI haemorrhage associated with diverticulosis is often painless and of abrupt onset. Patients should be managed as for any major GI haemorrhage with resuscitation, provision of blood and products and exclusion of an upper GI source of blood loss; as 10–15% of patients with overt rectal bleeding will have an upper GI cause. For most patients, diverticular bleeding is self-limited. For patients with ongoing bleeding, lower GI endoscopy may be diagnostic or therapeutic. Modern CT mesenteric angiography is helpful in locating occult

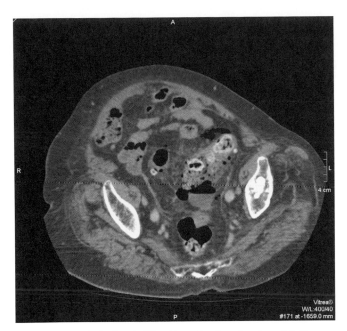

Figure 6.3 Colonic diverticulitis with perforation. Courtesy of Dr Ben Miller, Consultant Radiologist, Heart of England NHS Foundation Trust, Birmingham.

sources of lower GI bleeding and occasionally, embolisation of a colonic bleeding source can be successful in avoiding the need for surgery. Surgery in lower GI bleeding is only undertaken if endoscopic or angiographic treatments fail (Figure 6.3).

Diverticular colitis

Diverticular colitis is a relatively recently described condition; it has been reported in about 1.5% of colonoscopies and flexible sigmoidoscopies. The hallmark of the condition mucosal inflammation is not a prominent feature of diverticulitis and can vary from mild mucosal inflammation to changes identical to those seen in chronic idiopathic inflammatory bowel disease. As with diverticular disease, diverticular colitis can present as left-sided abdominal pain and rectal bleeding with diarrhoea or constipation. A high-fibre diet and a short course of antibiotics, such as metronidazole or ciprofloxacin, might be all that is needed for diverticular colitis. Identification of diverticular colitis from its differential diagnosis, Crohn's disease, is important as corticosteroids and immunomodulatory agents are likely to be inappropriate in diverticular colitis.

Summary

Diverticulosis is a common condition; the elderly population is increasing and young, obese patients appear to be developing severe colonic diverticulosis in rising numbers. The diagnosis and stratification of patients with diverticulitis is now based on the clinical presentation and correlated with the CT scan appearance. The treatment of perforated diverticulitis is changing from the current standard of laparotomy with resection, Hartmann's procedure and colostomy to minimally invasive techniques. Percutaneous drainage of pericolic or pelvic abscess can be used as a bridge before definitive surgery but also as a treatment option in its own right in high-risk surgical patients.

Further reading

Simpson J, Humes DJ, Spiller R. Colonic diverticular disease. *BMJ Clin Evid Concise* 2006;**16**:191–193.

Stollman N, Raskin JB. Diverticular disease of the colon. *Lancet* 2004;**363**(9409):631–639.

Biliary Colic and Acute Cholecystitis

Tom Palser[1] & Mark Taylor[2]
[1]Royal College of Surgeons of England, London, UK
[2]Mater Hospital, Belfast, UK

Introduction

Approximately, 15% of people in the United States and Western Europe have gallstones. Although many of these patients will remain asymptomatic, up to a quarter will develop biliary colic and around 2–3% will develop more serious complications such as cholecystitis or pancreatitis. Between April 2005 and March 2006, there were more than 130,000 admissions to English hospitals with gallstone complications, roughly half of which were emergencies. Despite advances in critical care and surgical technique, there is still a significant mortality associated with acute cholecystitis, cholangitis and gallstone pancreatitis, so early recognition and treatment is essential. The most common emergency presentations of gallstones are biliary colic, acute cholecystitis, acute cholangitis, obstructive jaundice and acute pancreatitis. Cholangitis, obstructive jaundice and pancreatitis are discussed in separate chapters, so will not be discussed further here.

Clinical presentation

Gallstones present acutely with a varying combination of abdominal pain (mainly in the right upper quadrant/epigastrium), jaundice and systemic symptoms such as fever, nausea and anorexia. The exact presentation depends on the site and degree of obstruction and inflammation of the biliary tree. Table 7.1 outlines the symptoms and signs of the various presentations.

Biliary colic occurs when a stone obstructs the neck of the gallbladder (Hartmann's pouch). The pain is usually constant, deep and aching in nature (although this can vary), is of short duration and is not associated with any symptoms of inflammation such as fever. Note that the pain may well be severe enough to cause nausea and vomiting. The patient may describe previous similar attacks which are classically associated with eating fat containing meals. On examination the patient usually looks systemically well, is apyrexial, with only a mild tachycardia. Their abdomen is soft with mild tenderness in the right upper quadrant.

Acute cholecystitis occurs when a stone obstructs the neck of the gallbladder and the gallbladder becomes inflamed. Infection then occurs due to biliary stasis. The pain is often very similar to biliary colic, albeit usually more severe. The main differentiating factor between biliary colic and acute cholecystitis is the presence of symptoms and signs of inflammation, such as pyrexia, tachycardia and abdominal tenderness.

The differential diagnosis of right upper quadrant pain +/− jaundice is shown in Table 7.1. Other important factors in the history include a previous history of gallstone disease, a previous biliary stent (both of which predispose to cholangitis) and symptoms suggestive of malignancy such as weight loss, anorexia and lethargy.

Investigations

The main findings that help differentiate between biliary colic and acute cholecystitis are the presence of raised inflammatory markers, in particular a raised white blood cell count and neutrophilia. A raised alkaline phosphatase and bilirubin suggests an obstructed biliary system and points either to obstructive jaundice, cholangitis or pancreatitis as being the diagnosis, but it is important to note that patients with acute cholecystitis can also get mildly deranged liver function tests. In addition to the standard blood tests, all patients should have either a serum amylase or lipase taken to investigate for pancreatitis. If the patient is pyrexial, blood cultures should be taken and patients should have a chest X-ray to look for a lower lobe pneumonia or free air suggestive of a perforated ulcer, and an ECG to exclude myocardial ischaemia. In addition, particular attention should be paid to renal function and clotting profile due to the risk

Emergency Surgery, 1st edition. Edited by Adam Brooks, Peter F. Mahoney, Bryan A. Cotton and Nigel Tai. © 2010 Blackwell Publishing.

Table 7.1 Symptoms and signs that differentiate between the main causes of right upper quadrant pain.

	Biliary colic	Acute cholecystitis	Obstructive jaundice	Acute cholangitis
Pain type	Constant, RUQ/epigastric, $+ \rightarrow +++$	Constant, RUQ/epigastric, $++ \rightarrow +++$	Not always present. Mild aching RUQ	Constant, RUQ/epigastric, $+++$
Nausea/vomiting	Yes	Yes	Possible	Yes
Pyrexia	No	Yes	No	Yes
Tachycardia	No/mild	Yes	No/mild	Yes
RUQ tenderness	No/mild	Yes	No/mild	Yes
Jaundice	No	Possible	Yes	Likely

RUQ, right upper quadrant.

of hepatorenal syndrome and impaired clotting secondary to impaired liver function.

The main imaging technique used to investigate right upper quadrant pain is transabdominal ultrasound. This may detect gallstones, signs of inflammation of the gallbladder (such as a thickened gallbladder wall or surrounding fluid), evidence of a common bile duct stone (either by actually visualising the stone or that the duct is dilated to >8 mm) or other more rare pathologies such as liver metastases. Note that the sensitivity of ultrasound is unknown and the absence of stones on ultrasound does not exclude their presence (e.g. small stones or sludge can easily be missed). It is also operator-dependent, so the best investigation for suspected gallstones in the presence of a negative ultrasound is another ultrasound a couple of weeks later. In the acute setting, if the diagnosis is unclear, a computed tomography (CT) scan or magnetic resonance cholangiopancreatogram (MRCP) may be helpful. MRCP is particularly useful in the investigation of suspected common bile duct stones. Endoscopic retrograde cholangiopancreatography (ERCP) should be reserved as a therapeutic procedure due to its risks of pancreatitis, perforation and haemorrhage.

Initial management

Patients with acute cholecystitis or cholangitis can potentially be extremely septic. If the patient is septic and shocked, prompt resuscitation and early discussion with critical care is vital as cholangitis and gangrenous cholecystitis are still associated with significant mortality and morbidity.

Once initial resuscitation has been completed, the initial management varies depending on the suspected diagnosis and patient's clinical picture. If acute cholecystitis is diagnosed, broad spectrum antibiotics should be started and the patient should be allowed clear fluids only until reviewed by a senior. A centrally acting anti-emetic such as cyclizine is usually required.

If the patient's pain has completely resolved, their observations are normal and they have no abdominal tenderness, they can potentially be discharged and be investigated as an outpatient. If there is any doubt, however, admit them overnight for observation, reassessment and senior review.

Definitive management

The definitive management of gallstones is either surgical removal of the gallbladder or percutaneous drainage followed by interval cholecystectomy for a suspected empyema or in a septic, high risk patient. Although ursodeoxycholic acid can reduce the formation of gallstones in at-risk patients (e.g. those undergoing obesity surgery), there is no evidence that it reduces symptoms once gallstones have developed.

Percutaneous drainage

Percutaneous drainage is very useful in patients who are septic and shocked who would therefore be at high risk for early surgery. This includes patients with an empyema or a pericholecystic abscess, the decision is primarily guided by the patient's clinical state and co-morbidity. Its purpose is to drain the source of infection and allow resolution of the disease. Definitive management can then be planned at later stage when the patient's acute disease has resolved.

Surgery

The definitive treatment of gallstones remains surgery. A Cochrane Database systematic review comparing the traditional open approach to the laparoscopic approach found no differences in mortality, postoperative complications or operating time. However, it was found that the length of hospital stay and overall recovery time was significantly shorter when the laparoscopic approach was used (with a mean difference of 3 and 22.5 days respectively). The potential need for conversion must always be borne in mind; however, many of the complications of laparoscopic cholecystectomy are caused by surgeons persisting with the laparoscopic route when the anatomy of Calot's triangle is unclear, rather than converting to an open operation at an earlier time.

The timing of surgery for acute cholecystitis has historically been controversial because of a perceived increased risk of complications when performed early. However, a Cochrane review comparing early (within 7 days of admission) with delayed (more than 6 weeks) surgery found no difference in complication rates and a shorter length of stay in the early group. Further studies have shown that up to 30% of people scheduled for delayed surgery are readmitted with further gallstone-related complications before their operation. **Surgery should therefore be performed at the time of the first admission, ideally within 72 hours of symptom onset.**

If there is any evidence from preoperative investigations that the patient may have a stone in the common bile duct, they should either undergo an MRCP to confirm it followed by an ERCP and stone removal before surgery, or a laparoscopic bile duct exploration at the time of surgery, depending on local expertise. When consenting the patient for a laparoscopic cholecystectomy, they should be warned about the risks of conversion (up to 5%), bile leak (0.5%), bile duct injury (0.2%), bowel injury, a retained stone in the common bile duct, and the possibility of further surgery to correct these complications.

Summary

Biliary colic and acute cholecystitis are common emergency presentations. Patients should be resuscitated expediently and receive adequate analgesia. Laparoscopic cholecystectomy should be undertaken in all who are fit for surgery with the timing of surgery being determined by the presentation and clinical course.

Further reading

Hirota M, Takada T, Kawarada Y, et al. Diagnostic criteria and severity assessment of acute cholecystitis: Tokyo Guidelines. *J Hepatobiliary Pancreat Surg* 2007;**14**(1):78–82.

Sanders G, Kingsnorth A. Gallstones. *BMJ* 2007;**335**:295–299.

Williams EJ, Green J, Beckingham I, Parks R, Martin D, Lombard M, for British Society of Gastroenterology. Guidelines on the management of common bile duct stones (CBDS). *Gut* 2008;**57**(7): 1004–1021.

8 Perforated Peptic Ulcer

A. Morris & Mark J. Midwinter

Derriford Hospital, Plymouth, UK

Introduction

The term *peptic ulcer* is used as a general term for a gastric or duodenal ulcer and this chapter will summarise the epidemiology, pathology and current evidence-based management of non-bleeding perforated peptic ulcers.

Currently in the Western world, ulcer perforation incidence is stable or in slight decline with duodenal ulcers developing in 0.8% of the population per year and gastric ulcers in 0.2% of the population per year. The peak age for duodenal ulcer is increasing in developed societies (25–50 years worldwide but higher in developed countries).

Duodenal ulcer perforation is a serious complication of peptic ulcer in 5–10% of duodenal ulcer patients and accounts for more than 70% of deaths associated with peptic ulcer disease (PUD). A previous history of PUD is present in 60–70% of patients presenting with perforated peptic ulcer. The incidence of this complication is 7–10 cases/100,000 adults per year.

Despite a dramatic decrease in developed countries over the past hundred years overall worldwide incidence is increasing. In the Western world, gastric ulcers occur in older age groups, there is a 3-to-1 male-to-female ratio for gastric ulcers and a 4-to-1 male-to-female ratio for duodenal ulcers and mortality is higher in the poor.

Rauws et al. suggest that there has been no change in incidence despite the discovery of *Helicobacter pylori* and subsequent increase in use of medical ulcer treatment. However, others have found a decrease in incidence of perforation attributing it directly to the discovery of this aetiological factor and subsequent medicalisation. Some opinions suggest that any improvement in prognosis lies with general advances in acute surgery such as operative technique and laparoscopy. Prescription of non-steroidal anti-inflammatory drug (NSAID)-induced ulcers is increasing with the result that perforated peptic ulcers will continue to present despite modern medical management of PUD.

Smoking is believed to be one of the most important aetiological factors in the development of peptic ulcers especially in the young and increases the risk tenfold in both men and women. It is estimated that smoking may account for 77% of all ulcer perforations in those younger than 75 years, whereas in the older population, smoking is of much less importance.

The use of NSAIDs is another well-documented and important risk factor for ulcer perforations. It has been estimated to increase the risk by 5–8 times. However, the use of NSAID is less common in the population than smoking and therefore accounts for a smaller number of perforations.

The role of *H. pylori* infection in ulcer perforation cannot be confirmed but this continues to be a well-debated subject. Current evidence shows that treatment for eradication of *H. pylori* significantly reduces the peptic ulcer recurrence rate. Recurrent ulcer rates were 6 and 4% for duodenal and gastric ulcers when *H. pylori* was eradicated compared with 67 and 59%, respectively, when the organism was not eradicated.

Other risk factors include alcohol, stress with burns leading to Curling's ulcer, neurological insult (Cushing's ulcer) and major surgery.

There are also some associated diseases that include alcoholic cirrhosis, chronic renal failure (CRF), chronic obstructive pulmonary disease (COPD) and hyperparathyroidism which increase serum calcium and subsequent gastrin production.

There is a familial association with a threefold increase in incidence of duodenal ulcers in relatives and duodenal ulcers are most common in HLA-B5 and people with blood group O.

Clinical presentation

The acute onset of epigastric pain is the usual initial symptom. Subsequent passage of gastroduodenal contents along with the paracolic gutters may cause pain in the lower

Emergency Surgery, 1st edition. Edited by Adam Brooks, Peter F. Mahoney, Bryan A. Cotton and Nigel Tai. © 2010 Blackwell Publishing.

abdomen. Ten per cent of patients may have an associated episode of melaena.

Signs include decreased bowel sounds, tympanic percussive note over the liver and signs of peritonitis. The older age groups (>50 years) commonly perforate in the prepyloric and pyloric areas. Anterior duodenal perforation leads to free air in the peritoneum. Posterior duodenal erosion/perforation leads to bleeding from the gastroduodenal artery and possibly acute pancreatitis.

Differential diagnoses include acute pancreatitis, acute cholecystitis, perforated acute appendicitis, colonic diverticulitis, myocardial infarction and any perforated viscus.

Blood tests commonly reveal a leucocytosis and, on occasions, an elevated serum amylase secondary to absorption into the blood stream from the peritoneum.

Diagnostic tests include an erect chest radiograph showing air under the diaphragm or in the lesser sac. If an erect chest X-ray is not possible then a left lateral decubitus can be performed as air will be seen over the liver and not confused with the gastric bubble. Ten per cent of patients will have no radiological evidence of free gas on erect chest X-ray. Plain abdominal X-ray may reveal free gas by the presence of gas on both sides of the bowel wall (Rigler's sign).

Initial treatment includes resuscitation with intravenous fluids, passage of a nasogastric tube and placing the patient nil by mouth. Monitoring of vital signs including pulse, blood pressure, temperature, oxygen saturation and urine output by a urinary catheter should be instigated. Antibiotics, a proton pump inhibitor (40 mg omeprazole or isomeprazole IV) and appropriate analgesia should be commenced with concomitant intravenous fluid resuscitation and supplemental oxygen.

Management

The principal decision to be made in the management of a perforated peptic ulcer is whether the approach is to be operative or non-operative.

A non-operative management approach with nasogastric suction, intravenous fluids, antibiotics and acid suppression and oxygen may be adopted in high-risk patients but this seems to be less successful in the over 70 year olds. A confounding factor in this approach is mis-diagnosis with the perforation being non-peptic in nature.

Open operative repair is usually performed through an upper midline incision. Repair of a perforated duodenal ulcer is performed by oversewing with an omental patch using a 2/0 synthetic absorbable suture. If the site of perforation is not immediately obvious the lesser sac must be opened and inspected. A thorough irrigation of the peritoneal cavity must be performed. Multiple perforations can also occur. Postoperative drainage is not required if the closure of the perforation is secure and adequate peritoneal lavage has

been performed. Prepyloric ulcers behave as duodenal ulcers. All gastric ulcers require biopsy. Surgical management is usually by excision and sutured closure.

All patients should be considered for *H. pylori* eradication therapy. More definitive anti-ulcer procedures such as partial gastrectomies with truncal or selective vagotomy are now rarely necessary.

Studies have so far not demonstrated the superiority of laparoscopic versus open surgery for closure of perforations in terms of morbidity. A Cochrane review found no difference in septic complications or pulmonary complications between open and laparoscopic repair for perforated peptic ulcer. However, only two randomised controlled trials were eligible for inclusion in this review. In 2006, a European Association of Endoscopic Surgery consensus' statement supported laparoscopy for abdominal emergencies including for perforated PUD. It was suggested that laparoscopically treated patients experienced less pain postoperatively after symptoms of peritonitis had diminished. Decreased pain levels also accounted for a shorter inpatient stay and an earlier return to normal activities.

The patient is placed in a 10–15° reverse Trendelenburg position. The operating surgeon stands between the legs or on the patient's left. The assistants stand on each side of the patient. Through a supraumbilical or infraumbilical incision a carbon dioxide pneumoperitoneum (up to 12 mm Hg) is established. A laparoscope is introduced though a suitably sized trocar. The whole of the abdomen should be inspected. Other trocars are placed under laparoscopic guidance, including a trocar in the epigastrium used for liver and gallbladder retraction and two other trocars; one in the upper left quadrant in the subcostal region and the second where the midclavicular line meets with the inferior border of the left upper quadrant. Failure to locate the perforation site is one of the most common reasons to convert to an open repair.

Sutureless techniques for closing the perforation site have been described. Examples are a gelatine sponge fibrin glue repair and application of omentum using fibrin glue alone to close the perforation. An automated stapler device and a running suture closure are other alternatives.

Conservative management with nasogastric suction, circulatory support and antibiotics can be an effective treatment of perforated ulcer and warrants serious consideration in the elderly patient. However, if a Gastrograffin upper gastrointestinal series shows continuing free perforation despite conservative management then surgery must be considered.

It is worth considering that with perforated peptic ulcer which occurs more commonly in elderly patients, mortality increases with three risk factors: the presence of severe comorbidity, perforation longer than 24 hours and the presence of hypotension on admission (systolic <100 mm Hg).

Postoperative mortality has been associated with concomitant diseases, shock on admission, delayed surgery and postoperative abdominal infections in patients undergoing emergency surgery for perforated peptic ulcer.

Boey risk factors

The Boey score can be used for risk stratification in patients undergoing open repair for perforated duodenal ulcer as well as being valid for laparoscopic repair. Boey score is defined as the sum of the Boey risk factors scoring one point for the presence of each of the following:

– Shock on admission (systolic blood pressure < 90 mm Hg)
– Severe medical illness (ASA III-IV)
– Delayed presentation (duration of symptoms over 24 hours)

Postoperative mortality rates of patients with various Boey scores have been documented as follows:

0–1.5%
1–14.4%
2–32.1%
3–100%

Prognosis is also dependent on the patient's age, the site of perforation and the delay in treatment. Svanes noted that patients with a long history of ulcer perforation have a lower survival rate.

Summary

The aetiology of perforated duodenal ulcers appears to be multifactorial but most often is associated with *H. pylori*. Simple patch closure alone with postoperative assessment for *H. pylori* is thought to be suffice. The treatment and subsequent eradication of *H. pylori* infection results in a very low risk for further recurrent ulceration.

It is important to remember that a small percentage of patients may have other aetiologies of ulcer disease such as Zollinger–Ellison syndrome and Crohn's disease.

Limiting time to treatment within 12 hours from onset of symptoms improves survival.

9

Fulminant Colitis

Deborah Nicol[1] & Richard L. Wolverson[2]
[1]West Midlands, Worcester, UK
[2]City Hospital Birmingham, Birmingham, UK

Introduction

Ulcerative colitis (UC) is a disease of unknown aetiology characterised by diffuse mucosal inflammation which is limited to the large bowel. The incidence of UC is 10–20 per 100,000 per year. In active UC, the colonic mucosa will be thickened and therefore ulcerated patients most commonly present with bloody diarrhoea. They may also complain of abdominal pain, weight loss, mucus secretion, urgency of defecation or tenesmus. Medical treatment can control the disease in most cases, but a severe attack of UC is still a potentially life-threatening condition.

Fulminant colitis is an acute, severe episode of UC where the disease may no longer be confined to the mucosa of the colon. Ulceration and inflammation may be extensive and involve the muscularis propria. This can lead to thinning of the musculature of the colon with the risk of colonic dilatation and perforation. About 5–10% of patients with UC present initially with acute severe colitis and a number of patients within the first 2 years of diagnosis will fail to respond to medical management and develop fulminant colitis.

The initial management of acute, severe UC is medical but a significant number of patients will develop fulminant colitis despite aggressive medical therapy and these patients require urgent surgery. Clinical assessment of these patients, therefore, aims to identify those patients who require colectomy at an early stage, as an inappropriate delay in surgery can be fatal.

Clinical presentation

Acute onset of UC should be considered as a diagnosis in all patients presenting with bloody diarrhoea. A full his-

tory should be taken and include the details outlined in Table 9.1.

A full examination of the patient requires careful assessment of their general state and fluid status to guide resuscitation. Pulse, blood pressure and temperature should be monitored regularly. Abdominal examination should assess the patient for evidence of colonic dilatation or impending perforation. The abdomen should be reassessed regularly for increasing tenderness, rebound tenderness and distension.

An accurate stool chart should be kept from admission to record the number, volume and consistency of bowel movements and the presence of blood.

Investigation

At admission blood should be sent for full blood count, urea and electrolytes (U&Es) and erythrocyte sedimentation rate (ESR) or C- reactive protein (CRP). These should all be repeated daily. Stool samples should be sent for microbiology testing including *Clostridium difficile* toxin to exclude an infective cause or superadded infection.

Plain abdominal X-ray (AXR) should be performed at admission (Figure 9.1). Radiological criteria that suggest severe disease and may predict the need for surgery include:
• Colonic dilatation >5.5 cm
• Mucosal islands
• Distended small bowel loops suggesting an ileus

AXR should be repeated daily if the initial film shows evidence of colonic dilatation (>5.5 cm). If there is evidence of colonic dilatation initially, there should be a low-threshold for repeating the AXR; however, the AXR should be repeated at any stage if there is clinical evidence of deterioration.

Endoscopic evaluation of the rectum and sigmoid colon plus biopsy may be appropriate in some cases to confirm the diagnosis and exclude cytomegalovirus infection.

Emergency Surgery, 1st edition. Edited by Adam Brooks, Peter F. Mahoney, Bryan A. Cotton and Nigel Tai. © 2010 Blackwell Publishing.

Table 9.1 Important symptoms to elicit during the history.

History
- Stool frequency and consistency
- Rectal bleeding
- Abdominal pain
- Urgency
- Weight loss
- Fever
- Symptoms of extraintestinal manifestations (joint, skin and eye)
- Previous episodes
- Recent travel
- Medication
- Family history

Table 9.2 Truelove and Witts' criteria.

• Bloody diarrhoea	>6 per day
Plus at least one of the following:	
• Temperature	>37.8°C
• Pulse	>90 bpm
• ESR	>30
• Hb	<10.5 g/dL

Management

Resuscitation and medical management

Patients with known UC who have failed to respond to maximal oral therapy or those with severe disease as defined by Truelove and Witts' criteria (Table 9.2) should be admitted for resuscitation, monitoring and treatment.

Patients should be managed jointly under the care of a gastroenterologist and colorectal surgeon, so that surgical

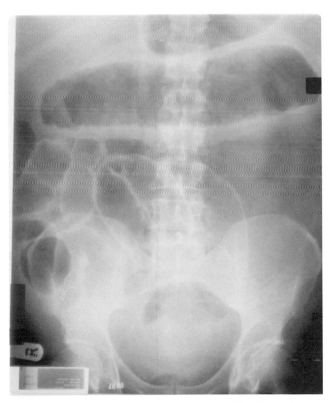

Figure 9.1 AXR in acute, severe UC showing toxic dilatation of the colon, thickened colonic wall, free gas within the abdomen indicating perforation and dilated small bowel loops. Kindly provided by Dr C. Winkles, City Hospital, Birmingham.

intervention is not unnecessarily delayed in those patients who fail to improve or show signs of impending perforation.

Intravenous (IV) fluid resuscitation and correction of electrolytes should begin immediately. This should be guided by a clinical assessment of the fluid status of the patient and the U&Es. In general, IV normal saline with potassium supplementation as required should be started as soon as possible. Potassium supplementation of at least 60 mmol/day is invariably required as hypokalaemia can increase the risk of toxic dilatation. A urinary catheter to monitor hourly urine output is helpful to guide fluid resuscitation in patients with evidence of dehydration. Patients with a haemoglobin <10 g/dL may require blood transfusion.

IV corticosteroids are the mainstay of medical treatment. IV hydrocortisone 400 mg daily or IV methylprednisolone 60 mg daily should be started at admission. Acute UC may be difficult to distinguish from an infective diarrhoea but IV steroids should *not* be withheld until stool culture results are available.

Non-steroidal anti-inflammatory drugs, opiates and antidiarrhoeal drugs should be stopped as these may increase the risk of colonic dilatation. Deep vein thrombosis prophylaxis should be started as usual unless there is severe haemorrhage.

Nutritional support by enteral or parenteral routes may be required if the patient has evidence of malnutrition. The enteral route is preferred as long as surgery is not imminently required and has been shown to be associated with fewer complications in acute colitis.

Indications for surgery

Despite the best medical therapy, 25–30% of patients with acute, severe colitis will require surgery and patients need to be kept informed of their prognosis. It is important to identify at an early stage those patients who are likely to require colectomy. The gastroenterologist and surgeon should review the patient on a daily basis to determine whether there has been improvement, deterioration or no change in clinical, biochemical and radiological markers.

It has been suggested that an objective re-evaluation of the patient should be performed on the third day of intensive medical therapy. A stool frequency of >8 per day or CRP >45 at this stage will predict a need for surgery in 85% of cases. There is no benefit in giving IV steroids for more than 7–10 days.

Indications for surgery include:
- Deterioration or failure to improve despite IV steroids
- Colonic dilatation (toxic megacolon)
- Colonic perforation
- Severe haemorrhage
- Recurrent severe attacks

Some gastroenterologists advocate the use of 'rescue' medical therapy in those patients who fail to respond to steroids by day 3 of treatment. The two main options for rescue therapy are calcineurin inhibitors (cyclosporin or tacrolimus) or infliximab. However, surgery must not be delayed in those patients who continue to deteriorate and is urgently indicated in those with evidence of megacolon or perforation. Perforation is a life-threatening development with a 40% mortality. It is important to maintain a high level of suspicion in patients on high-dose steroids where clinical signs may be obscured and perforation may be silent. Recurrent severe attacks with repeated hospital admissions may indicate a failure of medical management and these patients should be offered surgery at a fairly early stage.

The decision to operate should be made jointly by the gastroenterologist, colorectal surgeon and the patient. Preoperative counselling and marking of potential stoma sites should by performed by a clinical colorectal nurse specialist.

Anaesthetic issues

Patients requiring emergency colectomy for fulminant colitis are by definition critically unwell and about to undergo major surgery. Therefore, it is vital that the general condition of these patients is optimised prior to their transfer to the operating theatre. These patients may be severely dehydrated with grossly deranged electrolytes and these should be corrected as far as possible with aggressive IV fluid and electrolyte replacement. An up-to-date U&E result is vital to guide IV resuscitation. This may be adequately performed through large bore peripheral IV access but severely ill patients may require central access and resuscitation in a high-dependency setting. Patients who have been on high-dose steroids for prolonged periods preoperatively may need extra IV steroid replacement perioperatively.

Patients undergoing emergency colectomy may need to be cared for in a high dependency or intensive care setting postoperatively.

Surgery

The procedure of choice in fulminant colitis is subtotal colectomy with an end ileostomy and preservation of the rectal stump (Figure 9.2). The rectal stump may be closed or

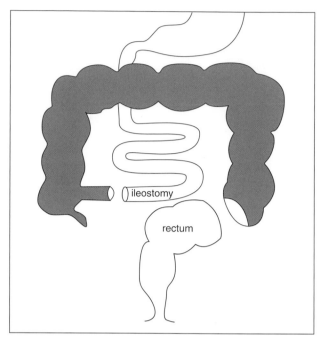

Figure 9.2 Endoscopic view of severe rectal UC. Kindly provided by Dr P. Wilson, City Hospital, Birmingham.

brought out as a mucus fistula. The patient should be placed on the operating table in a Lloyd-Davis position to allow access to the rectum and a urinary catheter inserted if not already in place. Access to the abdominal cavity should always be through a midline incision in patients with inflammatory bowel disease to allow easy placement of stomas as required. Anastomoses should not be performed in patients with fulminant colitis as malnutrition, sepsis and the use of preoperative steroids make anastomotic leaks a likely complication. The preservation of the rectal stump gives the patient the option of a subsequent elective restorative proctocolectomy (excision of the rectal stump and formation of a ileal pouch) thereby avoiding a permanent stoma. The rectum should not be excised in the acute situation except in rare circumstances for life-threatening rectal bleeding.

Summary

Fulminant colitis is an acute, severe episode of UC where ulceration and inflammation may be extensive and carries a risk of colonic dilatation and perforation. Patients present with severe bloody diarrhoea and evidence of systemic toxicity. Initial management involves fluid and electrolyte resuscitation and the commencement of IV steroids. However, despite medical therapy 25–30% of patients will require surgery. Indications for emergency colectomy include failure to improve with IV steroids, toxic megacolon and colonic perforation. The procedure of choice in fulminant colitis is subtotal colectomy with an end ileostomy and preservation of the rectal stump.

Further reading

Carter MJ, Lobo AJ, Travis SPL on behalf of the IBD section of the BSG. Guidelines for the management of inflammatory bowel disease in adults. *Gut* 2004;**53**(Suppl V):v1–v16.

Chew CN, Nolan DJ, Jewell DP. Small bowel gas in severe ulcerative colitis. *Gut* 1991;**32**:1535–1537.

Gan SI, Beck PL. A new look at toxic megacolon: an update and review of incidence, etiology, pathogenesis and management. *Am J Gastroenterol* 2003;**98**:2263–2271.

González-Huix F, Fernández-Bañares F, Esteve-Comas M, et al. Enteral vs parenteral nutrition as adjunct therapy in acute ulcerative colitis. *Am J Gastroenterol* 1993;**88**:227–232.

Loftus EV, Jr. Clinical epidemiology of inflammatory bowel disease: incidence, prevalence and environmental influences. *Gastroenterology* 2004;**126**:1504–1517.

Melville DM, Ritchie JK, Nicholls RJ, Hawley PR. Surgery for ulcerative colitis in the area of the pouch: St Marks Hospital experience. *Gut* 1994;**35**:1076–1080.

Travis SPL, Stange EF, Lémann M, et al., for the European Crohns and Colitis Organisation. European evidence-based consensus on the management of ulcerative colitis: current management. *J Crohns Colitis* 2008;**2**:24–62.

Truelove SC, Witts LJ. Cortisone in ulcerative colitis: final report on a therapeutic trial. *BMJ* 1955;**ii**:1041–1048.

10

Mesenteric Ischaemia

Justin Manley[1] & Tracy R. Bilski[2]
[1]University of Mississippi, Medical Center, Brandon, MS, USA
[2]Mary Washington Hospital, Fredericksburg, VA, USA

Introduction

Mesenteric ischaemia is the inability to deliver the nutrients and metabolites required to meet the metabolic demands of tissues supplied by the mesenteric circulation. Although uncommon, the ability to quickly recognise and make the diagnosis is essential to reduce the high morbidity and mortality that is associated with this condition. The initial signs and symptoms of mesenteric ischaemia are typically vague and therefore a high index of clinical suspicion is warranted. Patients at particular risk include those with advanced age, atherosclerosis, cardiac arrhythmias, low cardiac output states, severe cardiac valvular disease, recent myocardial infarction and intra-abdominal malignancy. Mesenteric ischaemia most commonly involves the small intestine and can be classified as acute or chronic. Acute mesenteric ischaemia (AMI) can be due to occlusive or non-occlusive obstruction of arterial or venous blood flow. Arterial obstruction is most commonly due to emboli or thrombosis. Venous outflow obstruction is most commonly due to thrombosis.

Chronic mesenteric ischaemia, also known as intestinal angina, is due to mesenteric atherosclerotic disease which causes chronic intestinal hypoperfusion. Several types of AMI exist (Table 10.1) yet the mainstays of therapy are fluid resuscitation and prompt restoration of blood flow. Restoration of blood flow can be accomplished via surgical or medical means depending on the underlying aetiology.

Anatomy

Mesenteric blood supply

1 Celiac axis
2 Superior mesenteric artery (SMA) – most common vessel involved
3 Inferior mesenteric artery (IMA)

Emergency Surgery, 1st edition. Edited by Adam Brooks, Peter F. Mahoney, Bryan A. Cotton and Nigel Tai. © 2010 Blackwell Publishing.

Collateral vessels

Extensive collaterals within the splanchnic distribution make mesenteric ischaemia uncommon:
1 Pancreaticoduodenal arcade – celiac axis to SMA
2 Marginal artery of Drummond – SMA to IMA
3 Arc of Riolan – SMA to IMA

Acute mesenteric ischaemia

Clinical presentation

Patients with AMI typically present with severe generalised abdominal pain. The pain is characteristically out of proportion to physical examination findings in the early stages. The location of pain may vary but as ischaemia progresses to infarction, the patient will develop generalised peritonitis. Patients can also present with symptoms of nausea, vomiting and diarrhoea early in the course of the disease. Progression of intestinal ischaemia to transmural bowel infarction may be signalled by fever, bloody diarrhoea and shock. At this point in the progression of AMI, when transmural bowel infarction has occurred, the mortality has been reported as high as 70–90%.

Early diagnosis of AMI requires a high index of clinical suspicion in any patient that is at high risk for embolic or thrombotic events. Patients at particularly high risk include those with cardiac disease, peripheral vascular disease, cardiac arrhythmias or recent history of myocardial infarction. Important clues to help distinguish small bowel ischaemia from colonic ischaemia can be elicited from features of the abdominal pain. Extreme pain is typically not a feature of colonic ischaemia, whereas lower abdominal pain associated with haematochezia is more common with colonic ischaemia. Pain will often precede emesis in obstruction of small bowel mesenteric blood flow. Physical examination of the abdomen may reveal relatively normal findings or only slight abdominal distention in the early stages of AMI. As the disease progresses from bowel ischaemia to transmural bowel infarction, the abdomen becomes grossly distended with absent bowel sounds and peritoneal signs will develop.

Table 10.1 Types of acute mesenteric ischaemia.

Type of AMI	Typical features
Acute embolic mesenteric ischaemia	Acute onset abdominal pain with bowel evacuation; risk factors include: A-fib, recent MI, prosthetic heart valve, ventricular aneurysm etc.
Acute thrombotic mesenteric ischaemia	Acute abdominal pain usually with recent history of dehydration
Non-occlusive mesenteric ischaemia	Less acute onset abdominal pain usually in patient taking digitalis, alpha-adrenergic agents, diuretics or patient in shock
Mesenteric venous thrombosis	Vague abdominal complaints but can be acute in onset; usually in patient with hypercoagulable disorder

Clinical investigation

Laboratory

The initial laboratory workup of a patient with suspected AMI should include routine bloods for abdominal pain workup including a complete blood count with differential, basic chemistry, amylase, liver function tests and lactate. **No single laboratory value is specific for AMI.** Findings may include an elevated white blood cell count with a left shift and a metabolic acidosis. AMI should be included in the differential diagnosis of any patient presenting with acute abdominal pain and unexplained metabolic acidosis. Unfortunately, laboratory values that prove to be of use are only elevated once bowel infarction has occurred. These laboratory values include elevated lactate, amylase and lactate dehydrogenase. AMI can occur in the setting of normal laboratory values and therefore one should not delay possible diagnosis in a patient with clinical suspicion for mesenteric ischaemia given the absence of abnormal laboratory values.

Radiography

Plain abdominal X-rays may help exclude other causes of acute abdominal pain. Often, they are non-specific and/or may be completely normal in the setting of AMI. X-ray findings suggestive of intestinal ischaemia include distended loops of bowel, bowel wall thickening ('thumbprinting') and pneumatosis intestinalis (Figure 10.1). Unfortunately, bowel wall thickening and pneumatosis intestinalis are generally associated with bowel infarction.

Computed tomography scan

Traditional spiral computed tomography (CT) with intravenous contrast typically demonstrates non-specific findings for intestinal ischaemia but may help to rule out other causes of generalised abdominal pain. CT findings consistent with intestinal ischaemia include focal or segmental bowel wall

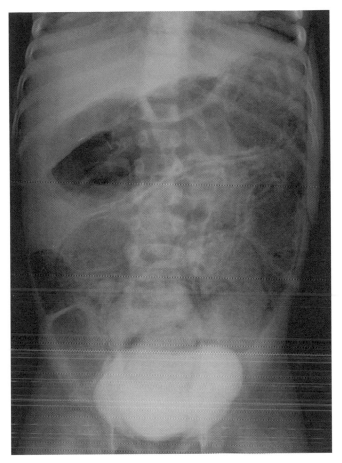

Figure 10.1 Abdominal X-ray showing pneumatosis intestinalis. Note the air within the bowel wall.

thickening, pneumatosis intestinalis or portal venous gas (Figures 10.2 and 10.3). These tend to be late findings, most commonly demonstrated in the late stages of intestinal ischaemia when bowel infarction has occurred. CT has a high sensitivity and specificity for mesenteric venous thrombosis when demonstrating a failure to opacify the mesenteric veins with contrast.

Angiography

Angiography remains the gold standard for the diagnosis of mesenteric ischaemia, with a very high sensitivity and specificity. Infusion of vasodilators and thrombolytic agents can be initiated during the procedure and may help to improve the outcome. Preoperative angiography also has the advantage of defining anatomy to help guide surgical intervention. Patients presenting with peritoneal signs are not candidates for angiography and one should proceed directly to the operating room for emergent laparotomy.

Conventional angiography

Conventional angiography has the highest sensitivity and specificity but may not be available at all institutions. Also,

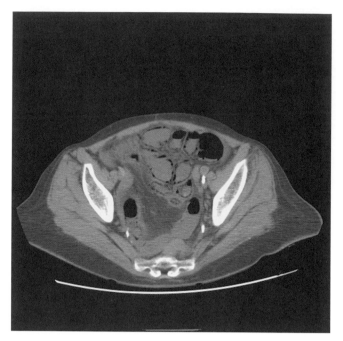

Figure 10.2 Multi-detector CT scan coronal section of abdomen showing pneumatosis intestinalis.

care must be taken in the patient with renal insufficiency as the use of contrast may induce acute renal failure. Patients with renal insufficiency should be well hydrated prior to the procedure. The use of renal protective infusions such as N-acetylcysteine and bicarbonate prior to the procedure may reduce the incidence of renal failure in these patients.

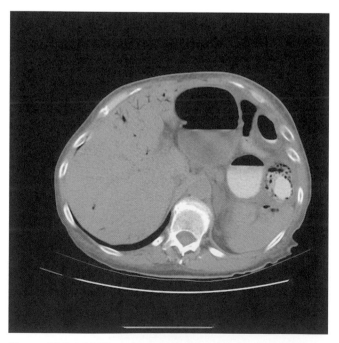

Figure 10.3 Axial CT scan image of abdomen showing gas in portal venous system from mesenteric infarction of small bowel.

In centres with the availability of intraoperative fluoroscopy, the delay from diagnosis to definitive treatment is virtually eliminated.

Magnetic resonance angiography

Magnetic resonance angiography is an evolving technology and has limited availability in certain regions, yet may be an alternative to conventional angiography in the patient with renal insufficiency or allergy to iodinated contrast agents. Magnetic resonance angiography tends to overestimate the degree of stenosis and is limited to the proximal celiac artery and SMA.

CT angiography

CT angiography is performed on newer generation multi-detector scanners and may eventually lead to a change in the diagnostic gold standard for mesenteric ischaemia. These scanners provide high resolution and three-dimensional reconstruction to aid in the visualisation of the mesenteric vessels (Figure 10.4).

Diagnoses

Acute embolic mesenteric ischaemia

Cardiogenic embolic events affecting the SMA remain the most common underlying cause. The classic presentation is acute onset of severe abdominal pain discordant with physical examination accompanied by abrupt vomiting or severe diarrhoea. Specific risk factors include atrial fibrillation, recent myocardial infarction, ventricular aneurysm and prosthetic heart valve. The treatment of choice is open surgical embolectomy, although endovascular techniques are being employed with varying degrees of success. Systemic anti-coagulation should be initiated to prevent thrombus propagation. All questionably viable small bowel is resected at the time of initial operation and frequently a second-look laparotomy is performed to reassess bowel viability in 24–48 hours.

Acute thrombotic mesenteric ischaemia

Acute thrombotic mesenteric ischaemia results from thrombus formation on a ruptured plaque therefore most patients will carry the diagnosis of, or have symptoms consistent with chronic mesenteric ischaemia (see below). The classic patient is a woman with a history of tobacco use and hypertension who presents with acute abdominal pain out of proportion to physical examination and frequently is suffering from recent dehydration due to postoperative fluid loss, vomiting, diarrhoea or pancreatitis. Any patient with a history of postprandial abdominal pain and weight loss who presents with an acute exacerbation of abdominal pain should undergo prompt mesenteric angiography.

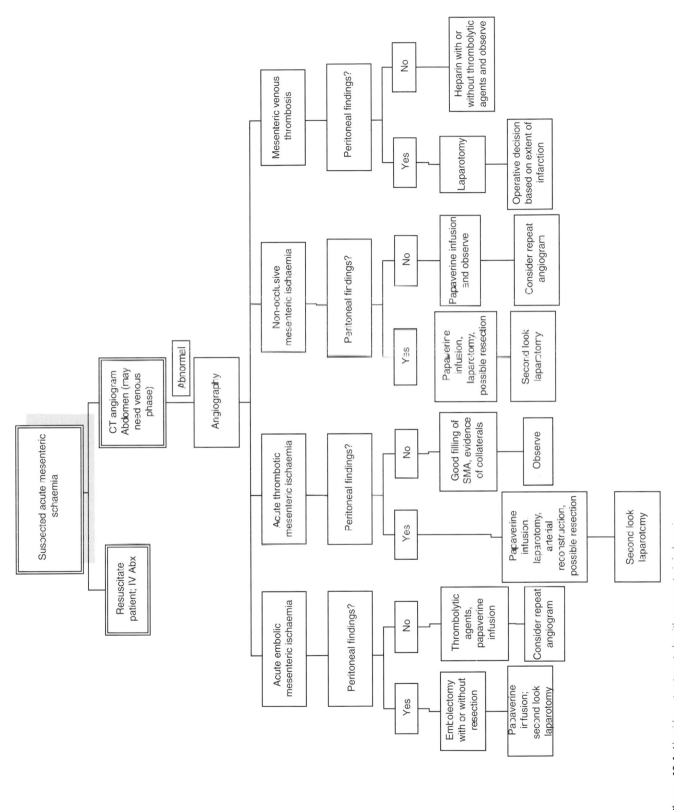

Figure 10.4 Algorithm – treatment algorithm mesenteric ischaemia.

Fluid resuscitation and prompt surgical revascularisation are the treatment goals. Open endarterectomy and multivessel bypass are the traditional therapies although endovascular thrombolysis or angioplasty with stent placement has been employed with varying degrees of success.

Non-occlusive mesenteric ischaemia

This is characterised by a low flow state in the mesenteric arterial distribution. Specific causes include shock (cardiogenic, hypovolemic or septic) or administration of drugs known to reduce intestinal perfusion (e.g. digitalis, alpha-adrenergic agents or diuretics). The pain associated with non-occlusive mesenteric ischaemia is not as pronounced as with other causes of AMI and may be variable in character and location. The typical patient is an elderly man or woman with known cardiovascular disease who suffers a life-threatening insult and demonstrates abdominal distention, progressive acidosis and peritonitis of unknown aetiology. The diagnosis is typically made by mesenteric angiography which may demonstrate segmental vasospasm of the SMA. Treatment is generally non-operative and supportive as long as the patient remains stable and does not develop peritonitis. Direct infusion of papavarine into the SMA may help resolve the arterial spasm and limiting vasopressor infusions may hasten the resolution of this condition.

Mesenteric venous thrombosis

This condition most commonly involves the superior mesenteric vein and commonly occurs in patients with hyper-coagulable disorders. Patients typically present with vague abdominal complaints such as decreased appetite, dull abdominal pain with abdominal distention, vomiting and diarrhoea. Some patients may present with signs and symptoms mimicking acute arterial mesenteric ischaemia. Diagnosis is made with CT scanning which demonstrates a hypo-dense thrombus ('filling defect') in the superior mesenteric vein (CT has near 100% sensitivity for mesenteric venous thrombosis). Non-operative management strategy would include bowel rest, prompt fluid resuscitation, broad spectrum antibiotics and systemic anti-coagulation. Superior mesenteric vein thrombectomy and thrombolytic therapy have met with little success and high rates of complications.

Management

Initial and preoperative resuscitation

Prompt fluid resuscitation and electrolyte correction should be initiated along with administration of broad-spectrum antibiotics in the immediate preoperative period. Underlying conditions such as hypotension, cardiac arrhythmias or dysfunction, renal failure, pulmonary insufficiency and metabolic acidosis should be addressed with the goal of op-

timising the patient's preoperative status. A Foley catheter should be placed to precisely monitor urinary output. Gastrointestinal decompression via a nasogastric tube should be instituted. A baseline electrocardiogram should be obtained, as the finding of atrial fibrillation would support the diagnosis of acute mesenteric embolic ischaemia.

Critical care

All patients should have a central venous catheter placed for fluid and medication administration as well as monitoring the central venous pressure to guide fluid resuscitation. The use of vasoconstrictive agents should be avoided if possible as they may exacerbate the intestinal ischaemia. Dobutamine, low-dose dopamine and milrinone may be used as they should have less vasoconstrictive effect on the mesenteric arteries. Systemic anti-coagulation is important to prevent thrombus formation or propagation unless anti-coagulation is clinically contraindicated.

Operative management

Patients with overt peritonitis should undergo emergent laparotomy with the goal of quickly identifying the cause and gaining prompt control. Visual inspection of the bowel can identify areas of infarction. Any segments of bowel that appear to be infarcted should be resected. The decision to restore bowel continuity should be made only if one is certain that the viability of all remaining bowel is not in question. This can often be difficult to ascertain by visual inspection alone. Various techniques to assess bowel viability may include intraoperative Doppler examination of the bowel/mesentery or intravenous injection of flurescein dye with examination under a Wood's lamp. If one is uncertain of the viability of remaining bowel, a second look laparotomy should be employed. In this situation, one can leave the bowel in discontinuity after resection and perform reanastomosis at the time of the second look. In addition, in cases in which large vessel occlusion is suspected or known, one must be prepared to perform mesenteric embolectomy or bypass surgery.

Postoperative critical care

Patients with AMI are critically ill. This group of patients will often require a second-look laparotomy to determine bowel viability and therefore many patients are left with an open abdomen. After closure of the patient's fascia, one should be astute to the potential development of abdominal compartment syndrome. Many of these patients will still be intubated and on mechanical ventilatory support. Any patient in which abdominal closure has been performed that demonstrates an increase in peak airway pressures not explained by mucus plugging or bronchospasm should undergo bladder pressure monitoring to rule out abdominal compartment syndrome. Total parenteral nutrition should be started on postoperative day 1 and continued until bowel function returns. The progression to multiple organ dysfunction syndrome (MODS) is unfortunately high in the postoperative period following mesenteric revascularisation. Individual organ function should be supported to optimise outcomes. These supportive modalities may include mechanical ventilation to support the lungs; continuous renal replacement therapy or haemodialysis to support the kidneys; and the use of chronotropic or inotropic agents to maintain haemodynamic stability.

Pitfalls

- The benign nature of the physical examination in AMI often leads to a delay in diagnosis and therefore a progression from ischaemia to infarction.
- Failing to provide adequate fluid resuscitation can hasten the progression from ischaemia to infarction.
- Lactate is a key laboratory value in AMI and often not tested in the initial evaluation of these patients.
- Failing to illicit a comprehensive history could delay diagnosis of AMI as certain symptoms and medical problems are frequent precursors.
- AMI can occur in the setting of normal laboratory values and normal physical examination.

Summary

AMI is a disease associated with a high mortality. The presenting signs and symptoms are vague and non-specific, therefore a high degree of clinical suspicion is essential to early diagnosis. Prompt diagnosis and definitive treatment can help reduce the high mortality associated with the disease. Every patient that presents with the acute onset of abdominal pain that is out of proportion to the physical examination findings should be suspected of having AMI. The diagnostic standard remains mesenteric angiography although newer generation CT scanners may eventually change the diagnostic algorithm for AMI. All patients should undergo prompt fluid resuscitation and be given parenteral broad-spectrum antibiotics prior to surgical intervention. All patients presenting with peritonitis should forgo further diagnostic evaluation and proceed directly with emergent laparotomy. These patients are critically ill and require a high level of care both pre- and postoperatively.

Further reading

Burns BJ, Brandt LJ. Intestinal ischemia. *Gastroenterol Clin North Am* 2003;**32**:1127–1143.

Fox CJ, Irwin Z. Emergency and critical care imaging. *Emerg Med Clin North Am* 2008;**26**:787–812.

Herbert GS, Steele RS. Acute and chronic mesenteric ischemia. *Surg Clin North Am* 2007;**87**:1115–1134.

Huber TS, Lee WA, Seeger JM. Chronic mesenteric ischemia. In: Rutherford RB (ed) *Vascular Surgery*, 6th edn. Elsevier Saunders, Philadelphia, PA, 2005, pp. 1732–1747.

Shanley CJ, Weinberger JB. Acute abdominal vascular emergencies. *Med Clin North Am* 2008;**92**:627–647.

Wyers MC, Zwolak RM. Physiology and diagnosis of splanchnic arterial occlusion. In: Rutherford RB (ed) *Vascular Surgery*, 6th edn. Elsevier Saunders, Philadelphia, PA, 2005, pp. 1707–1717.

11

Acute Upper Gastrointestinal Haemorrhage

John S. Hammond

Department of Surgery, Nottingham Digestive Diseases Centre, University of Nottingham, Nottingham, UK

Introduction

Acute upper gastrointestinal (GI) haemorrhage is a common gastroenterological emergency leading to approximately 2500 new admissions each year in the UK. It has a mortality rate of 11% in patients admitted to hospital with bleeding and when it occurs in patients that are already in hospital, the mortality rises to 33%.

Clinical presentation

Bleeding from the upper GI tract may present with a range of symptoms. Patients usually vomit fresh (haematemesis) or altered (coffee-ground) blood. They may pass dark tarry stool (melaena) and whilst the passage of red blood per rectum (haemochezia) is more commonly associated with lower GI bleeding, a massive upper GI bleed may also be responsible (see Chapter 13). Depending on the size of the bleed there may be symptoms and signs of haemodynamic instability (Table 11.1). Biochemically a disproportionate rise in the serum urea may be detected (blood urea nitrogen (BUN)-to-creatinine ratio >30), due to the increased uptake and metabolism of amino acids that results from haemoglobin breakdown. There may be risk factors for bleeding in the patient's history (varices and non-steroidal anti-inflammatory drug [NSAID] use), but even in the absence of clinical signs, upper GI bleeding should always be suspected in the unstable patient with an unexplained drop in their haemoglobin.

Table 11.1 presents the major causes of upper GI bleeding.

The most common cause is peptic ulceration (35%). Here bleeding may be preceded by dyspeptic symptoms (20%) and there is often a recent history of NSAIDs or aspirin use. The ulceration is an inflammatory process, with simple oozing caused by damage to submucosal vessels and more se-

Emergency Surgery, 1st edition. Edited by Adam Brooks, Peter F. Mahoney, Bryan A. Cotton and Nigel Tai. © 2010 Blackwell Publishing.

vere bleeding because the ulcer has eroded into an artery. The majority of peptic ulcer bleeding will stop spontaneously but those ulcers with a diameter >1 mm are more likely to require endoscopic or surgical intervention. The location of the ulcer also influences its natural history with ulcers on the posterior wall of the duodenum involving the gastroduodenal artery or on the lesser curve of the stomach being more likely to rebleed and require surgical intervention.

Bleeding from a Mallory-Weiss tear is usually self-limiting although occasionally endoscopic intervention is required. The tears are caused by retching or vomiting, there is often a history of alcohol consumption and they may be associated with other GI pathology (gastroenteritis or peptic ulceration) or a non-gastroenterological cause of vomiting. Acute haemorrhagic gastritis may be associated with physiological stress (liver failure, burns and head injury) or NSAID use. It is also usually self-limiting as is bleeding associated with oesophagitis, vascular malformations or an underlying malignancy.

Bleeding from oesophageal or gastric varices is the other important cause of upper GI bleeding. It should be suspected in patients with a history or peripheral stigmata of liver disease and should be detected early. Bleeding from oesophageal or gastric varices is often severe, may be torrential and a third of patients will die, with prognosis related to the severity of liver disease rather than the severity of the bleed.

Other rare causes of upper GI bleeding include Dieulafoy's lesions which are nodules of vascular tissue with macroscopically normal mucosa overlying. They are classically difficult to diagnose and treat and should be considered in patients with recurrent undiagnosed upper GI bleeding. Aortoenteric fistula may complicate aortic grafting but may also arise spontaneously. Small 'herald' bleeds may precede catastrophic haemorrhage. Bleeding from a duodenal diverticulum may occur due to erosion of ectopic gastric mucosa, an ulcer into a major vessel, an intra-diverticular inflammatory process or polyp. Haemobilia (bleeding from the biliary tract) occurs when there is an abnormal communication between blood vessels and the bile ducts. It can be caused by iatrogenic trauma (liver biopsy, endoscopic retrograde

Table 11.1 Risk factors for death and the Rockall's scoring system.

Oesophagus	Stomach	Duodenum	Small bowel
Oesophagitis	Peptic ulcer	Peptic ulcer	Peptic ulcer
Barret's ulcer	Gastritis	Aortoenteric fistula	Crohn's
Varices	Dieulafoy lesion	Neoplasia	Meckel's
Neoplasia	Varices	Haemobilia	Neoplasia
Mallory-Weiss tear	Vascular malformation	Post-ERCP	
	Neoplasia		

ERCP, endoscopic retrograde cholangiopancreatography.

cholangiopancreatography [ERCP] and percutaneous tran-shepatic cholangiography cholecystectomy), hepatic artery aneurysms or more rarely in the UK amoebic infection. It can usually be diagnosed by selective hepatic artery angiography after upper GI endoscopy has excluded another more common cause of bleeding.

Rockall's 1995 prospective, multicentre audit of upper GI haemorrhage admissions in the UK identified patient, clinical and endoscopic factors which predicted death. Increasing age (Figure 11.1) and the number and severity of their co-morbid illnesses, those patients who were shocked or who rebled following endoscopic intervention (Table 11.2) and those patients who had recent stigmata of bleeding seen at endoscopy (see below) were all more likely to die. This led to the development of an eponymous scoring system (the Rockall's score) in which age, co-morbidity, shock, endoscopic stigmata of recent bleeding and rebleeding were used to predict mortality from upper GI haemorrhage (Table 11.2).

The need for endoscopic findings to accurately measure the Rockall's score precludes its use in early risk stratifica-

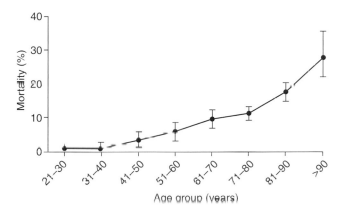

Figure 11.1 Mortality for emergency admissions with acute non-variceal upper GI haemorrhage by age with 95% confidence intervals.

tion of patients on admission (i.e. pre-endoscopy). However recognising the presence of shock, the patients' age and their co-morbidity as well as the history of their presentation still allows the clinician to determine if they have had a mild, moderate or severe bleed (Table 11.3). Rockall's scoring can

Table 11.2 The Rockall's scoring system.

Variable	Score 0	1	2	3
Age (years)	<60	60–79	≥80	
Shock	No shock (systolic BP>100, pulse < 100)	Tachycardia (systolic BP>100, pulse > 100)	Hypotension (systolic BP<100, pulse > 100)	
Co-morbidity	Nil major		Cardiac failure, ischaemic heart disease, any major co-morbidity	Renal failure, liver failure, disseminated malignancy
Diagnosis	Mallory Weiss tear, no lesion, and no SRH	All other diagnoses	Malignancy of upper GI tract	
Major SRH	None or dark spot		Blood in upper GI tract, adherent clot, visible or spurting vessel	

Each variable is scored and the total score calculated by simple addition.
SRH, stigmata of recent haemorrhage; GI, gastrointestinal.

Table 11.3 Differentiating low- and high-risk patients.

Rebleeding is defined as fresh haematemesis and/or melaena associated with:	the development of shock a fall in CVP >5 mm Hg a >20 g/L drop in Hg over 24 hours
Low risk (mild/moderate bleeding)	High risk (severe bleeding)
<60 years	>60 years
No co-morbidity	Significant co-morbidity
Haemodynamically stable	Haemodynamically unstable

CVP, central venous pressure.

then be used to stratify risk post-endoscopy or as a tool for data analysis.

Early management

The focus of early management in all patients with acute upper GI haemorrhage should be to correct fluid losses and restore haemodynamic stability. Oxygen should be given. Intravenous access must be obtained, routine laboratory tests and in the high risk patient arterial blood gas analysis should be performed. Bleeding severity and clinical risk can then be determined based on the patient's haemodynamic status, age and co-morbidity. This can be used to determine timing of endoscopy and the most appropriate level of care. In line with the British Society of Gastroenterology guidelines for the management of non-variceal and variceal upper GI haemorrhage all new admissions should be cared for by specialist medical or surgical gastroenterologists at a centre where a specialist endoscopy service is available.

Intravenous access, fluid replacement and monitoring

Initially two large bore venous cannulae should be sited in each ante-cubital fossa. The choice and volume of fluid and the rate of its infusion must be titrated to the individual's needs. In cases of refractory or profound hypotension rapid infusion of volume expanders, including at the earliest opportunity blood, should be commenced. In those patients with significant coexistent liver, cardiovascular or respiratory disease early insertion of a central venous catheter should be considered to more accurately gauge fluid replacement. Replacement of clotting factors and/or reversal of anti-coagulation in those patients receiving a massive transfusion (>10 units of packed red blood cells), who have abnormal clotting or who are on anti-coagulation therapy should also be initiated.

Patients should then be transferred to an appropriate level of care. Those with mild or moderate bleeding if stable can be transferred to a general ward, where pulse, blood pressure and urine output should be monitored hourly and

endoscopy performed on the next available list. Those patients with severe haemorrhage or who have significant co-morbidity should be cared for in a monitored bed. A urinary catheter to measure hourly urine output should be inserted and a central venous pressure (CVP) line sited where appropriate. The patient should then undergo an urgent endoscopy. In the unstable patient, resuscitation and investigation must happen simultaneously.

Endoscopic therapy

Patients with mild or moderate bleeding who have responded to fluid replacement and who remain haemodynamically stable can have their endoscopy as a semi-elective procedure, ideally within 24 hours of admission. In those patients who have major sustained haemorrhage endoscopy should be performed urgently. The endoscopy should be performed in an endoscopy unit unless the patient is very unstable or the bleed occurs 'out of hours' when a well-staffed operating theatre with resuscitation equipment and anaesthetic support may be preferable. In the very unstable patient endotracheal intubation to prevent pulmonary aspiration should be considered.

There are three aims for the endoscopy in cases of upper GI haemorrhage: to determine the cause of bleeding; to identify those patients at risk from rebleeding; and to treat the underlying cause. Identification of the cause for the bleeding (variceal versus non-variceal) allows appropriate treatment to be initiated. In the case of non-variceal bleeding there are a number of recent stigmata of recent bleeding that may be observed (Table 11.4). It is important to be aware that there can be considerable inter-observer variation in how these appearances are interpreted making it difficult to accurately estimate re-bleeding risk.

A range of endoscopic techniques for non-variceal (most commonly peptic ulcer) bleeding are available. These fall into three categories: injection, heat treatment and clipping (Table 11.5). It is difficult to determine which modality is the best and local practice will be determined by local expertise and resources. In cases where one modality fails to control bleeding a second modality can be used during the same endoscopy. Endoscopic haemostasis is effective in controlling initial active bleeding, it leads to a reduction in clinical rebleeding and reduces the need for emergency surgical or non-surgical intervention.

Table 11.4 Stigmata of recent haemorrhage identifiable at endoscopy.

Arterial bleeding
Visible vessel with oozing
Adherent clot with oozing
Non-bleeding visible vessel
Non-bleeding adherent clot

Table 11.5 Strategies for endoscopic haemostasis for non-variceal haemorrhage.

Modality	
Injection	Adrenaline
	Fibrin glue
	Sclerosants
	Alcohol
Heat	Heat probe
	Laser photocoagulation
Clip	Endoclip

Medical therapy

Three classes of drug have been used in the treatment of non-variceal bleeding: acid suppressants, somatostatin and antifibrinolytics. Acid suppression using high dose proton pump inhibitors (e.g. omeprazole 80 mg stat followed by infusion 8 mg hourly for 72 hours) following successful endoscopic haemostasis of major ulcer bleeding has been shown to reduce rates of rebleeding and should be commenced in all patients with a confirmed non-variceal upper GI bleed. There is no convincing evidence for the use of H_2 receptor antagonists. Somatostatin may be of benefit in reducing acid secretion and splanchnic blood flow but there is no evidence to support its routine use. Similarly, antifibrinolytic therapy may have a benefit but further studies are required.

Indications for surgery

Active non-variceal upper GI haemorrhage that cannot be stopped by endoscopic intervention needs an urgent surgical operation. In cases of rebleeding the decision to operate can be more complex. Surgery for GI haemorrhage carries a high morbidity and mortality but so does a delay to surgical intervention. The decision of whether or not to operate must therefore be made on a patient-by-patient basis.

Table 11.6 presents a list of indications for surgery. In those patients that are high risk (>60 years, shocked, haemodynamically unstable) or with an ulcer that has been difficult to treat endoscopically (e.g. a large chronic posterior duodenal ulcer with multiple bleeding points) early surgery should be undertaken. In lower risk patients (<60 years, no

Table 11.6 Indications for surgery in acute upper GI haemorrhage.

Absolute indications	Relative indications
Active bleeding not responsive to endoscopic haemostasis	First rebleeding in a high-risk patient
Profuse bleeding preventing visualisation and treatment	Second rebleeding in a low-risk patient
Endoscopic rebleed	

co-morbidity, haemodynamically stable), a more expectant policy can be employed.

Surgical management

In most cases endoscopy will provide the surgeon with the site of bleeding. The most common site of ulcer bleeding to require surgical intervention is a chronic posterior duodenal ulcer involving the gastroduodenal artery. The principle of surgical management for a bleeding posterior ulcer is to under-run the bleeding vessel.

The duodenum can be accessed through an upper midline incision. A longitudinal duodenotomy is made just distal to the pyloric ring. If there is active bleeding this can then be controlled with finger pressure. The vessel should then be under-run above and below the bleeding point using a 2–0 absorbable suture (PDS, dexon or vicryl) on a small round-bodied or semicircular needle whether or not active bleeding is present at the time of surgery. Care should be taken when doing this not to damage underlying structures. The duodenotomy can then be closed longitudinally to prevent narrowing. In cases where reconstruction of the duodenum is not possible because it has been destroyed by the ulcer a partial gastrectomy may be required.

It is now rare to encounter gastric ulcer bleeding that requires surgical intervention. If this does occur it is most likely to be from a chronic ulcer high on the lesser curve of the stomach involving the left gastric artery. The treatment options are to under-run the bleeding vessel and then biopsy the ulcer or to excise the lesser curve (Pauchet's manoeuvre). If these techniques fail, a formal gastrectomy may be required. In cases where there are multiple erosions throughout the stomach a total gastrectomy may be required. Rarely does oesophageal bleeding require surgical intervention. In cases when it does it is usually in patients with a Mallory-Weiss tear. In these cases the oesophagus can usually be accessed through the abdomen. Again the principle of surgical management is to under-run the mucosal tear.

Radiological intervention

Selective arterial angiography can be used to investigate and treat upper GI bleeding. When endoscopy has failed to identify the site of bleeding, coeliac artery and mesenteric artery angiography can be used to locate and treat the site of bleeding by embolisation or coiling. Selective angiography has also been used to treat ulcer bleeding following failed endoscopic haemostasis. For patients with significant medical co-morbidities who are unfit for surgery an endovascular approach may offer an alternative to repeat endoscopic intervention in the haemodynamically stable patient. However, further studies are required.

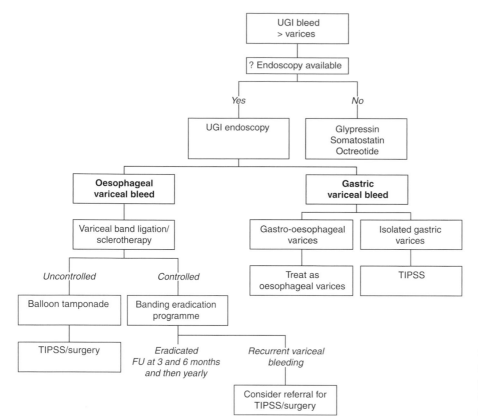

Figure 11.2 Algorithm for the management of variceal haemorrhage. UGI, upper gastrointestinal; FU, follow-up; TIPSS, transjugular intrahepatic portosystemic stent shunt.

Follow-up

Following a confirmed ulcer bleed patients should receive a treatment dose of proton pump inhibitor plus *Helicobacter* eradication. In those patients where there is associated NSAID or aspirin use of these drugs should be stopped. If essential, future NSAID and aspirin therapy must be undertaken in conjunction with a proton pump inhibitor. Those patients who have bled from a gastric ulcer should be re-endoscoped to confirm healing and to exclude a malignancy. Routine re-endoscopy of a non-surgically treated bleeding duodenal ulcer is not necessary unless evidence of arterial bleeding was seen at endoscopy in which case endoscopic evidence of resolution prior to discharge is desirable.

Variceal bleeding

The average mortality from the first episode of variceal bleeding is 50% in most studies. As with non-variceal bleeding it is crucial that these patients are cared for in centres with the resources and expertise to manage this challenging problem. The most important step in the emergency management of acute oesophageal or gastric variceal haemorrhage is effective resuscitation and airway

protection to prevent aspiration. Endoscopy should then be performed urgently to confirm the diagnosis, identify the site of bleeding (oesophageal versus gastric) and to plan treatment. In the acute setting a range of strategies can be employed to stop bleeding, these include endoscopic band ligation and sclerotherapy and transjugular intrahepatic portosystemic shunting (TIPSS). Figure 11.2 shows a treatment algorithm suggested by the British Society of Gastroenterologists for the management of acute variceal haemorrhage.

Further reading

Committee BSoGE. Non-variceal upper gastrointestinal haemorrhage: guidelines. *Gut* 2002; **51**(Suppl IV):iv1–iv6.

Jalan R, Hayes P. UK guidelines on the management of variceal haemorrhage in cirrhotic patients. *Gut* 2000; **46**(Suppl III):iii1–iii15.

Rockall T, Logan R, Devlin H. Incidence of and mortality from acute upper gastrointestinal haemorrhage in the United Kingdom. *BMJ* 1995; **311**:222–226.

12 Lower Gastrointestinal Bleeding

J. Alastair D. Simpson

Queen's Medical Centre, University Hospitals Trust, Nottingham, UK

Introduction

Acute lower gastrointestinal (LGI) haemorrhage is defined as acute bleeding emanating from the gastrointestinal tract, distal to the ligament of Treitz. As a proportion of all cases of acute gastrointestinal haemorrhage, LGI bleeding constitutes 20% and in the USA hospitalisation due to LGI bleeding was estimated to be 20–30 per 100,000 persons. The majority of LGI bleeds occur in the elderly and male populations. The correlation with age is likely explained by the increase in incidence of colonic diverticular disease and angiodysplasia in these groups. Typically, LGI haemorrhage is self-limiting with a reported mortality rate of 2–4%; however, increased mortality and stratification for risk of rebleed can be made, based on whether the patient presents with cardiovascular instability, significant associated co-morbidities or take regular anticoagulant, anti-platelet or non-steroidal anti-inflammatory medications.

Clinical presentation

Initial evaluation should constitute a thorough history and examination with ongoing resuscitation as necessary. To this end, initial triage is critical and patients should be managed in an appropriate environment for the severity of their disease. This may require transfer to a critical care setting before formal investigations commence.

The duration, frequency and colour of blood passed per rectum may help determine the severity and location of bleeding. Clinically, the most common presentation of LGI bleeding is haematochezia, though maelena, haemodynamic instability, anaemia and abdominal pain can be seen. Haematochezia is defined as gross blood seen either on toilet paper after defecation or mixed with stool and can occur in apparently well individuals. Maelena is defined as black stools resulting from the oxidation of haematin in the bowel originating from a proximal source in the gut. Occult bleeding is slow and chronic, frequently leading to anaemia as a first sign of blood loss. The stability of the patient and the rate of bleeding dictate the order in which various diagnostic procedures should be conducted. Resuscitation efforts should take place concurrently with the initial evaluation of the patient to prevent complications of blood loss. An initial haematocrit of less than 35%, the presence of abnormal vital signs 1 hour after initial medical evaluation, and gross blood on initial rectal examination are independent predictors of severe LGI bleeding and adverse outcome.

The past medical history may also help to elucidate the bleeding source. Abdominal pain tends to occur in the presence of ischaemia or inflammatory bowel disease and therefore risk factors for thrombus should be identified. A history of antecedent constipation or diarrhoea, the presence of diverticulosis, previous radiation therapy, recent polypectomy and a family history of colon cancer should all form part of the enquiry.

Physical examination should focus on assessment of loss of intravascular volume, a possible bleeding source and co-morbid conditions (which may affect suitability for investigation or intervention at a later stage). All patients presenting with LGI bleeding should have a documented digital rectal examination, commenting on the presence of anorectal lesions and stool colour. Despite presenting features and findings on physical examination, most patients with LGI bleeding will warrant a full examination of the colon. A full list of differential diagnosis for LGI haemorrhage can be found in Table 12.1.

Diverticular disease

Diverticular disease is recognised as the most common aetiology of major LGI haemorrhage, comprising between 20–55% of all cases. Diverticulosis is rare under 40 years of age, but is seen in up to 65% of patients over the age of 85. Clinical presentation generally is acute, painless haematochezia and in most cases resolves spontaneously, although up to 25% of patients will rebleed and require emergent

Emergency Surgery, 1st edition. Edited by Adam Brooks, Peter F. Mahoney, Bryan A. Cotton and Nigel Tai. © 2010 Blackwell Publishing.

Table 12.1 Causes of LGI haemorrhage.

- Diverticulitis
- Ischaemic colitis
- Angiodysplasia
- Haemorrhoids
- Neoplasia
- Post-polypectomy
- Inflammatory bowel disease
- Infectious colitis
- NSAID-induced colitis
- Radiation colitis
- Dieulafoy's lesion
- Colonic ulceration
- Meckel's diverticulum
- Rectal varices
- Aortoenteric fistula
- Small bowel sources

LGI, lower gastrointestinal; NSAID, non-steroidal anti-inflammatory drug.

intervention. The pathophysiology of diverticular bleeds is thought to be due to repeated trauma to the vasa recta which run across the diverticular dome. As bleeding frequently stops spontaneously the diagnosis is often presumptive, made following exclusion of other pathologies. Preventative strategies include a high-fibre diet and avoidance of non-steroidal anti-inflammatory drugs (NSAIDs).

Ischaemic colitis

Ischaemic colitis accounts for up to 20% of LGI bleeding. Typical presentation is with bloody diarrhoea and associated abdominal pain. The colon is predisposed to ischaemic insult because of its poor collateral circulation. Watershed areas including the splenic flexure and rectosigmoid junction harbour a particularly tenuous blood supply. Patients tend to be elderly with advanced atherosclerosis or cardiac disease. Colonic endoscopy has replaced barium enema as the investigation of choice for colonic ischaemia. Colonoscopic findings include oedema, haemorrhage and ulceration with a sharp line of demarcation between normal and abnormal mucosa. Most cases resolve spontaneously with supportive treatment over several days. About 15–20% of patients will develop gangrene requiring surgical intervention and have a substantial risk of death.

Angiodysplasia

Angiodysplasia are gastrointestinal vascular ectasias, estimated to be the source of LGI bleeding in approximately 11% of cases. They can occur anywhere along the gastrointestinal tract but are predominantly found in the caecum and ascending colon. Lesions can be multiple and incidental findings in 2% of non-bleeding patients over 65 years of age, where the classical endoscopic appearance is of a red, flat lesion, with ectatic blood vessels radiating from a central feeding vessel. However, angiography is considered more sensitive than colonoscopy for detecting angiodysplasia. The clinical presentation includes iron deficiency anaemia with faecal occult blood, maelena or painless haematochezia that may be intermittent and clinically indistinguishable from diverticular bleeding.

Anorectal disease

Haemorrhoidal disease is a common (5–10%) source of fresh LGI bleeding. It is usually intermittent, associated with bowel movements and rarely significant but highlights the importance of proctoscopy as an early assessment tool. Most haemorrhoidal bleeding will stop with conservative measures. Patients with significant refractory haemorrhage may require endoscopic or surgical intervention.

Rectal ulcers may be the result of faecal impaction, rectal trauma and/or rectal prolapse, resulting in significant rectal bleeding requiring endoscopic therapy. Radiation colitis is most often seen in the rectum following radiation therapy for prostate or gynaecological cancer and typically results in chronic, low-grade bleeding. It can however present with more overt blood loss.

Neoplasms

In most cases the bleeding associated with neoplasia is occult. Patients present with anaemia, weight loss and change in bowel habit. Laboratory values usually demonstrate a hypochromic, microcytic anaemia associated with iron deficiency. Massive haemorrhage is uncommon, accounting for 10–15% of LGI bleeds.

Post-polypectomy

Clinically relevant bleeding occurs in 1–6% of patients undergoing colonoscopic polypectomy. Bleeding at the time of polyp excision is amenable to immediate endoscopic haemostasis. Delayed bleeding typically occurs within a week but can occur up to 3 weeks following the original procedure. Risk factors for post-polypectomy bleeding include large polyps, sessile morphology and right colon location. As with other sources of LGI haemorrhage most patients with post-polypectomy bleeding present with mild-to-moderate blood loss, allowing for conservative management.

Small bowel

Up to 15% of LGI haemorrhage is the result of small bowel pathology. Angiodysplasia is the commonest cause, followed by lymphoma, erosions/ulcers and Crohn's disease. Diagnosis is difficult due to the inability of common investigative procedures to adequately visualise the small intestine. Enteroscopy, barium contrast radiography and capsule endoscopy are appropriate diagnostic tools. However, as a result these patients will often have more diagnostic procedures, blood transfusions and days in hospital when compared to either upper or lower GI bleeds.

Diagnostic procedures

The diagnostic and therapeutic approach to patients with severe LGI haemorrhage remains controversial, with patients often being managed in accordance to site-specific protocols. Several strategies are available but largely depend on staff experience and skills. The clinical signs and symptoms associated with LGI bleeds are notoriously inaccurate. Patients should be managed in accordance with the ABCDE algorithm of assessment and resuscitation.

A nasogastric tube may be placed in an attempt to exclude an upper GI source. If following gastric lavage frank blood is aspirated this is an indication of upper GI bleeding, however, a clear aspirate does not exclude an upper GI lesion. In severe LGI bleeding, particularly where there is evidence of cardiovascular instability, many clinicians would argue the merits of upper GI endoscopy to either exclude this region as a source or potentially halt the life-threatening haemorrhage. The relative value and appropriate order in which further investigations should be performed has been hotly debated. Below we highlight the merits and drawbacks of computed tomography (CT) angiography, colonoscopy, radionuclide scintigraphy and mesenteric angiography (Table 12.2).

Colonoscopy

Colonoscopy is considered the best test for confirming the source of LGI bleeding and excluding ominous diagnoses, such as malignancy. Advances in technique have significantly improved its diagnostic accuracy, which ranges from 72 to 86% in the setting of LGI bleeding, and allowed it to largely supersede barium enema as the investigation of choice. Caecal intubation rates for colonoscopy are greater than 95% and it is relatively safe with low morbidity and mortality rates. In subjects undergoing only diagnostic procedures, the major complication rate was 0.1%. Perforation of the colon, which requires surgical intervention more frequently than bleeding, occurs in less than 1% of patients who undergo diagnostic colonoscopy and may be seen in up to 3% of patients who undergo therapeutic procedures such as polyp removal, dilation of strictures, or laser ablative procedures.

Uncertainty remains regarding the optimal timing of colonoscopic intervention for LGI haemorrhage. Endoscopy performed within 24 hours of presentation potentially improves diagnostic and therapeutic opportunities and reduces length of stay. However, a 24-hour emergency endoscopy service is often difficult to provide and good bowel preparation is required to ensure adequacy and sensitivity of the procedure. Good bowel preparation is difficult to achieve in the acute setting but colonoscopy remains an efficient and cost-effective approach to LGI bleeding. Flexible sigmoidoscopy is an easier intervention to perform and yields all the diagnostic and therapeutic intervention of colonoscopy but only for left-sided lesions.

CT angiography

CT angiography has been shown to have a sensitivity and specificity of 90.9–99% respectively in patients assessed for LGI haemorrhage. It requires active bleeding at the time of

Table 12.2 Advantages and disadvantages of common investigative techniques of LGI haemorrhage.

Procedure	Advantages	Disadvantages
Colonoscopy	• Therapeutic possibilities • Diagnostic for all sources of bleeding • Efficient/cost-effective	• Bowel preparation required • Requires on-call endoscopy service • Invasive
Angiography	• No bowel preparation • Therapeutic possibilities • May be superior for patients with severe bleeding	• Requires active bleeding for successful examination • Serious complications are possible • False positives
Radionuclide scintigraphy	• Non-invasive • Sensitive to low rates of bleeding • No bowel preparation	• Variable accuracy • Not therapeutic • May delay therapeutic intervention • Diagnosis must be confirmed with endoscopy/surgery
CT scan	• Non-invasive • Efficient/cost-effective • Diagnostic • May localise source for future angiography/surgery	• Not therapeutic • May delay therapeutic intervention

LGI, lower gastrointestinal.

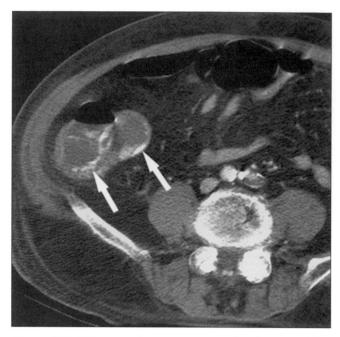

Figure 12.1 White arrows demonstrate extravasation of contrast within the ascending colon.

the examination but is now an accessible investigation and relatively efficient to perform. It is diagnostic in many cases but perhaps more importantly it allows localisation of the source of bleeding. This significantly improves the accuracy of subsequent procedures (angiography/surgery) and thus reduces the time taken to perform these procedures and reduces complication rates (Figure 12.1).

Mesenteric angiography

Angiography is an invasive procedure involving selective catheterisation of the arterial supply to the gastrointestinal tract. The introduction of contrast allows localisation of the bleeding point and the chance at therapeutic intervention. Success requires a rate of ongoing arterial bleeding of at least 0.5 mL/minute to demonstrate extravasation of contrast into the bowel lumen. In addition to its diagnostic role, angiographic localisation allows for vasopressin infusion and selective microembolisation, and therefore may reduce the need for surgical resection. Angiography is an invasive procedure, which can result in complications including contrast-induced renal failure, arterial injury and mesenteric ischaemia. In the worst case, patients can develop ischaemic segments of bowel which require surgical resection. This cohort will have a significantly higher morbidity and mortality.

Radionuclide scintigraphy

Two methods exist, one using technetium-99m sulphur colloid and the other Tc-99m-labelled red blood cells. Sul-

phur colloid is simple to prepare and is rapidly cleared from the circulation. However, uptake in the spleen, liver and bone marrow compromise localisation of upper gastrointestinal bleeding sources. Radiolabelled red blood cells have a longer half-life, making it possible to perform repeat scans for recurrent bleeding following a single injection. It has a sensitivity for bleeding as low as 0.05–0.1 mL/minute and is non-invasive. However, radionuclide scanning has variable accuracy, cannot confirm the source of bleeding and may delay other diagnostic/therapeutic procedures. Radionuclide scintigraphy has been associated with poor accuracy and a high rate of false-positive examinations, as a result it has fallen out of favour as a first-line investigation (Figure 12.2).

Small bowel assessment

When upper GI and Lower GI investigations are normal, small bowel assessment is warranted. Traditionally, this was attempted using push endoscopy, small bowel contrast studies and enteroscopy at the time of surgery. However, video capsule endoscopy has proven superior to other modalities for identifying obscure sources of gastrointestinal bleeding. In the colon capsule endoscopy is inadequate because of retained stool, limited battery life and poor field of vision due to the colon's large diameter. Currently access to capsule endoscopy services is not widespread, limiting its usefulness, but this situation is likely to improve in the future.

Surgical management of lower gastrointestinal bleeding

Surgical intervention is required in a minority of patients with LGI haemorrhage. The surgical options depend on whether the bleeding source has been identified preoperatively. If the source is known, then it is possible to perform segmental resection. If the source remains unknown then an upper and lower GI endoscopy should be performed on the anaesthetised patient, assuming this has not been carried out preoperatively. At laparotomy, it is often difficult to identify the bleeding source as blood refluxes into the bowel proximally as well as distally. On-table colonic lavage and endoscopy/enteroscopy may help identify the source. If the bleeding source remains unclear, a subtotal colectomy with end ileostomy is the procedure of choice. Surgeons must be aware that blind segmental resection and emergency subtotal colectomy is associated with substantial rates of rebleeding (up to 33%) and mortality (33–57%). Anastomosis after resection for haemorrhage will depend on the stability of the patient and the site of potential anastomosis (Figure 12.3).

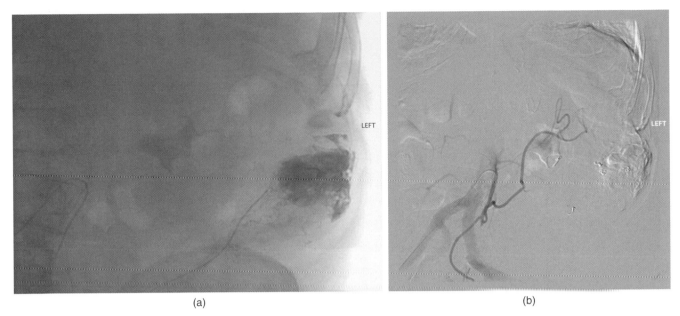

(a)   (b)

Figure 12.2 (a) Extravasation of contrast into descending colon following insertion of mesenteric angiography catheter. Also, note excreted contrast outlining the renal pelvis. (b) Contrast introduced in the same patient following placement of embolic coils, demonstrating no extravasation of contrast.

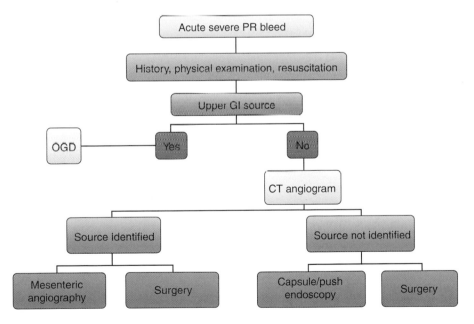

Figure 12.3 Management algorithm for acute severe LGI haemorrhage that does not resolve spontaneously. Resuscitation should remain ongoing through each of these steps.

Summary

- LGI haemorrhage is bleeding originating within the bowel, distal to the ligament of Treitz.

- LGI haemorrhage poses a significant burden on health care resources.

- It is a symptom of the elderly with multiple aetiologies.

- In the majority of cases it is self-limiting but in a small number of cases can lead to overt blood loss.

- A thorough history and physical examination may indicate the severity and potential source of bleeding.

- In the majority of patients assessment of the entire colon is warranted.

- Suitability of diagnostic procedures is defined by the knowledge and skills held at individual centres.

- It is likely that CT angiography will play an increasing role in the diagnosis of LGI haemorrhage but therapeutic intervention will remain in the hands of the endoscopist, radiologist and surgeon.

Further reading

Davila RE, Rajan E, Adler DG, et al. ASGE guideline: the role of endoscopy in the patient with lower-GI bleeding. *Gastrointest Endosc* 2005;**62**(5):656–660.

Edelman DA, Sugawa C. Lower gastrointestinal bleeding: a review. *Surg Endosc* 2007;**21**:514–520.

Farrel JJ, Friedman LS. Review article: the management of lower gastrointestinal bleeding. *Ailment Pharmacol Ther* 2005;**21**: 1281–1298.

Fearnhead NS. Acute lower gastrointestinal bleeding. *Medicine* 2007;**35**(3):164–167.

Hoedema RE, Luchtefeld MA. The management of lower gastrointestinal hemorrhage. *Dis Colon Rectum* 2005;**48**(11):2010–2024.

Strate LL. Lower GI bleeding: epidemiology and diagnosis. *Gastroenterol Clin North Am* 2005;**34**(4):643–664.

Acute Pancreatitis

Euan J. Dickson, Colin J. McKay & C. Ross Carter

West of Scotland Pancreatic Unit, Glasgow Royal Infirmary, Glasgow, Scotland

Introduction

Acute pancreatitis (AP) is a common presentation to the emergency general surgeon. The incidence in Europe and the United States is approximately 200–400 per million population. The number of cases per year is increasing steadily and there has been a small reduction in overall mortality. AP is an acute inflammatory condition, which may have local or systemic manifestations, and is broadly classified as mild or severe. This simplistic division does not recognise the spectrum of disease, but is a useful arbitrary mechanism for guiding clinical decisions. Mild AP is also referred to as interstitial pancreatitis and there is preservation of pancreatic blood supply and microcirculation. Severe AP implies coexistent organ failure, pancreatic necrosis or local complications. In the majority of cases, AP resolves rapidly with simple conservative management, but approximately 20% of patients develop a marked systemic inflammatory response and organ failure. The mortality varies widely from less than 1% in mild, self-limiting episodes to approximately 60% in the context of persistent organ failure or infected necrosis.

Clinical presentation

The diagnostic features of AP can be subdivided as shown in Box 13.1 and Table 13.1.

Clinical

Pain: acute onset of severe epigastric pain radiating through to the back

Associated features: vomiting and dehydration

Haemodynamic compromise: tachycardia, tachypnoea and hypotension

Emergency Surgery, 1st edition. Edited by Adam Brooks, Peter F. Mahoney, Bryan A. Cotton and Nigel Tai. © 2010 Blackwell Publishing

Biochemical

Serum amylase: >3 times upper limit of normal identifies >95% of patients with AP

- Peaks early and therefore needs to be interpreted in context of time to onset of pain
- Inaccurate in patients with hyperlipidaemia
- Absolute values of amylase are not prognostic for severity

Serum lipase: pancreas is the only source of lipase

- Remains in serum longer than amylase after acute attack
- Not increased by extrapancreatic disorders
- Greater overall accuracy than amylase but used less frequently in clinical practice

Radiology

Computed tomography

- Useful if above features are not conclusive or in delayed presentation
- Can differentiate from similar clinical scenarios, e.g. visceral perforation or ischaemia

The following mnemonic summarises the most common causes of AP – I GET SMASHED:

Idiopathic – this is a diagnosis of exclusion after extensive investigation. Fewer than 20% of new cases of AP should be classified as idiopathic.

Gallstones – and other obstructive causes – e.g. pancreatic duct (PD) stricture (benign/malignant) or type I pancreatic sphincter of Oddi dysfunction. Gallstones are the most common aetiology of AP in most populations.

Ethanol – alcohol is the second most common cause of AP – usually in patients drinking in excess of 80 g ethanol/day.

Trauma – typically blunt abdominal trauma resulting in crush injury of the pancreas against the vertebral column.

Steroids

Mumps – mumps (paramyxovirus) and other viruses (Epstein–Barr virus and cytomegalovirus). Patients may have prodromal diarrhoea which can help differentiate from other aetiologies.

Box 13.1 Diagnostic criteria for acute pancreatitis

A diagnosis of AP requires two of the following three criteria:
1. Characteristic abdominal pain
2. Serum amylase or lipase ≥3 times upper limit of normal
3. Computed tomography (CT) findings consistent with AP

Box 13.2 Pathophysiology of AP

Phase I	Premature activation of trypsin in pancreatic acinar cells
↓	activation of destructive pancreatic enzymes
Phase II	Intrapancreatic inflammation (pancreatitis)
↓	activation of systemic inflammatory mediators
Phase III	Extrapancreatic inflammation (systemic inflammatory response syndrome; SIRS)
↓	balance between pro- and anti-inflammatory cytokines
Phase IV	Multiple organ dysfunction syndrome/pancreatic necrosis

---

Autoimmune pancreatitis – rare – presents with abdominal pain and hyperamylasaemia, a raised IgG4/IgG ratio, and a response to steroids is diagnostic.

Scorpion sting

Hypercalcaemia, hyperlipidaemia, hypertriglyceridaemia and hypothermia – these are relatively uncommon.

ERCP – hyperamylasaemia may occur after endoscopic retrograde cholangiopancreatography (ERCP) in the absence of AP. A raised serum amylase in the context of pain post-ERCP is usually diagnostic of iatrogenic AP. This is often self-limiting and resolves rapidly with conservative measures. Patients with severe symptoms or physiological deterioration should have an urgent CT to exclude duodenal perforation as a result of sphincterotomy or direct endoscopic injury.

Drugs: S – sulphonamides
A – azathioprine
N – NSAIDs
D – diuretics

The pathophysiology of AP is summarised in Box 13.2.

In phase I, there are several proposed mechanisms which may result in premature trypsin activation: disruption of calcium signalling, cleavage of trypsinogen to trypsin by the lysosomal hydrolase cathepsin-B and decreased activity of the intracellular pancreatic trypsin inhibitor. Phase II and phase III share some common steps: activation of inflammatory cells, chemoattraction of these activated cells to the microcirculation, binding of inflammatory cells to endothelium by activated adhesion molecules and subsequent migration into inflamed areas. In the 20% of patients who develop severe AP, the pathways driving intra- and extrapancreatic inflammation may involve a genetically determined imbalance between pro- and anti-inflammatory mediators. This results in a marked SIRS and subsequent pancreatic necrosis and organ failure.

Table 13.1 Differential diagnosis.

Clinical features	
Inflammatory	Acute cholecystitis
	Gastritis
Perforation	Hollow viscus
Vascular	Mesenteric ischaemia
	Leaking aneurysm
Obstructive	Biliary colic
	Renal colic
	Intestinal obstruction
Medical	Pneumonia
	Myocardial Infarction (MI)
	Diabetic Ketoacidosis (DKA)
Aetiology	
Symptoms	
Alcohol	<40 years old, male > female
Biliary	>40 years old, female:male (3:1)
Pain	Rapid onset and epigastric
	Radiates through to back
	Eased by sitting forward
Nausea/vomiting	90% of cases
Signs	
General	Agitated
	Shock and respiratory failure if severe
Abdomen	Generalised tenderness and guarding
	Rigidity may mimic visceral perforation
	Distension to ileus
Chest	Pleural effusion
Skin discoloration	Retroperitoneal haemorrhage
	– Flanks – Grey Turner's sign
	– Umbilicus – Cullen's sign
Temperature	Pyrexia common, hypothermia if advanced

Pathophysiology – specific aetiology

The mechanism of gallstone related pancreatitis is not clearly established. There is little evidence to support the bile reflux theory. PD obstruction alone can cause AP with no biliary reflux. PD obstruction induces activation of pro-enzymes within the acinar cell by intracellular lysosomal enzymes – probably initiated by a rise in intracellular calcium.

Alcohol increases the sensitivity of acinar cells to cholecystokinin hyperstimulation, resulting in enhanced intracellular protease activation. Alcohol also influences acinar cell calcium homeostasis.

Management of AP

The initial management of patients presenting with AP is conducted in two stages. Stage 1 applies to the resuscitation of any critically ill surgical patient and is directed at identifying and correcting immediate life-threatening issues. This is done systematically. Stage 2 focuses on maintaining tissue perfusion and oxygen delivery, identifying the SIRS and recognising coexisting organ dysfunction. SIRS on admission identifies patients at risk of multiple organ failure, particularly when more than two criteria are present. Resolution of organ failure within 48 hours is associated with improved outcome and early intervention should therefore be directed at aggressive correction of hypoperfusion. There are several validated systems for quantifying the degree of organ dysfunction, e.g. multiple organ dysfunction syndrome (MODS) and Sequential Organ Failure Assessment Score (SOFA). Whilst these are too cumbersome for the assessment of organ failure in the resuscitation room, the concepts can be simplified in order to rapidly determine how many, and which, organ systems are involved. An approach using this system is outlined in Box 13.3.

In general, patients with AP require supplemental oxygen to maintain a pO_2 of >10 kPa or saturation of >95%; volume resuscitation to maintain adequate tissue perfusion evidenced by both a urine output of >0.5 mL/kg/hour and normal acid–base homeostasis; supportive therapy for organ dysfunction; and appropriate analgesia which is usually opiate-based (morphine). An arterial line is valuable if continuous blood pressure monitoring and blood gas analysis is required. A central venous catheter is useful for multiple infusions, including vasoactive agents; for central venous gas sampling as an estimate of mixed venous saturation; and the trend in central venous pressure (CVP) can be used as a guide to volume replacement. It should be recognised, however, that CVP (preload) is a poor surrogate marker for adequate tissue perfusion. Efforts should, therefore, be made to identify *occult hypoperfusion and cellular hypoxia* using acid–base markers, such as lactate and base deficit, even in the context of 'normal' haemodynamics including an apparently adequate filling pressure. Finally, review by the critical care service and discussion with a specialist unit should be considered at an early stage in the management of the patient with, or considered to be at risk of, severe AP.

Supportive management

This section will cover critical care, nutrition, prophylactic antibiotics and the role of ERCP in AP.

Critical care

Patients with mild AP and no complicating factors may be safely managed in a ward environment with close

---

Box 13.3 System for early management of AP

Stage 1
  Airway
  Breathing
  Circulation
  Disability
  Exposure

Stage 2
  Assessment of tissue perfusion and oxygen delivery:

Conventional	Blood pressure, pulse, respiratory rate, temperature and oxygen saturation
Physiological	H^+, base deficit, lactate, central venous saturation and urine output

  SIRS – two or more of the following:

Temperature	>38 or <36°C
Heart rate	>90 beats/min
Respiratory rate	>20/min or $PaCO_2$ <32 mm Hg (<4.3 kPa)
WBC	>12 × 10³/mm³, <4 × 10³/mm³ or >10% immature (band) forms

  Rapid recognition of organ dysfunction:

Respiratory	PO_2 <10 kPa on room air
Renal	Creatinine >170 mmol/L, or urine output <0.5 mL/kg/hour
Cardiovascular	MAP <70 mm Hg, or requiring vasopressors
Haematological	Platelets <120 × 10³/mm³
Neurological	GCS <15
Hepatic	Bilirubin >20 mmol/L (not applicable in *obstructive* jaundice)

---

monitoring. Patients with severe AP should be managed in the high dependency unit. Patients with severe AP and deteriorating organ function, particularly an indication for invasive respiratory support, should be managed in the intensive care unit. Patient physiology, not pancreatic necrosis per se, dictates the need for a higher level of critical care facility. All patients with severe AP should be discussed with, but not necessarily transferred to, a specialist pancreatic unit at an early stage.

Nutrition

Patients with mild AP do not usually require additional nutritional support. The enteral route is preferred over total parenteral nutrition (TPN) in patients with severe AP who require nutritional support for several reasons: (1) enteral feeding stabilises gut barrier function which may in turn reduce the incidence of infected pancreatic necrosis and organ failure; (2) gastric colonisation by pathogenic bacteria, which may also increase the risk of septic complications, is reduced with enteral nutritional support; (3) there are more complications associated with TPN including line sepsis; and (4) enteral nutrition is significantly cheaper.

Some patients may not tolerate enteral nutrition (delayed gastric emptying and ileus) – if this situation is likely to persist for >5 days, TPN should be considered. At present, there is little evidence to support the use of 'immuno-nutrition' preparations to modulate the disease course.

Key points

Patients with mild AP do not usually require dietary restriction or support.

If nutritional support is required, the enteral route should be used whenever possible.

Nutritional support should be considered *early* in the disease process.

Up to 80% of patients will tolerate nasogastric feeding, the majority of the remainder will tolerate *nasojejunal* feeding and a minority will require *TPN*.

Prophylactic antibiotics

There is no indication for prophylactic antibiotics in mild AP. Infected pancreatic necrosis is the most significant late complication in patients who survive the initial physiological insult of severe AP, and has a mortality of at least 40%. The risk of infected necrosis is greatest in patients with >30% necrosis. This has resulted in considerable interest in the role of systemic antibiotics to prevent secondary infection of pancreatic necrosis. Antibiotics do not appear to reduce the incidence of infected pancreatic necrosis nor extrapancreatic infection. The available data at present do not support the use of prophylactic antibiotics in the context of pancreatic necrosis.

Patients with deteriorating organ function and *culture-proven sepsis* may require antibiotics as an adjunct to percutaneous or surgical drainage of infected collections, but this should be for a defined period of time (7–10 days), is guided by culture results and must be viewed as *treatment* rather than *prophylaxis*. It is important to recognise that patients with severe AP, and particularly necrosis, may appear septic as a result of a marked SIRS response even in the absence of local or systemic infection. These patients do not require antibiotics. Patients with culture-proven sepsis should also be thoroughly evaluated for extrapancreatic septic foci, such as central venous catheters, prior to assuming the presence of infected necrosis. Repeated courses of antibiotics will increase the risk of developing resistant organisms and fungi.

Role of ERCP

The available evidence is conflicting regarding the role and timing of ERCP for AP. There is no role for early ERCP in mild AP. Patients with severe biliary AP and jaundice may have coexistent cholangitis and should have urgent ERCP and sphincterotomy regardless of whether stones are identified in the common bile duct. This should preferably be performed within 24 hours of admission, and certainly before 72 hours after which the procedure may become technically more difficult as a result of the inflammatory process and oedema in the duodenum and ampulla. Endoscopic ultrasound (EUS) or magnetic resonance cholangiopancreatography (MRCP) may be used in certain situations to determine the need for ERCP.

The three phases that describe the severity of AP are *predicting* severity, *early* determination of severity and *late* determination of severity.

Predicting severity – at the time of admission

Predicting the severity of an episode of AP may have clinical implications for the initial management of the patient, for example managing the patient in a higher level critical care facility. Severity prediction may be based upon the following features:
- Clinical impression of severity ('the end of the bed test')
- High body mass index
- Age >55 years
- C-reactive protein (CRP) >150 mg/L
- APACHE II score >8

Early determination of severity – within the first 48 hours of admission

APACHE II, serum haematocrit and persistence of organ failure beyond 48 hours appear to be the most useful early markers for severity of AP. Earlier multifactorial scoring systems for 'predicting' disease severity, for example the Ranson and Glasgow scores, in fact, described *existing* organ dysfunction.

APACHE-II score (>8) associated with severe AP should be measured on admission and every 24 hours for the first 72-hour trend which is more useful than the absolute value increasing score in the first 48 hours strongly suggestive of severe AP.

Ranson criteria <3 (3% mortality) and >6 (40% mortality) available only after 48 hours are shown in Box 13.4.

Box 13.4 Ranson criteria

At admission	At 48 hours
Age >55 years	Haematocrit decrease >10%
WBC >16,000/mL	BUN increase >5 mg/dL
LDH >50 IU/L	Calcium <8 mg/dL
AST >250 IU/L	PaO$_2$ <60 mm Hg
Glucose >200 mg/dL	Base deficit >4 mg/dL
	Fluid sequestration >6 L

Box 13.5 Glasgow (Imrie) criteria

	At admission	At 48 hours
G	Glucose >10 mmol/L	
L		LDH >600 IU/L
A	Age >55 years	Albumin <32 g/L
S		AST/ALT >200 IU/L
C		Calcium <2 mmol/L
O	Oxygen <60 mm Hg	
U	Urea >16 mmol/L	
W	WCC >15 × 109 mmol/L	

Glasgow (Imrie) scores available only after 48 hours. The original system had nine elements, but now eight (transaminases removed) may be remembered with GLASCOUW (Glasgow) and are shown in Box 13.5.

Haematocrit
Massive third-space fluid losses may occur in the retroperitoneum as a result of the local inflammatory process, and into distant extrapancreatic tissues as a result of increased vascular permeability via cytokine-mediated pathways. The reduction in effective circulating intravascular volume leads to end-organ hypoperfusion and results in pancreatic necrosis and organ failure. This haemoconcentration may be detected by increase in serum haematocrit – haematocrit of >0.44 on admission and failure of haematocrit to reduce after 24 hours of volume resuscitation are associated with pancreatic necrosis.

C-reactive protein
CRP is an acute phase reactant. Plasma levels >150 mg/L during the first 72 hours of admission are associated with pancreatic necrosis with sensitivity and specificity of >80%. CRP usually peaks between 36 and 72 hours and admission levels may be unhelpful.

Late determination of severity – after the first 48 hours of admission
Differentiating mild (interstitial) from severe (necrotising) AP during hospitalisation is dependent upon identifying the two most important and clinically relevant markers of disease severity: pancreatic necrosis and organ failure. The presence and extent of necrosis are most frequently determined by contrast-enhanced CT scan, although MRI may have some advantages particularly in differentiating necrosis from fluid collections. The presence, nature and duration of organ failure should be determined using validated organ failure scores such as MODS or SOFA. Patients with multisystem organ failure and *persistent* organ failure have the highest mortality. As it is not clear at the onset of organ failure whether it is going to be transient or sustained, these patients should be managed in an appropriate level of critical care facility.

Imaging in AP

Plain X-rays
Plain radiology is of value at the time of admission. A chest X-ray can exclude free intraperitoneal gas as a result of visceral perforation as alternative diagnosis, and may demonstrate pulmonary complications of AP (pleural effusions and acute respiratory distress syndrome). Plain abdominal X-ray helps exclude other causes of abdominal pain (e.g. obstruction), but in AP it is usually either normal, or demonstrates ileus. Plain radiology is of limited value following admission and has been replaced by axial imaging in the context of clinical deterioration, or for disease follow-up.

Ultrasound
Transabdominal ultrasound (US) should be performed in all patients with AP within 24 hours of admission to identify gallstones. If the initial US is negative for gallstones, at least one more US should be performed prior to discharge. This is mandatory prior to considering a diagnosis of idiopathic pancreatitis.

Computed tomography
CT helps to confirm the diagnosis when doubt exists, but it is not required in every patient with AP. The role and timing of CT are determined by clinical condition and can be divided into:
- On admission to exclude other acute pathology, e.g. mesenteric ischaemia
- Early to differentiate interstitial from necrotising AP if condition deteriorates
- Late to detect local complications of AP, e.g. fluid collections and necrosis
- Follow-up to monitor local complications and assess response to therapy

Dynamic contrast-enhanced CT scanning is the modality of choice, and there is a low threshold for serial scans if the clinical condition deteriorates. If there is significant renal impairment or contrast allergy, a non-contrast scan may still yield useful information but will not distinguish interstitial from necrotising AP. There is no evidence to suggest that intravenous contrast agents cause extension of pancreatic necrosis.

The CT severity index of Balthazar may be used to radiologically grade the severity of AP and may be used to compare treatment outcomes in different patient groups, but is of limited value in guiding individual patient management (Table 13.2).

Table 13.2 Balthazar CT severity index.

CT grade description	Score
A – normal	0
B – interstitial pancreatitis	1
C – B plus mild extrapancreatic changes	2
D – severe extrapancreatic changes including one fluid collection	3
E – multiple or extensive extrapancreatic collections	4

Necrosis	Score
None	0
30%	2
50%	4
>50%	6

CTSI score (0–10) = CT score (0–4) + necrosis score (0–6)

CTSI	Complications (%)	Mortality (%)
0–3	8	3
4–6	35	6
7–10	92	17

Endoscopic ultrasound

EUS is of increasing value in AP for both assessment and intervention. The role of EUS is rapidly evolving, but presently the main diagnostic indication is the detection of microlithiasis in patients otherwise labelled as 'idiopathic pancreatitis', and the therapeutic indications include definitive management of selected fluid collections and necrosis. Patients requiring this level of management should be referred to a specialist unit.

Further management

The complications of AP can be broadly divided into loco-regional and systemic. Systemic complications are essentially extrapancreatic end-organ dysfunction and have been dealt with previously. This section will focus on the further management of loco-regional complications.

Gallstones

There are two issues to address in acute biliary pancreatitis to prevent recurrent episodes: (1) management of duct stones and (2) cholecystectomy. Patients with mild AP should have definitive management of gallstones during the admission for the index attack, and no later than 2 weeks post-discharge from hospital. Patients with severe AP should have an interval laparoscopic cholecystectomy when clinical condition permits and the inflammatory process has resolved. From this point their management should

be as outlined below for those with mild AP. ERCP with endoscopic sphincterotomy may be definitive management if age or co-morbidity preclude safe cholecystectomy, but this is less effective in preventing recurrent biliary AP.

Non-gallstone pancreatitis

Idiopathic AP should be a diagnosis of exclusion to avoid missing a potentially treatable cause. The majority of non-gallstone AP will be secondary to alcohol. The remaining minority of patients should be investigated as follows, aiming to achieve a diagnosis in at least 80–90%:

History	Family history
	Drugs
	Features of viral aetiology including exposure
Initial investigations	Amylase/urinary amylase/lipase
	LFT
	Transabdominal US
Follow-up investigations	Fasting plasma lipids
	Fasting plasma calcium
	Viral antibody titres
	Second transabdominal US
	MRCP
	CT
Further investigations	Usually for recurrent idiopathic AP
	Further transabdominal US
	EUS – microlithiasis and evaluation of pancreatic parenchyma
	Autoimmune markers (IgG4:IgG ratio)
	ERCP – biliary, pancreatic cytology and manometry
	Pancreatic function tests

Pancreatic necrosis

The management of pancreatic necrosis should be in a specialist unit. The timing and nature of intervention (if any) are determined by (1) duration since onset of AP, (2) sterile versus infected necrosis and (3) coexistent organ dysfunction. The management of pancreatic necrosis has changed dramatically over the past decade, and rigidly held dogma has been successfully challenged.

Sterile pancreatic necrosis

Sterile pancreatic necrosis is not an absolute indication for intervention and can be managed conservatively. If intervention is required, it should be delayed as long as possible and then managed using the least invasive modality in a stable patient. The relative indications to intervene are:
- Static organ dysfunction/failure to progress clinically
- Loco-regional complications (e.g. gastric outlet obstruction; GOO)

Infected pancreatic necrosis

Infected pancreatic necrosis, even gas-containing collections, do not require intervention if the patient is well and progressing with conservative treatment. Management algorithms are determined by sepsis-driven organ failure rather than simply the presence of infected pancreatic necrosis. Diagnostic Fine Needle Aspiration (FNA) does not, therefore, influence management, may infect previously sterile pancreatic necrosis, and should be avoided. Patients with deteriorating organ function secondary to infected necrosis require drainage of the septic focus, with minimal debridement initially to avoid provoking further complications (bleeding, increased systemic inflammatory 'hit'). Further management is determined by physiological response and guided by serial axial imaging. The various methods for dealing with infected necrosis are beyond the scope of this chapter, but can be divided into open and minimally invasive techniques including:

Open	Laparotomy with debridement	– drainage + closed packing – drainage + open packing – closed lavage system
Minimally invasive	Percutaneous drainage	drains usually block
	Endoscopic drainage Percutaneous necrosectomy	– via EUS cystogastrostomy – radiological drain – drain tract dilatation – continuous lavage – staged debridement

Fluid collections

Peripancreatic fluid collections are common after AP. Many do not require intervention and will resolve spontaneously. The indications for intervention are collections which are infected or symptomatic. In general, the transgastric (EUS) or transpapillary (ERCP) routes are preferred for drainage. Percutaneous drainage carries the risk of an external pancreatic fistula and is reserved for the patient with an infected collection and organ dysfunction.

Haemorrhage

Bleeding may be secondary to pancreatic necrosis itself, or to surgical intervention for necrosis. The treatment of choice is urgent angiography and endovascular embolisation. Surgical control is rarely required and associated with a high mortality.

PD stricture

PD stricture occurs as a result of post-inflammatory fibrosis after AP. Isolated PD stricture may present with pain and recurrent AP. PD stricture associated with duct disruption may present with a pseudocyst or pancreatic fistula. Management options include:

| Endotherapy (ERCP) | Dilate or stent the stricture |
| Surgery | Distal pancreatectomy to include the stricture, or Pancreatico-jejunostomy to drain the PD |

Gastric outlet obstruction

GOO occurs in up to 10% of patients with AP, and can prevent effective nasogastric feeding. Nasojejunal nutrition allows the local oedema to settle in the majority of patients who can then resume oral intake. Few patients require a gastro-jejunostomy for chronic GOO as a result of AP.

Further reading

American College of Gastroenterology. Practice guidelines in acute pancreatitis. *Am J Gastroenterol* 2006;**101**:2379–2400.

UK Working Party on Acute Pancreatitis/British Society of Gastroenterology. UK guidelines for the management of acute pancreatitis. *Gut* 2005;**54**:1–9.

14 Small Bowel Obstruction

J. Edward F. Fitzgerald
Department of Gastrointestinal Surgery, Nottingham University Hospital, Nottingham, UK

Introduction

Small bowel obstruction (SBO) remains a common condition for surgical teams to manage. Despite this, variable presentations and difficulties in correctly timing appropriate surgical intervention give rise to considerable challenges. Balancing conservative treatment against operative, guided by a range of diagnostic aids with numerous management options, presents a significant clinical dilemma.

SBO has been estimated to represent 5% of all acute general surgical admissions in the United Kingdom, with previously reported mortality rates ranging from 4% in patients managed conservatively to 28% in high-risk groups undergoing surgery. The complexity of managing these patients should not be underestimated and an absence of high level evidence to guide this means that many strategies remain controversial. An understanding of the underlying pathophysiology, early diagnosis, meticulous fluid balance and close observation together with timely surgical intervention, if required, are all essential components of a successful outcome.

Aetiology and pathophysiology

The underlying causes of SBO vary considerably with geographical region. In 'developed' countries, postoperative adhesions are the most common cause, whereas strangulated hernia are more commonly responsible in other areas of the developing world. The range of possible causes are described in Table 14.1.

More generally, the aetiology can be considered in terms of the underlying abnormality: mechanical or paralytic obstruction.

Emergency Surgery, 1st edition. Edited by Adam Brooks, Peter F. Mahoney, Bryan A. Cotton and Nigel Tai. © 2010 Blackwell Publishing.

Paralytic obstruction

Also known as adynamic or postoperative ileus, paralytic obstruction is characterised by disordered or absent peristalsis. Although considered an almost inevitable consequence of gastrointestinal surgery, it may also occur in association with other procedures (particularly orthopaedic), systemic infection and metabolic and neurological disorders. Whilst the exact aetiology is not fully understood, research suggests numerous contributing factors including pharmacological (e.g. anaesthetic and opioid analgesia), inflammatory causes (e.g. bowel manipulation and inflammatory mediator release) and neural reflexes (postoperative sympathetic over activity or other inhibitory neuronal actions). Management is typically supportive, with treatment of the underlying cause as appropriate. Diagnostic problems may arise with prolonged postoperative ileus (>3 days) as differentiating this from postoperative mechanical obstruction can be difficult.

Mechanical obstruction

This is characterised by initial episodes of vigorous peristalsis attempting to overcome a physical obstruction. If this cannot be overcome, bowel proximal to the obstruction dilates leading to decreased peristalsis and ultimate flaccidity, whilst distal bowel empties as normal, ultimately collapsing. Appreciating the cause of this pathological proximal dilation is vital to understanding both the clinical course and the profoundly disordered physiology that can occur in SBO.

Initially, bowel dilation occurs secondary to swallowed air and intestinal secretions collecting within the bowel proximal to the obstruction. Approximately, 8–9 L/day of digestive juices are secreted and reabsorbed within the gastrointestinal tract; any interference to this process leads to rapid intraluminal stasis. This in turn allows bacterial overgrowth, with resulting fermentation of undigested bowel contents contributing to the accumulation of gas. Oxygen within this gas is absorbed across the bowel wall, leaving the relatively poorly absorbed atmospheric nitrogen, increasing levels of carbon dioxide and the gaseous products of fermentation. This further establishes a gradient for gaseous diffusion

Table 14.1 Causes of small bowel obstruction.

- Adhesions
- Hernias external/internal
- Intussusception
- Crohn's disease
- Gallstone ileus
- Tumour
- Foreign body
- Tuberculosis
- Radiation enteritis
- Sclerosing peritonitis

from the bowel wall into the lumen. Similarly, fermentation within the luminal fluid creates an osmotic gradient resulting in movement of fluid and electrolytes into the lumen. This can equate to several litres of fluid sequestered within the bowel, termed 'third space' losses from the intravascular space. Reduced or absent oral fluid intake together with defective intestinal absorption of the sequestered fluid further compounds these losses.

Numerous complications arise from this process of bowel dilation and fluid loss. Vomiting accentuates fluid and electrolyte losses, and patients are prone to developing hypokalaemia as the obstruction progresses. Urine output falls as the hypovolaemia worsens and accompanying volume changes in body fluid compartments adversely impact on morbidity and operative outcomes if inadequately corrected.

Pressure within the bowel wall also increases as a result of gas and fluid accumulation. If this continues unchecked, low-pressure venous return is eventually compromised and venous congestion develops. This creates a vicious cycle of further reductions in bowel wall perfusion, with further accompanying fluid losses. This eventually culminates in ischaemia, infarction and intestinal perforation, with failure of the mucosal barrier also allowing bacterial translocation to occur.

In addition to the typical course of mechanical obstruction, several specific types merit further consideration.

Simple versus strangulated obstruction

Strangulated obstruction is a term used to denote bowel with a compromised blood supply, either through venous congestion or arterial occlusion. The cause may be extrinsic or intrinsic, or related to interruption of mesenteric flow through intussusception or volvulus. Initial assessment and management of SBO aims to identify patients with strangulated bowel, or to intervene in those who fail conservative management in order to prevent this. Unless moribund, operative input is mandated with resection of the necrotic bowel. Untreated, the subsequent bowel perforation and resulting peritonitis are invariably fatal.

In simple obstruction the blood supply is intact, although with time the bowel may go on to become strangulated. In patients not responding to conservative therapy within the first 24 hours, the risk of bowel resection for necrosis or perforation increases markedly.

Closed loop versus open loop obstruction

Closed loop obstruction is a special case where both the proximal and distal points of a bowel segment are obstructed, as shown in Figure 14.1. By its very nature, this 'closed loop' is more prone to rapid strangulation, infarction and perforation without the typical symptoms of early proximal distension seen in open loop obstruction.

Clinical presentation

Symptoms and signs

The clinical presentation of SBO varies considerably between patients, according to the anatomical level of the obstruction and the underlying cause, together with the time course and presence or absence of strangulation. Despite this, the common clinical features are pain, distension, constipation, vomiting and dehydration.

Throughout the assessment it is essential to identify the patient with threatened or actual strangulation. This is suggested by the patient's pain being sharper and more constant than the central pain typical of obstruction and is likely to

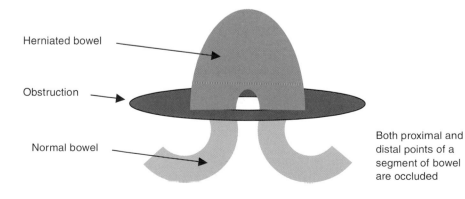

Herniated bowel

Obstruction

Normal bowel

Both proximal and distal points of a segment of bowel are occluded

Figure 14.1 Closed loop obstruction.

be more localised. On examination these patients are often peritonitic and have a fever. The patient may also have a raised white cell count and a raised lactate.

Abdominal pain

Mechanical obstruction is characterised by initial episodes of vigorous peristalsis attempting to overcome a physical obstruction. The typical picture of colicky pain arising from a luminal obstruction results. Stimulation of stretch receptors in the visceral peritoneum refers pain to areas relating to the embryonic fore-, mid- or hind-gut, which are poorly localised. As the obstruction progresses and flaccidity develops peristalsis ceases and the colicky pain becomes a less predominant feature. It is usually absent in paralytic ileus.

Regular serial reassessment of the abdomen is important to note any change of symptoms. Colicky pain becoming more localised and constant, or the presence of signs indicating peritonism, both suggest simple obstruction may have progressed to infarction or perforation. Detection of an underlying abdominal mass may also help suggest the cause of the obstruction.

Abdominal distension

The degree of abdominal distension depends on the extent of dilated bowel proximal to the obstruction, and may be pronounced in low distal obstruction and absent in high or closed loop obstruction. Similarly, vomiting may be an early symptom in high obstruction and much later in low distal obstruction.

Constipation

Digital rectal examination should be performed; however, the findings resulting from this are less useful than for suspected colonic obstruction. Bowel distal to the SBO will empty as normal and the presence or absence of rectal contents will therefore depend on the duration of symptoms. Hence, the patient may not give a history of absolute constipation with an early presentation, as the distal bowel continues to empty.

Vomiting and dehydration

Non-specific signs of dehydration may help indicate the degree of accompanying hypovolaemia. Tachycardia, hypotension and oliguria are important to note as, in addition to hypovolaemia, these may also suggest strangulation with systemic toxicity. As discussed earlier, vomiting may not be a predominant feature in a patient with more distal SBO.

Other clinical features

History or evidence on examination of previous abdominal surgery is important to note, raising the possibility of postoperative adhesions as the underlying cause.

Examination of the hernial orifices is always mandated in order to exclude an obvious incarcerated or strangulated hernia. Erythema, tenderness, non-reduction and absence of cough impulse over a hernial mass suggest strangulation may be present.

Auscultation of the abdomen can be helpful, but the 'tinkling' high-pitched bowel sounds described in many surgical texts are not always present. When heard without a stethoscope, these classical sounds are termed borborygmi. In advanced or strangulated obstruction, the paralysed, flaccid bowel no longer peristalses and bowel sounds are absent.

Pyrexia is not typically seen with simple SBO and this may herald the onset of infarction and perforation. Alternatively it may be associated with the underlying cause if this is associated with an inflammatory process. Hypothermia may be associated with septic shock if bacterial translocation and/or perforation has occurred.

Investigations

Whilst identification of the patient with strangulated bowel remains a largely clinical diagnosis, thorough assessment of the patient requires further investigation.

Blood tests

Monitoring the trend in white cell count is important to identify the deteriorating patient. Whilst this may initially be normal or slightly raised, marked elevation suggests infarction and perforation.

Careful monitoring of renal function is essential, with daily or even twice daily biochemistry. Gastrointestinal fluid losses deplete sodium and chloride levels, which will need correction. Hyperkalaemia may indicate infarcted bowel. Urea will rise, reflecting the degree of dehydration. In cases with profound hypovolaemia the patient is at risk of pre-renal failure and early identification of this is vital.

Radiological imaging

Plain radiograph

Radiological diagnosis starts with an erect chest radiograph to exclude perforation. This is usually taken in combination with a supine plain abdominal radiograph, which may show the cardinal signs of SBO. Dilated loops of small bowel may be seen centrally on the film, although air is required within the lumen in order to identify these (Figure 14.2). With fluid alone the distended loops may not be obvious. The jejunum can be distinguished by valvulae conniventes across the width of the bowel, whereas the ileum is relatively featureless. Bowel distal to the obstruction may be collapsed and difficult to visualise. Rarely a plain radiograph may suggest the cause of the obstruction, such as through identifying a calcified ectopic gallstone.

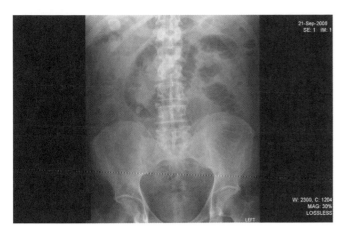

Figure 14.2 Plain abdominal radiograph showing small bowel obstruction with multiple distended loops of small bowel clearly visible.

Contrast studies

Recent research suggests an important role for contrast studies in identifying patients suitable for conservative treatment. Water-soluble contrast instilled through a nasogastric tube is tracked on serial radiographs in order to identify a clear obstruction or eventual passage into the caecum. Meta analysis of the published studies in relation to adhesive SBO indicates that the appearance of contrast in the caecum within 24 hours of administration is highly sensitive (97%) and specific (96%) for non-operative resolution. Given the current difficulty in selecting patients for conservative management it is likely that contrast studies will play an increasingly important role in the diagnosis and management of SBO in the future.

Computed tomography

Computed tomography (CT) with or without contrast is useful in identifying the level of the obstruction and suggesting the likely cause. It gives useful information relating to structures outside the bowel and in so doing can prepare the surgeon for potential unexpected findings, allowing the procedure to be planned accordingly. Although identification of gas within the bowel wall may suggest infarction and impending perforation, this is unreliable and CT does not necessarily aid the clinical decision to operate in these patients.

Management

The key principles underlying the management of mechanical SBO centre on resuscitation and correction of physiological and electrolyte abnormalities, decompression of the bowel and surgery, if appropriate. This has historically been described as the 'drip and suck' regimen. Supportive measures are also required, including analgesia and addressing nutritional requirements in those with prolonged periods of minimal oral intake. Many clinicians also advocate antibiotics in order to reduce bacterial colonisation within the obstructed bowel lumen.

An overview of the principle management decisions for a patient with mechanical bowel obstruction are shown in Figure 14.3.

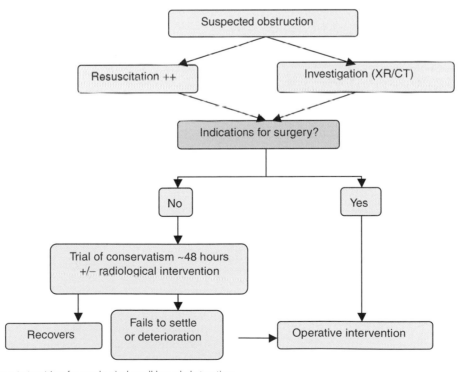

Figure 14.3 Management algorithm for mechanical small bowel obstruction.

Resuscitation

Resuscitation is a priority, irrespective of the need for surgery. In the event that surgery is required, hypovolaemic patients with SBO have a significantly higher morbidity and mortality. Replacement of losses should be delivered through intravenous fluid infusion. Large volumes of crystalloid may initially be required. Meticulous monitoring of fluid balance, including urinary catheterisation, should be used to guide further fluid therapy. In patients with profound hypovolaemia or a history of congestive heart failure central venous catheterisation may be required to fine-tune treatment. Overall, losses must be replaced in addition to normal daily requirements.

Bowel decompression

Resting the bowel and decompression through passage of a nasogastric tube reduces the risk of aspiration from vomiting and allows measurement of gastrointestinal losses. These should be measured hourly with regular aspiration and free-drainage.

Subsequent management centres on identifying those patients requiring operative intervention and those that can be managed conservatively. The old adage 'Don't let the sun set and rise on intestinal obstruction' remains important in emphasising the need for early surgical intervention to prevent more serious complications arising from infarcted or perforated bowel. However, this should be treated as a guide rather than an absolute as there is a risk of unnecessary surgery in some patients in whom SBO would resolve with conservative management.

In addition to several firm indications, a number of symptoms and signs have been described that help direct the need for surgery. Despite their usefulness, several large studies have failed to prove the value of these in predicting prognosis. Generally, patients with SBO and no history to indicate the presence of adhesions require an early laparotomy. Surgery is also indicated in those with suspected intestinal ischaemia, those with an irreducible hernia and those in whom conservative management fails.

Surgical principles

In the appropriately resuscitated patient, surgery is undertaken to decompress the bowel, release the cause of obstruction, careful assessment of bowel viability and undertake such secondary procedures as necessary. This may include resection of infarcted and perforated bowel, or further surgery relating to the primary cause of the obstruction. At the time of surgery distinguishing viable from non-viable bowel may not be clear cut. In cases of doubt, bowel should be wrapped in warm, moist packs for 10 minutes. During this period a more normal colour and peristalsis may return in viable bowel. Useful features for identifying viable and non-viable bowel are given in Table 14.2.

Table 14.2 Features suggestive of viable and non-viable bowel.

Viable bowel	Non-viable bowel
Visible peristalsis	No visible or inducible peristalsis
Pulsatile vessels	Failure to recover colour following release of constriction
Sheen	

Specific conditions

Adhesions

In the case of previous abdominal or pelvic surgery and in the absence of firm indications for operative intervention then a period of close observation for ~48 hours may be appropriate. Many cases of adhesional obstruction will settle with conservative management alone. Contrast studies should be requested to identifying patients for whom this is unlikely to be the case (see *Radiological imaging* section).

Hernia

In the case of an obvious recently obstructed inguinal hernia (<24 hours duration) gentle pressure combined with postural treatment (raising the foot of the bed) may reduce this and avoid the need for further treatment. Care must be taken to avoid simply reducing the hernia still inside the hernial sac, termed 'reduction en masse'. Forceful attempts at reduction are not recommended.

Surgery for an obstructed hernia depends on the anatomical site. In all cases the sac must be identified and opened with careful examination of its contents. Release within 24 hours of onset will usually avoid infarction. Viable bowel can be returned directly to the abdominal cavity, whereas infarcted bowel must be resected. In the case of inguinal and femoral hernia this may require a further abdominal incision in order to obtain sufficient exposure. Finally, appropriate repair of the hernial defect should be undertaken to prevent recurrence.

Malignancy

Primary malignancy of small bowel is rarely encountered. More common is secondary malignant obstruction potentially arising from any intra-abdominal neoplastic process. Many cases respond to conservative management with a liquid diet and medication to reduce bowel secretions. If this fails, operative intervention is largely determined by the nature of the underlying primary and likely prognosis. Often a palliative bypass procedure will be the most appropriate procedure.

Volvulus

Volvulus occurs when a loop of bowel rotates through 360° on itself. With such a 'closed loop' obstruction the vascular supply may become rapidly compromised and the classical

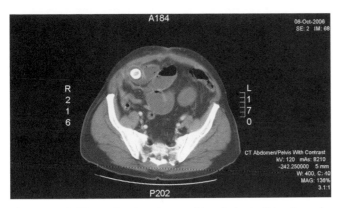

Figure 14.4 CT scan showing a large gallstone lodged within a loop of distal ileum.

signs of obstruction are absent. Volvulus of the colon is considerably more common than small bowel, and when this does occur it is typically related to congenital malrotation or persistence of the vitello-intestinal duct. Surgery involves untwisting the bowel segment.

Gallstone ileus

Gallstone ileus arises when an inflamed gallbladder adheres to adjacent bowel, forming a biliary-enteric fistula which allows a stone to pass into the intestinal tract. Classically a disease of elderly women, it remains an uncommon cause of SBO accounting for 1–3% of admissions for SBO. Often the stone periodically obstructs as it passes distally, presenting with episodic symptoms known as 'tumbling' obstruction, delaying diagnosis. Complete obstruction typically occurs when the stone lodges in the narrower terminal ileum (Figure 14.4). Rigler's triad, the classic radiological signs of air in the biliary tree, SBO and dystopic stone also allow for correct diagnosis but are seldom seen. Two surgical strategies have been described: enterolithotomy alone, allowing a delayed cholecystectomy after an inflammation-free period of 4–6 weeks (and therefore two-stage surgery) or enterolithotomy in combination with cholecystectomy and fistula division (one-stage surgery). Although the appropriate choice of procedure is controversial, a two-stage procedure is usually performed due to complexities of definitive one-stage surgery and the typically frail condition of the patients.

Intussusception

More common in children, intussusception occurs when a segment of bowel is invaginated inside the segment immediately adjoining this. Whilst typically idiopathic in children, in adults a nidus such as a bowel wall lipoma or intestinal polyp is usually the underlying cause. Treatment involves manual reduction of the bowel if possible, or resection of the offending segment.

Laparoscopic surgery

SBO has traditionally been considered a contraindication to laparoscopic techniques owing to the technical difficulty arising from distended bowel and the increased risk of iatrogenic injury and enterotomy. Advances in expertise and experience have now, in the right hands, enabled a laparoscopic approach to be considered in carefully selected patients. This typically includes those with no history of previous abdominal or pelvic surgery, minimal distension and higher obstruction. Conversion rates of 6.7–53% have been reported, and concerns remain that for those procedures completed laparoscopically inadequate bowel evaluation may be performed.

Postoperative management

Depending on the underlying cause of the obstruction, condition of the patient and severity of findings at surgery, careful postoperative management may be required in a high-dependency or intensive care setting. Treatment involves meticulous fluid balance management, nutrition and in severe cases addressing the systemic toxicity or sepsis resulting from infarcted or perforated bowel.

Further reading

Abbas SM, Bissett IP, Parry BR. Meta-analysis of oral water soluble contrast agent in the management of adhesive small bowel obstruction. *Brit J Surg* 2007;**94**:404–411.

Bickell NA, Federman AD, Aufses AH, Jr. Influence of time on risk of bowel resection in complete small bowel obstruction. *J Am Coll Surg* 2005;**201**:847–854.

Diaz JJ, Jr, Bokhari F, Mowery NT, et al. EAST practice management guidelines: guidelines for the management of small bowel obstruction. *J Trauma* 2008;**64**:1651–1664.

Fevang BT, Jensen D, Svanes K, Viste A. Early operation or conservative management of patients with small bowel obstruction? *Eur J Surg* 2002;**168**:475–481.

Foster NM, McGory ML, Zingmond DS, Ko CY. Small bowel obstruction: a population based appraisal. *J Am Coll Surg* 2006;**203**:170–176.

Jones K, Mangram AJ, Lebron RA, et al. Can a computer tomography scoring system predict the need for surgery in small bowel obstruction? *Am J Surg* 2007;**194**:780–784.

Margenthaler JA, Longo WE, Virgo KS, et al. Risk factors for adverse outcomes following surgery for small bowel obstruction. *Ann Surg* 2006;**243**:456–464.

Williams SB, Greenspon J, Young HA, Orkin BA. Small bowel obstruction: conservative vs surgical management. *Dis Col Rec* 2005;**48**:1140–1146.

15 Surgical Jaundice and Cholangitis

John S. Hammond[1] & Ian Beckingham[2]

[1]Department of Surgery, Nottingham Digestive Diseases Centre, University of Nottingham, Nottingham, UK
[2]Queens Medical Centre, Nottingham University Hospital, NHS Trust, Nottingham, UK

Introduction

Jaundice is the yellow discoloration of skin and sclerae caused by excess bilirubin deposition. Clinically, it becomes detectable when the serum bilirubin concentration is greater than 35 μmol/L (normal upper limit 17 μmol/L), and traditionally it is classified as either prehepatic, hepatic or posthepatic jaundice based on its aetiology and presentation.

Prehepatic jaundice

Prehepatic jaundice is characterised by a build up of unconjugated (water insoluble) bilirubin. Normally the liver can process up to six times the daily load of bilirubin before jaundice develops. Increased haemolysis from spherocytosis, thalassaemia and sickle-cell disease is the commonest cause. Other causes include haemolysis during the breakdown of a massive haematoma, inherited defects in bilirubin conjugation and Gilbert's syndrome.

Hepatic jaundice

A wide range of toxins, infections, metabolic and autoimmune conditions can cause hepatic jaundice. The patient may present with acute liver failure or with cirrhosis and the features of chronic liver disease. In hepatic jaundice, the serum bilirubin may be unconjugated because the damaged hepatocytes are unable to process bilirubin or it may be conjugated because of a failure to excrete bilirubin into the canaliculi. Often there is a mixed picture. Conjugated bilirubin is water soluble and therefore excreted in the urine. Surgery plays no role in the management of hepatic jaundice (except to transplant the failing liver).

Posthepatic (obstructive) jaundice

Posthepatic jaundice is often referred to as surgical jaundice. Bile duct obstruction causes a conjugated hyperbilirubinaemia with pale stools and dark urine. In complete obstruction of the biliary tract urobilinogen is absent from the urine. The commonest causes of posthepatic (obstructive) jaundice are bile duct calculi and malignancies of pancreas, bile duct and ampulla. Less common causes include chronic pancreatitis, sclerosing cholangitis, metastatic lymphadenopathy and choledochal cysts. In patients from the Far East and elsewhere in the developing world parasitic infection (*Ascaris lumbricodes* or *Clonoirchis sinensis*) should be considered.

Investigation of the jaundiced patient

History and examination

Investigation of the jaundiced patient begins with clinical history and examination. Recent travel (hepatitis and malaria), alcohol intake, prescription and recreational drug usage, previous blood products, occupational history and family history should all be established.

Obstructive jaundice typically presents with dark urine, pale stools and pruritis. Pruritis, which is related to bile salt deposition within the skin, is often a prominent feature in both hepatic and posthepatic cholestasis. Pain and rigors suggest the presence of stones in the common bile duct (CBD). Back pain and weight loss are suggestive of pancreatic cancer. Intermittent shoulder tip pain is suggestive of gallstone disease.

General examination should detect the stigmata of chronic liver disease (spider naevi, palmar erythema, finger clubbing, leuconychia, gynaecomastia and ascites) and the presence of splenomegaly and prominent abdominal wall veins suggest cirrhosis and portal hypertension. Bruising may be present indicating malabsorption of vitamin K or hypoprothrombinaemia due to hepatocellular damage.

Hepatomegaly may be detected and the character of the liver edge and surface may indicate malignant disease.

Emergency Surgery, 1st edition. Edited by Adam Brooks, Peter F. Mahoney, Bryan A. Cotton and Nigel Tai. © 2010 Blackwell Publishing.

Table 15.1 Differentiating prehepatic, hepatic and posthepatic jaundice.

	Prehepatic	Hepatic	Obstructive
Bilirubin	Unconjugated	Conjugated or unconjugated	Conjugated
ALT or AST	Normal	Raised	Normal or moderately raised
ALP	Normal	Normal or moderately raised	Raised
GGT	Normal	Normal or moderately raised	Raised
Urine	Urobilinogen	Urobilinogen	Bilirubin, no urobilinogen

Initial history and examination together with urinary, biochemical and serological tests allow classification of the jaundiced patient in around 70% of cases.

ALT, alanine aminotransferase; AST, aspartate aminotransferase; ALP, alkaline phosphatase; GGT, gamma glutamyltanspeptidase.

Gallbladder distension together with signs of sepsis and tenderness suggests acute cholecystitis or empyema of the gallbladder. Non-tender dilatation of the gallbladder may occur due to distal duct obstruction secondary to a cancer (Courvoisier's sign).

Blood and urine

Full blood count
Patients with prehepatic jaundice secondary to haemolysis usually have low serum haemoglobin and examination of their blood film identifies reticulocytosis and abnormal erythrocytes.

Alkaline phosphatase
Alkaline phosphatase (ALP) is expressed in liver and bone with smaller amounts derived from the kidney and intestine. Its levels are increased with bile duct obstruction.

Gamma glutamyltanspeptidase
Gamma glutamyltanspeptidase (GGT) is present in many organs but not in bone. It is elevated in bile duct obstruction and by many toxins including alcohol.

Alanine aminotransferase and aspartate aminotransferase
Transaminases are indicators of hepatocellular damage. Alanine aminotransferase (ALT) is localised mainly in the liver, and aspartate aminotransferase (AST) is found in liver, heart, kidney and muscle. An AST:ALT ratio (>2) is highly suggestive of alcohol as the aetiology of parenchymal liver disease. Transaminase levels are not specific and can be elevated in congestive heart failure and in biliary obstruction with or without cholangitis.

Clotting profile
The liver is the principle site for synthesis of clotting factors. Factors II, VII, IX and X are produced in the liver and rely on vitamin K absorption. A failure to absorb vitamin K or impaired synthetic capacity causes a coagulopathy. It is important to recognise and correct these clotting abnormalities before any interventional procedures are undertaken.

Albumin
Albumin is synthesised exclusively by the liver. Hypoalbuminaemia is seen in patients with chronic liver disease and hepatic malignancy and is a component of prognostic scoring systems for chronic liver disease.

Urinalysis
Normal urine contains small amounts of urobilinogen but no bile pigments. Elevated levels of conjugated bilirubin secondary to obstructive jaundice, hepatitis, or cirrhosis can lead to bilirubin in urine. Urobilinogen is absent in the urine of patients with complete biliary obstruction and is elevated in patients with non-obstructive jaundice. Urinalysis is a cheap test but has a low specificity due to the incomplete nature of most obstructions (Table 15.1).

Investigation of obstructive jaundice

When cholestatic jaundice is suggested by the biochemical, serological and urinary tests an ultrasound scan should be obtained to demonstrate duct dilatation, gallstones or intrahepatic lesions. An ultrasound scan is a very sensitive test for gallbladder stones and biliary duct dilatation. Its main limitation is in the assessment of the lower CBD when overlying bowel gas in the duodenum or colon can obstruct the view. Computed tomography (CT) should be considered when malignancy is suspected. It is a less sensitive test for gallstones in the gallbladder but does enable clear visualisation of the distal CBD and will usually determine the cause and level of obstruction.

Further management is determined by the level of obstruction, its cause, the degree of jaundice and locally available resources and expertise. Magnetic resonance cholangiopancreatography (MRCP) provides views of the biliary tract and because it is a non-invasive test it carries no risk to the patient (unlike endoscopic retrograde cholangiopancreatography [ERCP]). In patients with a high serum bilirubin (>150 μmol/L) it is reasonable to proceed directly to ERCP, as stone removal or stent placement is likely to be required. Hilar obstruction is generally better assessed and is more easily drained with percutaneous transhepatic cholangiography (PTC) than ERCP. Ideally all staging investigations should precede intervention to allow a single interventional treatment, surgical, endoscopic or PTC drainage. Patients with biliary sepsis or very high levels of jaundice (>300 μmol/L) require endoscopic or percutaneous drainage to achieve biliary decompression prior to definitive treatment or staging.

In patients with liver function tests indicative of cholestasis but in whom duct dilatation cannot be identified, a liver biopsy should be considered and the patient should be followed up by the local medical gastroenterology or hepatology service.

Gallstones

Gallstones are classified as cholesterol stones or pigment stones (black and brown). Cholesterol-rich stones are the commonest gallstones in Western society accounting for >80% of stones. Epidemiological studies have demonstrated a familial tendency in patients with cholesterol gallstones with 37% of patients having a first degree relative with stones. Black pigment stones occur commonly in patients with haemolysis (from any cause) or in patients with cirrhosis due to polymerisation and co-precipitation of unconjugated bilirubin to form sludge which then coalesces into stones. Brown pigment stones are found more often in the bile ducts than in the gallbladder and are rare in the Western hemisphere. They are most common in the Far East, where their formation is associated with parasitic infection of the bile ducts.

It is estimated that 10–15% of the adult population has gallstones with similar figures of 12% of men and 24% of women reported from postmortem studies. This equates to around 7.5 million people with gallstones in the United Kingdom. Of these less than 15% will experience symptoms attributable to gallstones (Williams et al. 2008).

Choledocholithiasis and jaundice

Gallstones can migrate from the gallbladder into the bile duct. Many patients remain asymptomatic and pass the stone spontaneously. Impaction of the stone within the dis-

tal CBD or ampulla may lead to the development of obstructive jaundice. The diagnosis is made on the basis of liver function tests confirming an obstructive or mixed picture together with the presence of dilated bile ducts on ultrasound. Common bile duct stones (CBDS) are only visible in 30–50% of patients with transabdominal ultrasound (Williams et al. 2008). MRCP, endoscopic ultrasound or ERCP can be used to confirm the diagnosis.

Management of gallstone disease

Cholecystectomy

The indications for cholecystectomy are documented cholelithiasis with symptoms attributable to the presence of gallstones or a diseased gallbladder. Cholecystectomy should not be performed for patients with asymptomatic gallstones unless there is a risk of gallbladder cancer or in young asymptomatic patients with gallstones associated with haemoglobinopathies (homozygous sickle-cell disease) where the majority will become symptomatic. Cholecystectomy is now performed routinely by the laparoscopic approach. Absolute contraindications for laparoscopic cholecytectomy are an inability to tolerate general anaesthesia, refractory coagulopathy and suspicion of gallbladder cancer (laparoscopy in patients has the risk of port site metastases). Relative contraindications are dictated primarily by the surgeon's philosophy and experience and include previous upper abdominal surgery with extensive adhesions, portal hypertension and third trimester of pregnancy. Severe cardiopulmonary disease and morbid obesity are associated with a lower morbidity when surgery is performed laparoscopically.

Intraoperative cholangiography using dilute non-ionic contrast media and an image intensifier may be performed routinely or on an occasional basis when a bile duct stone is suspected or there is uncertainty over the biliary anatomy. From this four pieces of information should be established: the entry point of the cholangiogram catheter must be through the cystic duct and not through the common hepatic duct; there must be cephalad and caudal flow along the main bile duct with opacification of right (anterior and posterior branches) and left ducts; the presence or absence of stones within the bile ducts; contrast should flow into the duodenum (Table 15.2).

Table 15.2 What to look for during intraoperative cholangiography.

Entry point of catheter
Filling of the intrahepatic ducts
The presence or stones or other filling defects
Flow into the duodenum

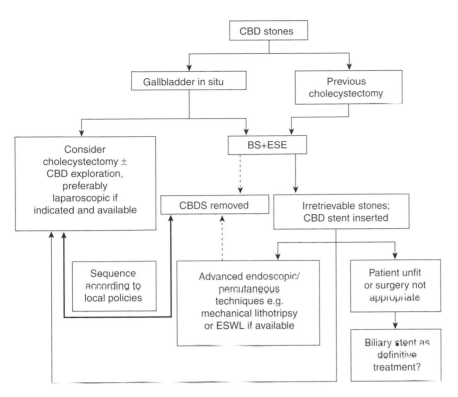

Figure 15.1 Algorithm for management of common bile duct stones. BS, biliary sphincterotomy; CBD, common bile duct; CBDS, common bile duct stones; ESE, endoscopic stone extraction, ESWL, extracorporeal shock wave lithotripsy. Reproduced by the courtesy of Williams et al. (2008).

Cholecystostomy

Cholecystostomy is a useful method of treating severe acute gallbladder disease in the critically ill patient. It can be carried out percutaneously using ultrasound guidance. The catheter should be left in situ for 4–6 weeks to ensure adherence to the abdominal wall prior to its removal. Premature removal carries the risk of bile leak and biliary peritonitis. If the patient is a candidate for surgery, a cholecystectomy should be performed once their condition has improved.

Management of choledocholithiasis

The management of CBDS has become increasingly complex in the last decade due to the wide range of diagnostic and therapeutic strategies available. The solution for many patients will therefore be dictated by the available expertise and resources in a particular unit. The British Society of Gastroenterology recently published some guidelines for the management of patients with bile duct stones. The algorithm from these guidelines is shown in Figure 15.1 (Williams et al. 2008).

Techniques for CBDS removal

Endoscopic retrograde cholangiopancreatography

ERCP is an endoscopic technique that uses retrograde injection through the duodenal papilla to investigate the bile ducts. Its role has now largely been replaced as a diagnostic test by MRCP; however, ERCP remains a valuable tool for treating biliary pathology. It allows visualisation of stones and strictures within the main bile ducts and intrahepatic ducts and allows removal of stones from the bile duct with baskets or balloons, or the insertion of plastic or metal wall stents to relieve biliary obstruction from stones or tumour. It also allows cytological and histological specimens to be obtained from pathology within the bile ducts, pancreas or duodenum. Prior to ERCP, patients should have coagulation studies and any abnormalities of their clotting corrected (INR < 1.5). There are a number of situations in which ERCP remains the best option for removal of CBDS· these include acute cholangitis; stones causing obstructive jaundice; severe acute gallstone pancreatitis in the presence of biliary obstruction; post-cholecystectomy CBDS; and bile duct stones in elderly patients considered unfit for cholecystectomy. The complications of ERCP are failure to cannulate the papilla (5–10%), acute pancreatitis (5% of which 20% is severe acute pancreatitis), bleeding and perforation (1%) (Williams et al. 2008).

Percutaneous transhepatic cholangiography

PTC is a radiological technique where the intrahepatic ducts are entered percutaneously. Once access to the ducts has been established antegrade injection of water-soluble contrast allows visualisation of filling defects, tissue sampling and drain and stent insertion. Like ERCP its role is now primarily therapeutic. Bacteraemia and occasionally septic shock are rare complications of the technique and are most common in patients with strictures or stones. Antibiotic prophylaxis and pre-procedure coagulation studies are essential (Williams et al. 2008).

Bile duct exploration

Bile duct exploration and stone removal can be performed as an open or laparoscopic procedure. At laparoscopy stones identified on the intraoperative cholangiogram can be removed either via the cystic duct or through a choledochotomy. The transcystic route has the advantage that it avoids performing a choledochotomy, but it requires an ultra-thin choledochoscope and is only effective for stones of a comparable diameter to the cystic duct. For larger stones a choledochotomy is required. A flexible choledochoscope is inserted through the choledochotomy and stones removed using a dormia basket, balloon catheter or lithotripsy. The choledochotomy can be closed primarily or over a T-tube and a drain left for 24–48 hours, then removed if no bile is present. Stone extraction rates of 70–95% are achievable using the laparoscopic approach (Williams et al. 2008).

To perform an open bile duct exploration a choledochotomy is performed in the distal CBD through which a flexible choledochoscope and dormia baskets or Fogarty balloon catheters can be inserted under direct vision with minimal trauma. To ensure duct clearance the scope must be passed into the intrahepatic ducts and down to the ampulla. The duct can then be closed primarily or over a T-tube and a drain left for a period of 24–48 hours, then removed if no bile is present (Williams et al. 2008).

Management of T-tubes

T-tubes should be managed meticulously. They should be sutured in place securely at the end of the procedure and should be carefully labelled to prevent inadvertent removal. Following insertion they should be left on free drainage and kinking of the tube should be avoided. Patients should have a T-tube cholangiogram performed before discharge from hospital to confirm that no stones are present; that there are no leaks and that there is good passage of contrast into the duodenum. The T-tube can then be spigotted and strapped to the abdominal wall to avoid unnecessary bile loss, and to reduce the risk of contamination, infection and accidental removal. The patient then returns on the ward 4–6 weeks later for T-tube removal. The T-tube should come out with gentle traction. If the tube will not dislodge it should be left for a further 2–4 weeks before attempting its removal again. If stones are found at T-tube cholangiography they may be removed by ERCP or endoscopically/radiologically via the T-tube tract.

Table 15.3 Overview of the causes and pathogens in acute cholangitis.

Causes of cholangitis	Bile duct stones
	Stents
Bacteria	Aerobic gram-negative bacilli (coliforms)
	Enterococci
	Anaerobes

Mirrizi syndrome

Mirrizi syndrome occurs when there is partial obstruction of the common hepatic duct from impaction of a large gallstone within Hartmann's pouch. The stone induces chronic fibrosis and this together with the obstruction by the stone causes obliteration of the cystic duct. The inflammatory process fuses the gallbladder to the common hepatic duct and obstruction of the main bile duct ensues. A cholecystocholedochal fistula may also develop. Mirrizi syndrome is usually associated with dense fibrosis in Calot's triangle and treatment is therefore challenging and depends on the extent of disruption to the normal biliary anatomy.

Acute cholangitis

Acute cholangitis is defined as acute infection of the biliary tree. It is a surgical emergency and must be recognised and treated early to prevent rapid progression of sepsis. Normal bile is sterile but the presence of stones or instrumentation of the bile duct (ERCP or PTC) is associated with bacterial colonisation. In the presence of partial or complete biliary obstruction, bacterial infection leads to acute cholangitis. The most common causes of this are bile duct stones and biliary stent occlusion and the commonest bacteria are enteric in origin and include *Escherichia coli*, *Klebsiella* spp. and Enterococci. Cholangiovenous reflux of these bacteria and their toxins into the systemic circulation is thought to be the cause of the rapid progression of acute cholangitis to severe sepsis and multi-organ dysfunction (Table 15.3).

Presentation

Acute cholangitis presents as a combination of right upper quadrant pain, rigors (swinging fever associated with shaking and chills) and jaundice. This combination is called Charcot's triad although the full triad is rarely present.

Initial management

Initial management is aimed at adequate resuscitation. Oxygen should be given, fluid resuscitation commenced, blood cultures performed, lactate and arterial gases performed (in line with the surviving sepsis guidelines) and broad spectrum antibiotics, such as a second generation cephalosporin and metronidazole, commenced. Where appropriate the patient should be assessed by the critical care team and transferred to a ward where hourly observations and urine output will be recorded or transferred to a monitored facility. The diagnosis should be confirmed by abdominal ultrasound examination and an early ERCP performed to decompress the bile ducts. A plastic biliary stent should be inserted if pus is present but definitive clearance of the bile duct should be delayed until the patient's condition has improved. In patients in whom ERCP is unsuccessful, PTC drainage offers an alternative.

Malignant bile duct obstruction

In patients presenting with suspected malignant obstructive jaundice the aim of investigation is to achieve early and accurate diagnosis and to identify which patients are candidates for resectional surgery. Early symptoms are non-specific (abdominal pain and discomfort, anorexia and weight loss and pruritis) and the usual presentation is with progressive jaundice. Cholangitis is uncommon in these patients unless there has been previous instrumentation of the ducts (bacterial contamination of the bile duct occurs in 100% in patients who have had ERCP or PTC compared with less than 30% who have had no previous intervention (Hochwald et al. 1999).

Transabdominal ultrasound is indispensable as the first-line investigation for malignant obstructive jaundice. It will demonstrate biliary duct dilatation and may identify the underlying cause of obstruction. However, it is less effective as a staging tool for hepatobiliary and pancreatic malignancy. The next step in the investigation of suspected malignant bile duct obstruction is therefore cross-sectional imaging either by spiral CT or by MRI. Ongoing management of malignant obstructive jaundice will be dictated by the results of these investigations. The British Society of Gastroenterology has provided detailed guidelines for the management of cholangiocarcinoma (Khan et al. 2002), pancreatic and peri-ampullary cancers (Gastroenterology 2005).

References

Gastroenterology PSotBSo, Ireland PSoGBa, Surgeons AoUG, Pathologists RCo, Radiology SIGfG-I. Guidelines for the management of patients with pancreatic cancer periampullary and ampullary carcinomas. *Gut* 2005;**54**(Suppl V):v1–v16.

Hochwald S, Burke E, Jarnagin W, Fong Y, Blumgart L. Preoperative biliary stenting is associated with increased post-operative infectious complications in proximal cholangiocarcinoma. *Arch Surg* 1999;**134**:261–266.

Khan S, Davidson B, Goldin R, et al. Guidelines for the diagnosis and treatment of cholangiocarcinoma: consensus document. *Gut* 2002;**51**(Suppl VI):vi1–vi9.

Williams E, Green J, Beckingham I, Parks R, Martin D, Lombard M. Guidelines on the management of common bile duct stones (CBDS). *Gut* 2008;**57**:1004–1021.

16 Large Bowel Obstruction

Igor V. Voskresensky[1] & Bryan A. Cotton[2]

[1]Department of Surgery, Vanderbilt University Medical Center, Nashville, TN, USA
[2]Department of Surgery and the Center for Translational Injury Research, The University of Texas Health Science Center, Houston, TX, USA

Introduction

Patients presenting with symptoms of abdominal pain accompanied by distention, obstipation/constipation and/or nausea and vomiting should be suspected of having gastrointestinal obstruction. Although symptoms of small bowel obstruction (SBO) and large bowel obstruction (LBO) are similar, aetiologies, diagnostic approach and therapeutic considerations are quite different. Sources of acute LBO can be separated into mechanical (colorectal carcinoma [CRC], diverticulitis, volvulus, faecal impaction, inflammatory bowel disease [IBD], anastomotic stricture and other pelvic malignancies), and non-mechanical causes (acute colonic pseudo-obstruction). Furthermore, obstruction can be complete or partial.

Evaluation of a patient with LBO in the acute setting must answer the following questions: (1) Is operative intervention indicated? (2) Can the operation be delayed for further resuscitation and planning without increasing risks of morbidity and mortality?

Clinical presentation

By carefully obtaining the history, one can often determine the particular cause of the obstruction prior to any imaging. Known history of abdominal malignancy or progressive complaints of constipation, decreasing stool calibre, haematochezia, vague abdominal pain, weight loss and general malaise raise suspicion of cancer. Recurrent, localised (usually left lower quadrant) pain radiating to the groin or perineum with defecation, and accompanied by fevers and constipation may represent diverticulitis. Colonic volvulus may not be associated with specific signs and symptoms aside from abdominal pain and distention most pronounced in the upper quadrants of the abdomen. Any of the aforementioned processes can also present with perforation leading to uncontrolled spillage of intestinal contents and progressive sepsis. Patients with faecal impaction are usually older with a long-standing history of constipation. Anastomotic strictures should be suspected in anyone with previous intestinal resections. Patients with IBD or history of radiation to the pelvis not infrequently present with obstruction; however, the possibility of strictures and/or malignancy should be entertained. Acute colonic pseudo-obstruction (Ogilvie's syndrome) should be considered in critically ill patients presenting with obstructive signs and symptoms. Finally, the possibility of a rectal foreign body should be entertained, especially in younger patients and those without pre-morbid complaints.

Initial attention should be focused on signs of systemic infection and haemodynamic compromise. These signs include altered mental status, hyper/hypothermia, tachycardia, hypotension and tachypnoea. Patients with the above findings cannot tolerate delay in operative intervention. Abdominal discomfort can be of various qualities depending on the process. In uncomplicated LBO abdominal pain is vague and periodic, occurring at 20- to 30-minute intervals corresponding to colonic smooth muscle activity. Localised abdominal findings occur from local irritation of peritoneum such as in perforated colon cancer or diverticulitis. Proximal bowel distention can be severe enough to lead to ischaemia and necrosis. In such cases, abdominal pain becomes progressively worse and is worse in the peri-umbilical region.

Generalised peritonitis occurs with perforation and spillage of faeculent contents. Abdominal distention and tympany on percussion are almost always present. Rectal examination must be performed to assess for low-lying causes of obstruction (e.g. mass, inspissated stool, stricture and foreign body). Furthermore, it is critical to assess the patient's cardiovascular and respiratory reserves to determine the appropriate approach to operative intervention if one is required. One should also identify patients who are candidates for palliative care as opposed to definitive therapy (involvement of patient and family in this decision is of utmost importance).

Emergency Surgery, 1st edition. Edited by Adam Brooks, Peter F. Mahoney, Bryan A. Cotton and Nigel Tai. © 2010 Blackwell Publishing.

The results of laboratory values along with physical examination can help guide decision making. Leucocytosis or pronounced leucopenia in the setting of peritoneal findings suggests systemic infection. Hyperglycaemia in non-diabetics further confirms suspicion of a septic picture. If the clinical condition allows, one should attempt to correct glucose values (to less than 200 mg/dL) and to reverse electrolyte and acid–base disturbances prior to surgical intervention. Additionally, anaemia and the presence of coagulopathy must be noted as these may need to be corrected prior to the operation. Patients who are immunocompromised may not show typical laboratory changes mentioned above.

Imaging

Plain film radiographs

Radiological findings on supine and erect films depend on the side of obstruction and competence of the ileocaecal valve. Typically, the images show dilated intestine proximal to the mechanical site of obstruction with an abrupt cut-off of colonic gas and distal paucity of air. Because ileocaecal valve incompetence is not uncommon, many patients may present with small bowel distention as well. Caecal volvulus can be identified by a large bowel loop with one to two haustral markings located in the left upper or right lower quadrants. In caecal volvulus, the distal large bowel is usually decompressed while the small bowel is distended. In sigmoid volvulus, a large inverted U-shaped bowel loop without haustral markings is seen in the upper abdomen (Figure 16.1). In acute colonic pseudo-obstruction the entire colon may appear dilated. However, findings can mimic mechanical obstruction, and a water-soluble contrast enema, computed tomography (CT), or endoscopy is needed to confirm the diagnosis. Severity of distention can be estimated by measuring caecal diameter; size greater than 12 cm leads to significant risk of perforation (Figure 16.2). Along with abdominal films, an erect chest X-ray should be obtained to evaluate for pneumoperitoneum in suspected cases of perforation.

Computed tomography

CT of the abdomen and pelvis with intravenous (IV) and oral contrast can aid in decision making in cases where plain films are inconclusive. CT can help identify the exact location of colonic and other intra-abdominal malignancies, their extent, presence of metastatic disease and other organ involvement. In suspected cases of diverticulitis, CT scan can localise areas of thickened, inflamed bowel, and identify an abscess or colonic perforation (Figure 16.3). Findings of pneumatosis intestinalis in the context of a concerning abdominal examination suggests bowel ischaemia and is an indication for a laparotomy. CT is diagnostic for acute colonic

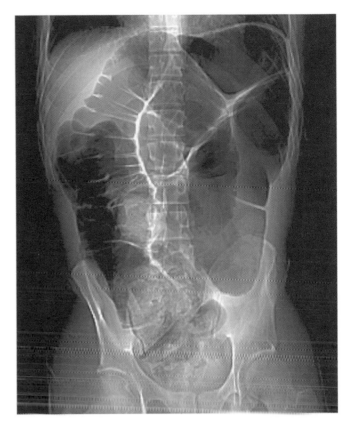

Figure 16.1 Sigmoid volvulus.

pseudo-obstruction as generalised distention is noted without the presence of obvious lesion. It is imperative to assess renal function to avoid contrast nephropathy. Ensure euvolemia prior to IV contrast. Once volume status is adequate, a sodium bicarbonate infusion (three ampules in 1 L of 5% dextrose) or enteral N-acetylcysteine may be administered to reduce the likelihood of renal injury.

Contrast enema

Water-soluble contrast enemas can be used if CT is not available. Intraluminal masses can be identified as a filling defect within the colon, or a classic apple core lesion in the case of circumferential cancers. Extraluminal compression is seen by deflected contours of colonic wall. Contrast extravasation into the peritoneal cavity is diagnostic of intestinal perforation although physical signs should obviate the need for a contrast examination in this scenario. In cases of volvulus the typical tapering ('bird beak' appearance) of contrast in proximal bowel is observed. Although barium is better visualised within the bowel its use is not recommended if intestinal perforation is suspected as it can lead to further peritoneal inflammation.

Endoscopy

Endoscopic evaluation can be both diagnostic and therapeutic. Colonic insufflation during endoscopy can lead to

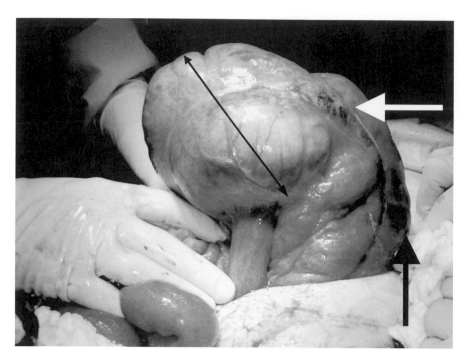

Figure 16.2 Markedly distended caecum exceeding 12 cm in diameter (thin double black arrow) with areas of ischaemia and threatened perforation (thick single black arrows).

perforation and is generally contraindicated in cases where it is already suspected. Flexible sigmoidoscopy can be the initial therapy for patients with non-toxic sigmoid volvulus. As well, it allows for assessment of mucosal viability, presence of inflammation (such as in IBD), and identification of unsuspected malignancy or stricture. Decompression can be achieved by simple suctioning, placement of colonic drainage tubes and mechanical stents, and performing laser photocoagulation or electrocoagulation of completely obstructing lesions.

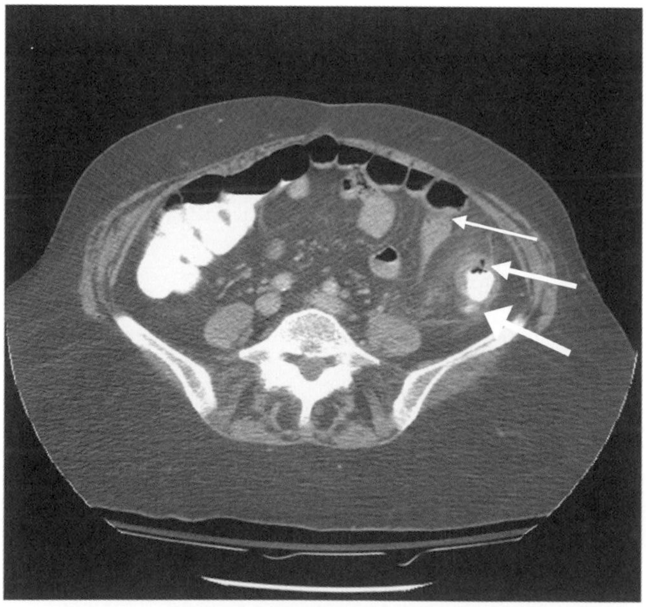

Management

The patient should have nothing by mouth (NBM), crystalloid-based IV fluids to correct the likely volume depletion, urinary catheter placement to measure exact urine output and a nasogastric tube (NGT) placement for proximal bowel decompression. Attention should be paid to correction of electrolyte deficiencies. Aforementioned signs of infection should be diligently thought out and IV broad-spectrum antibiotic coverage initiated when indicated. Patients taking adrenergic blockers may have a blunted haemodynamic response to volume depletion and infection. This population requires special attention during their resuscitation and in the interpretation of their physiological responses. Moreover, patients with a recent (within 6 months) history of corticosteroid use should be supplemented with stress IV steroids to avoid acute adrenal insufficiency. Necessary laboratory and imaging studies should be obtained.

Immediate operation

Patients presenting with uncontrolled perforation, generalised peritonitis, sepsis and complete bowel obstruction require emergent laparotomy. Exceptions to this rule are patients with terminal illness, non-toxic sigmoid volvulus (endoscopic decompression should be attempted first), and patients undergoing active cardiopulmonary resuscitation. Intraoperatively, all segments of compromised intestine should be identified and resected. Oncologic principles must

Figure 16.3 CT demonstrating complex diverticulitis with intraperitoneal fluid (thin white arrow), extraluminal air (medium white arrow) and pericolonic stranding with possible extraluminal contrast (thick white arrow).

be kept in mind as invasive carcinoma may be found later on pathologic examination. If the patient's clinical condition deteriorates or there is questionable bowel viability, the patient may be managed with an open abdomen and return when physiology allows for definitive intervention (anastomosis, stoma etc.). In the absence of peritonitis, antibiotics should be limited to the initial 24 hours postoperatively. Expected complications, especially in elderly patients with medical co-morbidities include sepsis, wound infections, abscess formation, respiratory failure, renal compromise, cardiac disturbances and malnutrition.

> If the patient is haemodynamically unstable or bowel viability is questionable, primary anastomosis should be avoided.

Colorectal carcinoma

CRC accounts for 50–80% of all causes of LBO. Ten to fifteen per cent of patients with CRC present with acute colonic perforation or occlusion. Left-sided obstructions occur more often than obstructions due to right-sided lesions (25–50% and 10–15%, respectively). Patients presenting with LBO due to CRC are usually older, have more medical co-morbidities, and have a higher mortality rate after emergency procedures. Furthermore, cancers that lead to obstruction and perforation are found to be more aggressive, have a shorter history of symptomatology, are more difficult to remove completely, and have worse overall outcomes.

Treatment

Therapy of LBO due to CRC depends on the side of the obstruction. Right-sided lesions (caecum to splenic flexure) can be successfully managed with right hemicolectomy and primary ileocolonic anastomosis even in the setting of perforation and contamination. Left-sided lesions (descending colon to rectum) in acute setting historically have been treated with avoidance of primary anastomosis and staged procedures. Preferred operations included segmental left colon resection with colostomy and mucous fistula, or low anterior resection with colostomy and Hartman's procedure. However, recent trends suggest that primary anastomosis, even with generalised peritonitis, may be a better alternative to staged procedures as preferred in the past. Subtotal/total colectomy is performed when known synchronous cancers exist (up to 7% of all CRC) or caecal perforation has occurred in the setting of left-sided obstructing lesion. As in emergent right colon operations, staged procedures and avoidance of primary anastomosis should be considered in haemodynamically unstable patients, those with carcinomatosis, malnutrition and immunologic compromise.

Colonic decompression with endoscopic tube placement, with or without lavage, prior to the operation has been suggested to decrease left colon faecal load. This approach may

lower incidence of postoperative infections and anastomotic leak rates, and further argues for single-stage procedures. Additionally, endoscopic laser photocoagulation (Nd-YAG) and electrocoagulation with partial removal of occluding lesions have led to successful intestinal recanalisation for poor operative candidates. Finally, use of self-expandable metallic stents (SEMS) has been suggested as effective and a safe means for decompression of left colonic obstruction due to CRC, and avoidance of immediate surgery.

Outcomes and complications

The 30-day mortality for patients undergoing emergency operations for CRC has been reported to be 6–34%, compared to less than 5% in elective setting. The mortality and morbidity rates are similar for right and left obstructing lesions. High American Society of Anesthesiology (ASA) class, poor performance status and cancer stage are the most important predictors of long-term survival. Patients undergoing single-stage procedure seem to have lower mortality (0–22% versus 3–33%), less complications (9–52% versus 11–64%) and shorter hospital stay when compared to 2- and 3-staged operations.

Diverticulitis

Diverticulitis accounts for approximately 5–10% of all cases of LBO, affecting the sigmoid colon in the vast majority of patients. Most of the cases of obstruction are partial. Recurrent inflammation leads to bowel wall thickening, fibrosis and stricture formation. Abscess formation can cause tethering of the colon to the pelvic sidewall. Pericolonic inflammation resulting in severe bowel oedema can lead to a dynamic obstruction. Moreover, close relationship with small intestine can cause SBO.

Treatment

Because CRC can present similarly to acute complicated diverticulitis, differentiation should be made if non-operative management is elected. CT with judicial use of endoscopy or contrast enemas is recommended. Non-operative management is similar to the initial approach in all patients with LBO. Placing the patient NBM, and initiating IV fluids and antibiotics with gram-negative and anaerobic coverage are the basic principles of non-operative management of uncomplicated diverticulitis. This approach allows resolution of obstruction due to intestinal oedema without a mechanical source. If a percutaneously accessible abscess is present, drainage using CT or US guidance is preferred.

Up to 25% of patients admitted with acute diverticulitis undergo emergent operations. Operative intervention is indicated in cases of peritonitis and sepsis, perforation, failure of medical management, and symptomatic abscess not amenable to percutaneous drainage. As with the management of CRC, debate exists as to whether primary anastomosis or a two-stage procedure should be performed.

Historically, sigmoid colectomy with colostomy and Hartman's procedure was the operation of choice in patients with generalised peritonitis. More recently, single-stage procedures have gained popularity based on data showing their outcomes to be quite similar.

Outcomes and complications

The two-stage approach of colostomy and Hartman's is associated with a postoperative mortality and morbidity of around 10 and 40%, respectively. Less than 70% of patients undergo eventual stoma takedown and anastomosis. Recent reviews show that mortality (10%), anastomotic leaks (6% versus 8%), abscess formation (4% versus 8%) and wound infections (14% versus 22%) are similar between one- and two-stage procedures. In light of these results, many authors argue that colostomy and Hartman's procedure should be reserved for patients with severe peritonitis and questionable integrity of bowel wall from inflammation and oedema.

Volvulus

Colonic volvulus accounts for up to 5% of all causes of LBO. Of these, sigmoid and caecal volvulus is responsible for 70 and 20% of all cases, respectively. Long mesenteric attachments allow for increased bowel mobility and subsequent twisting about the base of the mesentery. This leads to development of a closed-loop obstruction, intestinal ischaemia, necrosis and perforation. Once intestinal strangulation develops, mortality increases dramatically (as high as 80%). Caecal rotation can involve a simple cephalad fold over a fixed ascending colon (caecal bascule) or an actual twist of ascending colon, caecum and terminal ileum (more likely to lead to gangrene due to vascular compromise). Previous abdominal operations, pregnancy, left colon obstruction, malrotation and serious medical co-morbidities have been associated with caecal volvulus.

Treatment, outcomes and complications

Therapy for non-toxic sigmoid volvulus (lack of peritonitis, leucocytosis and haemodynamic instability) should begin with decompression via sigmoidoscopy and placement of a rectal drainage tube for 2–3 days. This approach is effective in up to 95% of patients. If initial endoscopic detorsion is unsuccessful, water-soluble contrast enemas can be attempted. However, sigmoidoscopic decompression and rectal tube placement alone is inadequate as a definitive procedure as recurrence is seen in up to 90% of cases.

Elective intervention requires bowel preparation and laparoscopic or open sigmoid colectomy with primary anastomosis. Sigmoidopexy is inadequate as recurrence is observed in 30–40% of patients. Upon endoscopic examination, if mucosal necrosis or bleeding is noted the procedure should be aborted and patient taken to the operating room for immediate sigmoid resection. Caecal bascule and volvulus are unlikely to respond to endoscopic colonic decompression. Caecopexy and caecal resection have similar results; however,

the former procedure is less invasive and can be performed if the intestinal wall is viable. Right hemicolectomy is suggested if extensive intestinal necrosis is suspected. Placement of caecostomy tube for decompression has been suggested in poor operative candidates. This procedure is associated with high incidence of intestinal spillage and enterocutaneous fistula formation.

Presence of bowel wall compromise dictates whether a primary anastomosis is feasible during the emergency operation.

Other mechanical causes of obstruction

Faecal impaction

Faecal impaction usually affects the elderly, with multiple medical, neurologic and psychiatric co-morbidities. This chronic problem can lead to severe obstruction with proximal colonic dilation. Low colonic pressure in response to dilation is one of the main mechanisms. Enemas and disimpaction should be attempted, unless signs of ischaemia and perforation are present. Eventual resection of sigmoid colon and rectum may be required.

Inflammatory bowel disease

Patients with IBD infrequently present with acute LBO. Recurrent inflammation leads to scarring and formation of fibrotic strictures; however, compression effect from an abscess should be ruled out. The mainstream therapy is to quell active inflammation with corticosteroids and 5-aminosalicylates. In cases of failed anti-inflammatory therapy resection of fibrotic strictures (stricturoplasty) or endoscopic balloon dilation can be attempted. It is imperative to rule out malignancy by multiple biopsies as reports suggest 7–50% of carcinoma in fibrotic strictures of IBD. Cancer is found more frequently in patients with ulcerative colitis. If bowel resection is undertaken pouch formation should be avoided in patients with malnutrition, severe inflammation or expected pelvic radiation.

Anastomotic strictures

Anastomotic strictures after colorectal resections are found in up to 30% of patients. Although partial obstruction is more frequent than complete, the overall incidence of acute LBO is not infrequent. History of anastomotic leak, abdominal sepsis and postoperative radiation increases risk for obstructive stricture formation. If bowel resection was performed for cancer recurrence should always be ruled out with biopsies. Balloon dilation, electrocautery resection, transrectal stapling or formal bowel resection are available options. The same principles of acute LBO management apply.

Hernias

Though typically considered to occur exclusively with small bowel, redundant colon may incarcerate into fascial defects throughout the abdomen and pelvis. These include through the diaphragm, femoral hernias, inguinal hernias and ventral defects as well. In addition, parastomal hernias may occur and are associated with bowel strangulation and, thus, high mortality rates.

Other malignancies

Advanced gynaecologic, prostate and bladder cancer can cause intestinal infiltration or mass effect and lead to LBO. When colonic involvement occurs it is likely that small intestine is also affected. Decompression with rectal tube placement or stenting has been successful. Intestinal resection generally leads to poor results with rapid recurrence of symptoms.

Acute colonic pseudo-obstruction

The signs and symptoms of acute colonic pseudo-obstruction are sometimes indistinguishable from mechanical LBO. Although the pathophysiology of acute colonic pseudo-obstruction is not completely understood, inhibition of colonic motility via sympathetic fibre activation may play an important role. The most common predisposing factors include pelvic fractures, prolonged mechanical ventilation, systemic infection, severe cardiac dysfunction and other types of critical illness. ACP should be distinguished from mechanical obstruction and megacolon caused by *Clostridium difficile* as initial therapies are markedly different. When plain films are non-diagnostic, CT, enema and endoscopy may be used for additional information. Up to 15% of patients with acute colonic pseudo-obstruction will experience spontaneous colonic perforation with mortality reaching 50%.

Treatment, outcomes and complications

The initial therapy for ACP is non-operative and includes NBM, NGT placement and IV fluids. As well, frequent ambulation, limiting opioids and anti-cholinergics, and placement of rectal decompression tube should be considered. Supportive therapy is effective in 80% of patients. Because colonic distention can progress to cause ischaemic bowel necrosis and perforation, frequent abdominal examinations should be performed to assess daily clinical status. Risk of perforation is increased substantially when caecal diameter is greater than 12 cm and distention has been present for more than 3–4 days.

If no improvement occurs over the first 24 hours then 2 mg of neostigmine can be infused intravenously over 3–5 minutes. Patients should be placed on continuous telemetry monitoring prior to infusion as the risk of bradyarrhythmia is not insignificant. Neostigmine can be repeated if a partial response or recurrence is observed. Administration leads to resolution in over 90% cases, with the majority of responses occurring within several minutes of infusion. Contraindications for neostigmine therapy include severe bronchospasm, pregnancy, cardiac arrhythmias and renal failure. The most common complication is bradycardia requiring atropine. In addition to having atropine immediately available, pre-treatment with an anxiolytic (many patients describe a feeling of 'impending doom') and a bronchodilator (ipratropium and beta-agonist) should be considered.

Patients who do not respond to medical therapy can undergo colonoscopic decompression with rectal tube placement under fluoroscopic guidance. Decompression has been reported to be effective in 60–95% of cases. Bowel perforation from endoscopy is much higher in patients with acute colonic pseudo-obstruction compared to those with 'normal' colon; 3% versus <0.01%, respectively. Operative intervention is indicated when the above attempts are failed or signs of intestinal necrosis or perforation are present. Placement of a percutaneous caecostomy tube should be considered in patients who are at high risk of surgery and when no bowel ischaemia is suspected. The mortality after surgical therapy for non-perforated acute colonic pseudo-obstruction is around 6%.

Summary

LBO is a frequent diagnosis on the surgical take and can arise from a wide range of aetiologies. It is important that all potential diagnoses are considered and that active management and resuscitation is commenced early. Those patients managed non-operatively need close ongoing assessment. The operative management continues to evolve towards single-stage procedures; however, the patient's physiology should be taken into account when planning surgical procedures.

Further reading

Abbas S. Resection and primary anastomosis in acute complicated diverticulitis: a systematic review of the literature. *Int J Colorectal Dis* 2007;**22**(4):351–357.

Cameron JL. *Current Surgical Therapy*, 9th edn. Elsevier Health Sciences, Philadelphia, PA, 2007.

Constantinides VA, Tekkis PP, Athanasiou T, et al. Primary resection with anastomosis vs. Hartmann's procedure in non-elective surgery for acute colonic diverticulitis: a systematic review. *Dis Colon Rectum* 2006;**49**(7):966–981.

Saunders MD. Acute colonic pseudo-obstruction. *Gastrointest Endosc Clin N Am* 2007;**17**(2):341–360.

Townsend C, Beauchamp RD, Evers BM, Mattox K. *Sabiston Textbook of Surgery*, 18th edn. Saunders, Philadelphia, PA, 2007.

17 Emergency Surgical Management of Herniae

John Simpson & David J. Humes

Department of Surgery, QMC Campus, Nottingham University Hospitals NHS Trust, Nottingham, UK

Introduction

A hernia is a protrusion of a viscus through an abnormal opening in the wall of its containing cavity. The most common types of spontaneous abdominal wall hernia are inguinal, femoral and umbilical. Epigastric herniae are seen less frequently and rarely obturator, spigelian, lumbar, gluteal, sciatic and diaphragmatic hernias. Incisional herniae are an acquired type, seen in up to 15% of abdominal incisions depending on the type of initial surgery performed. Most herniae are uncomplicated and are seen and managed as elective cases but the minority which do present as emergencies require prompt assessment and management.

In 2005–2006, there were more than 9000 emergency admissions to English hospitals for inguinal and femoral herniae. Up to 13% of external herniae require emergency operation and although the overall morbidity and mortality associated with hernia surgery as a whole is low, the majority of complications arise in this small group of patients. Complications can be reduced by prompt diagnosis, appropriate resuscitation and operative intervention. The first part of this chapter will focus on general considerations in the assessment and management of patients presenting to the emergency unit with a common hernia type. The second part will highlight general points in the operative management of these patients followed by highlighting specific points related to the more commonly seen hernia types.

Clinical presentation

History

Patients in the emergency setting will usually describe a tender irreducible swelling at the site of the hernia. This may be at the site of a previous reducible hernia or alternatively may represent a de novo presentation. Around half of patients presenting with strangulation are known to have a hernia at the time of emergency admission. A history of recent weight loss may predispose to the development of a femoral hernia as a result of loss of fat within the femoral sheath. Although an uncomplicated irreducible hernia may not require immediate management, careful assessment must be made for symptoms and signs of intestinal obstruction and strangulation.

Intestinal obstruction: Approximately, 25% of the cases of intestinal obstruction are caused by strangulated external hernia. The cardinal signs of intestinal obstruction are abdominal distension, colicky abdominal pain, absolute constipation and vomiting although the onset of each symptom will depend on the anatomical region of bowel involvement. Furthermore, with small herniae in obese patients and the rarer pelvic herniae, intestinal obstruction may be the only presenting symptom.

Strangulation: A hernia becomes strangulated when the blood supply of the contents within the sac becomes impaired to such a degree that gangrene becomes imminent. The intestine becomes obstructed, venous congestion followed by arterial compromise occurs which can result in gangrene as early as 5 or 6 hours following the first onset of symptoms. Alternatively the pressure of a tight constriction ring at the neck of the peritoneal sac may cause a localised necrosis of the bowel wall. A Richter's-type hernia is when there is only partial involvement of the bowel wall within the sac and as a result is not necessarily associated with bowel obstruction.

Examination

A general assessment must be made looking for any signs of systemic response resulting from a complicated hernia. As a result of third space losses, patients with intestinal obstruction can become dehydrated with loss of skin turgor, dry mucous membranes, tachycardia and, in advanced cases, hypotension. The cardinal signs of the systemic inflammatory response syndrome (SIRS) are listed below and the presence of these may also indicate strangulation and imminent perforation (Box 17.1).

Emergency Surgery, 1st edition. Edited by Adam Brooks, Peter F. Mahoney, Bryan A. Cotton and Nigel Tai. © 2010 Blackwell Publishing.

Box 17.1 Systemic inflammatory response syndrome

SIRS is considered to be present when the patient has more than one of the following clinical findings:

Temperature: $>38°C$ or $<36°C$

White cell count: <4000 or $>12,000$ cells/mm^3 or the presence of $>10\%$ immature neutrophils ('bands')

Tachycardia: heart rate >90 beats/minute

Tachypnoea or supranormal minute ventilation: respiratory rate >20 breaths/minute or $P_aCO_2 <4.3$ kPa

---

Box 17.2 Differential diagnosis

- Lump in groin
  Inguinal hernia
  Femoral hernia
  Lymph node
  Sapheno-varix
  Ectopic testes
  Femoral aneurysm
  Hydroceles of the cord or of the canal of Nuck
  Lipoma of the spermatic cord
  Psoas abscess
  Psoas bursa

- Anterior abdominal wall herniae
  Divarication of the rectus muscles. This occurs due to stretching of the linea alba allowing separation of the recti. Although the defect can appear impressive, it is not typically regarded as a hernia and no surgical intervention is required.

  Rectus sheath haematoma. This accumulation of blood in the sheath of the rectus abdominis, secondary a muscle tear or rupture of an epigastric vessel or. It could occur spontaneously or after trauma and is usually managed with conservative measures.

Abdominal distension secondary to obstruction may be present and specifically, there will be a tender irreducible lump at the site of the hernia without a transmissible cough impulse. Subcutaneous ecchymosis can also present as a feature of strangulated herniae. Although the history and examination can often be conclusive, differential diagnoses must always be considered (Box 17.2). This is especially true of femoral herniae which are seldom large and in an obese person may be difficult to identify. Whilst the patient is supine gentle manipulation of an irreducible hernia can be attempted although care must be taken not to hurt the patient. There is a slight but real risk that this may reduce the hernia 'en masse', i.e. the hernia reduces within its peritoneal coverings, the neck of which remains a constriction.

Investigations

The basis of initial investigations is to determine the current physiological status of the patient and to allow preparation for theatre. If the diagnosis is in doubt, radiological investigations may be required to aid diagnosis. Baseline haematological investigations include full blood count (FBC), urea and electrolytes (U&Es), clotting profile and group and save. Depending on the clinical condition, co-morbidity and age of patient, an electrocardiograph (ECG) and arterial blood gases (ABGs) may be required. An abdominal X-ray may show evidence of intestinal obstruction (Figure 17.1). Rarely a CT scan may be required to make the diagnosis.

Initial management

Fluid shifts and vomiting as a result of intestinal obstruction may result in severe dehydration which requires urgent management with replacement intravenous fluids. If there is evidence of intestinal obstruction, a nasogastric tube should be passed and a urethral catheter will allow assessment of fluid replacement. If there is evidence of toxaemia from is-

chaemia, broad spectrum antibiotics such as a cephalosporin and metronidazole should be commenced (Box 17.3).

Surgical management

If there is evidence of strangulation and therefore imminent ischaemia, the patient requires operative repair. Ideally the operation is performed under general anaesthetic in an adequately resuscitated patient although in extremely sick patients local or regional anaesthesia is sometimes appropriate.

The principles of operative technique are to define the defect, assess and manage the contents of the sac and finally to repair the defect and in general the operations employed in emergency cases are very similar to those described for non-strangulated cases although there are a few important differences.

The role of laparoscopic surgery in the emergency repair of hernia is less clear than its role in the elective setting and has not been the subject of a randomised controlled trial. The evidence so far is restricted to case series and individual case reports but repair has been effective for both incarcerated and strangulated incisional, ventral and inguinal herniae. A series with 220 patients demonstrated a comparable morbidity (3%) to elective surgery using the laparoscopic transperitoneal hernia repair. However, the European Association for Endoscopic Surgery consensus statement

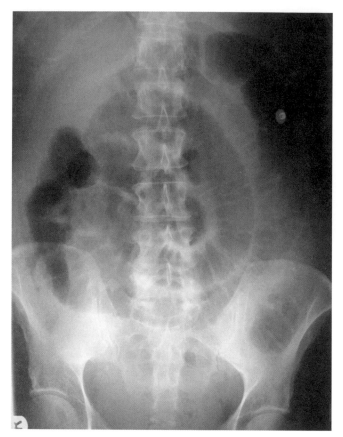

Figure 17.1 Abdominal X-ray showing dilated small bowel loops secondary to a strangulated right femoral hernia.

concluded that whilst initial reports were encouraging only surgeons with experience in laparoscopic hernia repair should attempt emergency repair.

General considerations

In cases of strangulated hernia, the hernial sac contains a variable amount of dark-coloured fluid derived from devitalised bowel or omentum. Depending on the duration of ischaemia, and viability of tissues within the sac, this fluid can be contaminated and spillage should be avoided. The sac should therefore be opened at the fundus of the sac and fluid removed with suction or swabs to prevent contamination of

---

Box 17.3 Initial management

Baseline blood tests (FBC, U&E, clotting, group and save)
Intravenous access and fluid resuscitation
Nasogastric tube
Urethral catheter
CXR, ECG, ABG
Broad spectrum antibiotics

---

the general peritoneal cavity. Samples should be sent for microbiological analysis.

Once the constriction has been divided, the contents of the hernial sac must be delivered into the wound and carefully examined prior to possible resection or delivery back into the abdominal cavity. If the contents spontaneously reduce during the preliminary dissection it is essential that the affected parts should be identified and thoroughly inspected.

Reconstruction of hernial defect

The past 20 years have seen increasing use of prosthetic material for the reconstruction of hernial defects. Although their use has been effective in reducing recurrence rates, introducing a foreign material can provide a nidus for infective complications which can cause significant morbidity. If there is gross contamination of the wound, the use of prosthetic material is best avoided. However, if the level of contamination is kept to a minimum and broad spectrum antibiotics are used throughout the perioperative period the use of mesh is not absolutely contraindicated.

Viability of bowel

When a loop of bowel has been strangulated, its viability must be assessed. The entire loop of bowel contained within the sac may be affected or the damage may be confined to the neck of the sac or to a section of wall (Richter's hernia). Even though the bowel may initially appear very congested and with dark red or purple discolouration, recovery may be possible and if viability is in question, the affected segment must be placed in warmed saline-soaked packs and left for 5–10 minutes before reassessing. This must be repeated if doubt persists. The presence of peristaltic waves is encouraging and these can often be stimulated by gentle flicking a healthy section of bowel just proximal to the questionable segment. When viability of bowel is more markedly impaired, the fluid within the peritoneal sac is likely to be turbid and offensive smelling. The bowel is ashen or even black and flaccid to touch and if infarction has been prolonged, perforation of the bowel wall may have occurred. Furthermore, there is likely to be thrombosis and lack of visible or palpable pulsation within the mesenteric vessels.

Treatment of necrotic intestine

The choice of procedure is dependent on the severity and extent of the damage. If the damage is localised and does not affect the entire circumference of the bowel wall simple infolding or partial resection may be acceptable if this does not compromise the bowel lumen. However, this is the exception and in most cases of intestinal necrosis, resection and anastomosis is the mainstay of treatment. In the majority of cases it is small bowel which is affected and following resection there are several methods of anastomosis. It is imperative that the surgeon is fully trained and competent

---

Box 17.4 Common techniques for repair of femoral and inguinal hernia

	Type of repair	Advantages	Disadvantages
Inguinal	Shouldice	No prosthetic mesh therefore reduced infection risk	Technically more demanding
	Mesh/Liechtenstein	Easier to perform Low recurrence rate	Prosthetic material may increase risk of infection
Femoral	Crural/low	Simple	Not recommended in strangulation as difficult to resect bowel
		Can be done under GA or LA Used in elective setting	
	High extraperitoneal approach (McEvedy approach)	Most useful approach in strangulation	Need to avoid damage to surrounding structures
		Allows small bowel resection	

---

in the method chosen. Strangulated omentum should also be excised.

Specific considerations in complicated herniae

Inguinal hernia

In the UK, there are approximately 100,000 inguinal herniae repaired annually and the cumulative probability of strangulation has been estimated at approximately 4% at 2 years. Operative repair should therefore be considered in all patients although a policy of watchful waiting is considered to be an acceptable option by some authors for elderly men with minimally symptomatic inguinal herniae. However, if presented with a strangulated inguinal hernia, it is approached through a standard groin crease incision (Box 17.4). The constriction is usually caused by the narrowed neck of the sac and is therefore situated at the level of the deep ring. Following dissection through the skin and subcutaneous tissues the tense sac is typically seen arising through this. The inguinal canal is opened, the sac is gently separated from surrounding structures using a combination of sharp and blunt dissection and the sac is delivered into the wound. The sac is opened with care to prevent spillage of contents and the opening is extended proximally through the constriction to allow a thorough examination of the contents of the sac which are dealt with appropriately. In the absence of gross contamination a mesh repair may be undertaken; however, where there is gross contamination the Shouldice operative repair technique is recommended to treat a strangulated inguinal hernia.

Femoral hernia

This risk of strangulation in femoral hernia is higher than inguinal and has been quoted as high as 50% within a month or as high as 45% at 2 years; therefore, prompt outpatient referral and repair for uncomplicated cases is recommended. In 2005–2006, 49.43% of all femoral herniae presented as emergency cases compared with just 8.6% of inguinal herniae. Femoral herniae are more likely to present in women compared to men (52.6% versus 6.5% of all groin hernia types presenting as an emergency) and require small bowel resection more frequently than inguinal hernia.

For strangulated cases, a high extraperitoneal approach is generally advised as it allows good exposure to the constriction at the level of the femoral ring and provides better access for the assessment and treatment of involved bowel (Figure 17.2a and b and Box 17.4). A unilateral Pfannenstiel-type incision is generally used nowadays rather than the classical McEvedy's vertical incision. The incision is continued through the anterior rectus sheath and the rectus muscle is retracted medially. The transveralis fascia is exposed and opened transversely allowing access to the preperitoneal space. The hernial sac is identified medial to the iliac vessels and is reduced if possible by gentle traction. For incarcerated herniae, the lacunar ligament can be incised to allow delivery of the sac into the wound. If an accessory obturator artery is present on the medial side of the femoral ring this can identified and avoided when using the high approach. The sac is then opened and contents managed as outlined above. The pectineal and inguinal ligament can then be approximated with non-absorbable sutures to narrow the defect or if the operative field has remained sterile a prosthetic mesh can be used.

Umbilical and paraumbilical herniae

In these cases, strangulation occurs not at the neck of the sac but more distally, near the fundus. The operation is approached as in elective cases but with reference to the specific points made above.

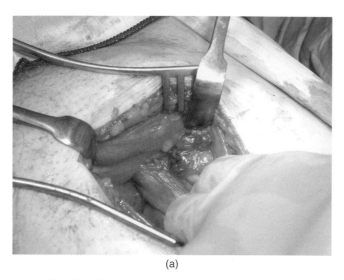
(a)

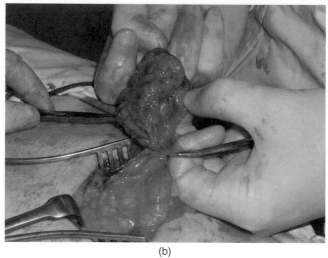
(b)

Figure 17.2 (a) A high approach for a tender right-sided femoral hernia. (Photograph taken from the patient's left side looking down into the operative field.) Note the peritoneal sac heading down into the femoral canal. (b) Following reduction of the hernia it was found that the hernia consisted of incarcerated preperitoneal fat. This was resected and the hernia repaired with prolene sutures and the patient made an uneventful recovery.

Epigastric hernia

These herniae are found in the midline between the xiphisternum and umbilicus. The hernia is approached through a transverse or vertical incision and although a slender peritoneal sac containing omentum or rarely intestine may be found, a protrusion of incarcerated extraperitoneal fat through the defect is the predominant finding. This can be resected or reduced and the defect closed with either simple sutures or a prosthetic mesh if the defect is larger.

Obturator hernia

These are most commonly found on the right side in elderly females and are a rare cause of mechanical bowel obstruction. The sac passes through the obturator canal which is bounded by the superior pubic ramus anteriorly and the obturator membrane posteriorly. The obturator nerve and vessels pass through the canal lying posterolateral to the hernial sac although position can be variable. The most common feature is intestinal obstruction and the patient may describe several milder antecedent episodes which settled spontaneously. Patients may describe referred pain down the inner side of the thigh resulting from compression of the cutaneous branch of the anterior division of the obturator nerve in the canal (known as the Howship-Romberg sign). There may be a palpable mass high in the medial aspect of the thigh which is most easily palpated with the thigh flexed, adducted and externally rotated. Although a femoral approach can be used, often obturator herniae are only discovered following laparotomy for intestinal obstruction. This approach allows easier access to contents of the sac and also permits assessment of the contralateral orifice. Either sutured repair or prosthetic mesh can be used to prevent recurrence.

Incisional hernia

It is estimated that approximately 10–15% of laparotomy wounds will result in an incisional hernia. As the location, size and presentation can vary widely a detailed outline for the individual management of such herniae is beyond the scope of this chapter. One feature, however, of incisional herniae is that there are often multiple defects within the scar, the so-called 'swiss cheese effect' and it is essential that these are sought and managed appropriately otherwise a further recurrence may ensue.

Outcomes from surgery

Those patients undergoing emergency hernia repair are older and have longer hospital stays than those undergoing elective repair. The median age of men undergoing emergency groin hernia repair is 67.9 years versus 58.6 years for elective repair (72.1 years versus 56.9 years in women).

General complications include bleeding, infection, haematoma, deep vein thrombosis, pulmonary embolus and cardiovascular events. Procedure-related complications for groin surgery include ischaemic orchitis, testicular atrophy, hydrocele, chronic pain, numbness and urinary retention. Recurrence does occur but no accurate data are available on outcomes in emergency repair but it is estimated to be higher than that seen in the elective setting.

Postoperative complications

The literature on outcomes following hernia surgery focuses on major complications and mortality. The majority of significant complications following surgery are principally cardiovascular and pulmonary and the duration of symptoms prior to admission has shown to be related to the incidence of complications following surgery. Surgical site infections have not been shown to be consistently significantly higher in those patients undergoing repair in the emergency setting although some data suggest they may be higher in those who undergo small bowel resection.

Mortality from elective groin hernia surgery is 0.1% compared to 2.9% with emergency cases, rising to over 12% in cases with bowel resection. The risk of death is greater in women but this is attributed to the fact that women have higher rates of femoral hernia which is associated with a higher mortality. Those patients with a high ASA grade preoperatively, high levels of co-morbid illness and suffering from at least one postoperative complication have the highest rates of mortality following surgery.

Postoperative care should include adequate analgesia, early mobilisation, thromboprophylaxis and early restoration to diet as clinically indicated. Data on return to work and normal activities following emergency surgery are limited. It is well established in the elective setting that return to normal activities should occur within 2–10 days. Driving following uncomplicated inguinal repair appears to be plausible during this time period. It is likely in the uncomplicated emergency setting that similar time frames should be used; however, due to the increased age, co-morbidity and subsequent increased hospital stay it is often longer before normal activity is resumed.

Summary

Presentation with an incarcerated hernia is common and associated with a substantial increase in mortality and morbidity compared with elective repair and prompt diagnosis and resuscitation are necessary to improve outcomes from surgery. The basic principles of operative technique are identical to elective repair namely to define the defect, assess and manage the contents of the hernial sac and finally to repair the defect.

Further reading

Fitzgibbons RJ, Jr, Giobbie-Hurder A, Gibbs JO, et al. Watchful waiting vs. repair of inguinal hernia in minimally symptomatic men: a randomized clinical trial. *JAMA* 2006;**295**(3):285–292.

Kingsnorth A, LeBlanc K. Hernias: inguinal and incisional. *Lancet* 2003;**362**(9395):1561–1571.

Koch A, Edwards A, Haapaniemi S, Nordin P, Kald A. Prospective evaluation of 6895 groin hernia repairs in women. *Br J Surg* 2005;**92**(12):1553–1558.

Nilsson II, Stylianidis G, Haapamaki M, Nilsson F, Nordin P. Mortality after groin hernia surgery. *Ann Surg* 2007;**245**(4):656–660.

3 Vascular

18 Ruptured Abdominal Aortic Aneurysm

Ross Davenport[1] & Nigel Tai[2,3]

[1]Trauma Clinical Academic Unit, Royal London Hospital, Whitechapel, London, UK
[2]Academic Department of Military Surgery and Trauma, Royal Centre for Defence Medicine, Birmingham, UK
[3]Defence Medical Services, Trauma Clinical Academic Unit, Royal London Hospital, Whitechapel, London, UK

Introduction

Abdominal aortic aneurysms (AAAs) occur as a result of a degenerative process of the abdominal aorta most often the result of advanced atherosclerosis. Ruptured AAA is a life-threatening surgical emergency with high mortality and morbidity rates. Rapid diagnosis, expedient open surgical or endoluminal repair and aggressive blood replacement therapy are required to ensure improved outcomes.

Clinical presentation

Definition

Aneurysms are defined as a focal dilatation of a blood vessel involving all three layers of the wall with at least a 50% increase over normal arterial diameter. An abdominal aortic aneurysm is thus usually greater than 3 cm in diameter. Most AAAs begin below the level of the renal arteries (95% are infra-renal) and end above the iliac arteries. They generally are spindle shaped; however, size, shape and extent vary considerably (Figure 18.1).

Incidence

Most AAAs are asymptomatic and are detected incidentally in routine radiologic investigation, i.e. ultrasound and computed tomography (CT) scan. Their true prevalence is therefore difficult to estimate but screening studies in the UK have estimated a prevalence of 1.3–12.7% depending on the age group studied and the definition of AAA. The incidence of symptomatic AAA in men is approximately 25 per 100,000 at age 50, increasing to 78 per 100,000 in those older than 70 years. In the UK frequency of rupture is 13 cases per 100,000 persons.

Emergency Surgery, 1st edition. Edited by Adam Brooks, Peter F. Mahoney, Bryan A. Cotton and Nigel Tai. © 2010 Blackwell Publishing.

Aetiology and risk factors

Atherosclerosis accounts for more than 90% of AAAs – other causes include infection, cystic medial necrosis, arteritis, trauma and inherited connective tissue (collagen) disorders, e.g. Marfan's syndrome.

AAAs are uncommon in non-Caucasian ethic groups. Primary risk factors are:
- Age (peak incidence at 70 years)
- Male gender (below the age of 80 years male-to-female ratio is 2:1 – no gender associative risk in older patients)
- Family history (approximately 25% of cases occur in persons with first-degree relatives with AAA)
- Peripheral aneurysms (femoral and popliteal)
- Smoking
- Coronary artery disease
- Hypertension

Pathophysiology

In general, AAAs gradually enlarge at a rate of 0.2–0.8 cm per year and all will eventually rupture if the patient lives long enough. The rate of growth and the risk of rupture increase exponentially with the diameter of the aneurysm (Table 18.1). Most elective repairs of AAA are carried out once the aneurysm is wider than 5.5 cm as the risk of rupture at this level outweighs the risks of surgery.

High haemodynamic arterial wall stress within the AAA correlates with the site of rupture. Computer-generated models suggest that aneurysm volume is a better predictor of areas of peak wall stress than aneurysm diameter. The balance between proteolytic degradation of aortic wall connective tissue, inflammation and immune responses, biomechanical wall stress, and molecular genetics all represent a dynamic process which leads to eventual AAA rupture. These factors in combination are likely to have implications for the future in determining which AAAs require early surgical repair.

Clinical assessment

The mortality rates of AAA rupture are approximate 80–90%. Of patients that make it alive to hospital to undergo

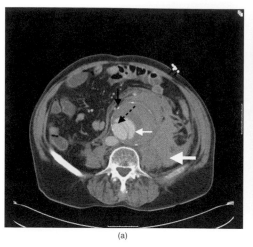 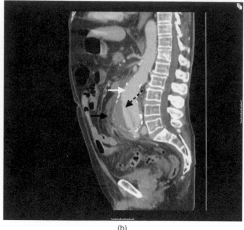

(a)   (b)

Figure 18.1 CTA (left: transverse section; right: saggital section) of a leaking infra-renal AAA. Note aneurysm sac (thin black arrow), aneurysm lumen (thin white arrow) and retroperitoneal haematoma (thick white arrow). The aneurysm is complicated by intimal dissection (hatched black arrow).

emergency surgery, only about half survive beyond 30 days. Patients with a leaking or ruptured AAA may present in many ways depending on the site of rupture. Intraperitoneal leaks (20%) are almost always associated with immediate death following exsanguination into the abdominal cavity. Retroperitoneal rupture is often contained and can give rise to the following symptoms with *or without* signs of haemodynamic compromise:

- Pulsating sensation (and/or mass) in the abdomen
- Abdominal, groin or back pain
- Vague-generalised symptoms

Clinically significant aneurysms can be missed on physical examination, especially if the patient is shocked. Detection largely depends on the experience of the examiner, the size of the aneurysm and the size of the patient. The key finding is a tender pulsatile mass in the upper abdomen above the umbilicus. Femoral pulses in one or both groins may be diminished or absent in the shocked patient.

Diagnostic pitfalls

1 When asked to see a patient with a suspected AAA this is a surgical emergency. Patients can deteriorate rapidly therefore early senior review is essential.

Table 18.1 Annual risk of AAA rupture.

AAA diameter (cm)	Rupture risk (% per year)
<4	0
4–5	0.5–5
5–6	3–15
6–7	10–20
7–8	20–40
>8	30–50

2 Symptoms of AAA may include groin pain, syncope, paralysis or flank mass. Be sure to exclude AAA with appropriate imaging before assigning the symptoms to other common conditions (renal calculi, diverticulitis, incarcerated hernia or lumbar spine disease).

Investigations

Laboratory studies

Patients with a ruptured AAA may present in varying degrees of circulatory shock through massive blood loss. At the time of blood sample draw insert two large bore cannula (12–16G) into both antecubital fossa. Blood should be sent for:

1 Full blood count – (poor) indicator of transfusion requirements

2 Urea and electrolytes – may demonstrate associated renal failure

3 Cross-match eight units of packed red blood cells (+/− blood products if patient actively bleeding)

4 Arterial blood gas analysis – best bedside indicator of tissue hypoperfusion and shock

Cardiac function

Formal cardiac function evaluation or echocardiology is not practical in the emergency setting and therefore an ECG is likely to be the only information available. Identification of cardiac ischaemia, atrial fibrillation and other conduction abnormalities are useful in evaluating overall operative risk.

Imaging

Radiographic studies are required to assess the site, size and degree of rupture in addition to determining pre-existing comorbidities which must be taken into account when planning high-risk surgical intervention.

1 Chest X-ray:
- Preliminary assessment of the status of the heart and lungs and any thoracic Aneurysmal disease.
- Severe concurrent pulmonary or cardiac disease may preclude emergency repair if anaesthetic, i.e. intraoperative risk of death is too high.

2 Abdominal ultrasonography:
- Operator dependent.
- Can determine aneurysm presence, size and extent in the emergency department at the bedside.
- The UK is currently embarking on a national ultrasound screening programme for men aged 65–79 years to identify AAA disease. Large meta-analyses have shown a significant decrease in mortality from men where AAA was detected early.

3 CT scanning:
- In patients without signs of haemodynamic compromise contrast-enhanced multidetector CT scanning of the abdomen and pelvis, with multi-planar reconstruction and CT angiography is the test of choice in order to answer the question: Is this aneurysm suitable for endovascular repair?
- Able to determine the anatomic relationships required for endovascular planning, i.e. location of the renal arteries, length of the aortic neck, condition of the iliac arteries.
- Can clearly define the anatomy of the aneurysm and other intra-abdominal pathologies and any important anatomic variants, e.g. horseshoe kidney, retro-aortic renal vein.

Patients in severe haemorrhagic shock are too unstable to be taken to the CT scanner. Following confirmation of an AAA clinically or by ultrasound the patient should be taken to the operating theatre for emergency open repair.

Preoperative considerations

Obtain a careful history from the patient and any next of kin available in addition to the standard investigations detailed above. From the information derived from these basic assessments, perioperative risk and life expectancy after the proposed procedure can be estimated. A senior vascular surgeon and anaesthetist must give careful consideration to the patient's current quality of life to justify the high-risk operative intervention. Emergency surgical repair of AAA has a 50% 30-day mortality rate and patients suffering from severe COPD, cardiac or renal disease are at a much greater risk.

Resuscitation of the shocked patient with an AAA rupture should adhere to the principles of permissive hypotensive. To reduce the risk of displacing the forming clot around the site of rupture, blood pressure should be maintained around 80–90 mm Hg or a palpable radial pulse. Fluid boluses administered in 250 mL boluses are required to prevent large spikes in blood pressure.

Operative management

Repair of elective and emergency AAAs has altered dramatically over the past 10 years. Techniques available for repair now include:

a Conventional (open) repair
b Laparoscopic (assisted) repair
c Endovascular aneurysm repair (EVAR – minimally invasive endoluminal technique)

EVAR is not suitable for all patients and largely depends on (a) the morphology and position of the aneurysm and (b) the institutional experience. Potential advantages of EVAR over open repair include reduced time under general anaesthesia, elimination of the need for aortic cross clamping, reduction of the pain and trauma associated with major abdominal surgery, reduced length of stay in the hospital and intensive care unit, and lowered blood loss. However, EVAR in the context of leaking AAA remains controversial. Mobilisation of the angiography team out of hours and a lack of theatre instruments/stocks required for open conversion is a limiting factor for the use of EVAR in the emergency setting. Most ruptured AAAs are managed by the conventional open approach. As expertise in EVAR develops and specialist vascular units able to provide 24/7 cover for vascular emergencies develop, open repair of ruptured AAA may be replaced by this technique.

Once a decision to operate has been taken and consent obtained the following must be in place prior to anaesthetic induction.

Preoperative checklist

✓ Large bore intravenous access
✓ Foley urethral catheter
✓ Cross-match eight units of packed red cells and four units of plasma
✓ Warmed intravenous fluids
✓ Two large bore Yankauer suckers
✓ Warming blanket to prevent hypothermia and limit coagulopathy
✓ Surgical prep of patient from nipples to mid thigh
✓ Deep vein thrombosis prophylactic compression devices
✓ Intraoperative cell saver use primed and ready for use if available
✓ Invasive arterial blood monitoring if clinical situation permits – do not delay surgery for insertion of monitoring lines

Operative approach (open)

Following induction of anaesthesia and paralysis of the abdominal wall musculature a precipitous drop in blood pressure may occur. For this reason the timing of the initial surgical incision must occur almost immediately after administration of the anaesthetic agents. Ensure that the intravenous prophylactic antibiotics are given prior to graft insertion.

Access

• Midline incision extending from xiphisternum to pubis.

• Lift omentum and large bowel superiorly and move the small bowel with its mesentery to the right.

• Confirm the presence of the aneurysm and note the site of haematoma (usually to left of midline as this is the leak usually occurs on the left side of the aneurysm sac).

• Dissect duodenum off sac.

• Open the posterior peritoneum and identify the neck of aneurysm beneath overlying left renal vein.

• Carefully develop a plane either side to accommodate a straight vascular clamp and apply immediately to gain proximal control in shocked patients, or defer clamping to identify the pulsatile iliac vessels (see below) as a prelude to distal control.

• Haematoma that projects anteriorly rather than laterally is a warning sign of anterior rupture, with the possibility of free uncontrolled bleeding during neck dissection.

• Such cases are best managed with application of a vascular clamp – unratcheted – around the supracoeliac aorta (via the lesser sac and the diaphragmatic crus) prior to neck dissection, ready to ratchet down should torrential bleeding be encountered.

• Distal control: access the right common iliac vessel by palpating the pulsatile vessel inferior and to the right of the aneurysm's inferior limit and dividing peritoneum and overlying retroperitoneal tissue, being wary for presence of ureter distally (crossing) bifurcation. Access the left common iliac vessel by palpating the pulsatile vessel inferior and to the left of the aneurysm's inferior limit. The mesentery of the sigmoid colon is draped across the distal common iliac artery (CIA) and its bifurcation – control distally can alternately be achieved by tracing the EIA proximally, mobilising the sigmoid off the lateral left pelvis by dividing peritoneal attachments.

Inspection

• Assess the aortic bifurcation and the iliac arteries – straight grafts can be used in 60–70% of patients as a minor degree of ectasia of the iliac vessels can be accepted.

• Assess the inferior mesenteric artery – in most cases is occluded from thrombus within the aneurysm sac. If it is patent, check the effect of temporary clamping on the distal bowel circulation.

Procedure

1 Once proximal and distal control of the aneurysm is achieved with vascular clamps to above the neck and across the iliac arteries you are ready to proceed to repair.

2 Apply sufficient clamp pressure to occlude blood flow and no more.

3 Open aneurysm sac longitudinally and remove thrombus and any atheromatous material (always send sample for microbiology and histology).

4 Back bleeding from lumbar vessels can be controlled with sutures from within the aneurysm sac.

5 An intraluminal foley catheter placed in the proximal aortic neck can be used to provide control if external (clamp) control is not possible.

6 Using a PTFE or Dacron graft with 3/0 monofilament nonabsorbable continuous sutures to construct an end-to-end anastomosis to the proximal aorta (this is done within the sac using the inlay technique).

7 Apply a soft clamp to graft in order to test the anastomosis.

8 Place additional sutures as required for haemostasis.

9 The graft should be cut to length, prior to commencement of the distal in-lay anastomosis using a 3-0 prolene suture.

10 Flush the graft with heparinised saline prior to completing the distal anastomosis to eliminate any blood clots and evaluate back bleeding from the recipient vessels – pass embolectomy catheters if this is not the case to remove distal debris.

11 Before releasing clamps on the iliac arteries inform the anaesthetist and re-perfuse one leg at a time to reduce the risk of circulatory collapse.

12 Once haemostasis is obtained at all anastomotic sites fold the anterior aneurysm sac over the graft and fix it in place to minimise the risk of graft infection and enteric fistula formation.

13 Repair and approximate the posterior peritoneum over the aneurysm sac.

14 Inspect colon prior to closure for viability and palpate femoral arteries.

15 Close abdominal walls in layers with clips to skin.

16 Before the patient leaves the operating room determine lower extremity circulation.

Complications

• Death (50%)

• Lower respiratory tract infection (5%)

• Myocardial infarction (2.5%)

• Graft infection (<1%)

• Colon ischaemia (15–20%)

• Renal failure – related to pre-morbid function and site of aneurysm

• Incisional hernia (10–20%)

• Amputation from major arterial occlusion

• Trash foot – multiple distal embolisation

• Impotence in males – erectile dysfunction and retrograde ejaculation (>30%)

• Late graft enteric fistula

Operative technique (EVAR)

Patients with an anatomically suitable AAA and stable haemodynamic parameters may be amendable to EVAR in an appropriately staffed and equipped vascular unit. Aneurysm morphology and availability of a suitable graft in conjunction with the patient's condition will ultimately determine if EVAR can be undertaken. In patients unfit for open surgery it is a viable alternative although procedural failure requiring open conversion to complete the repair is likely to be associated with poor outcomes.

Procedure

The preoperative work-up is the same for conventional open AAA repair:

1 Gain access to both femoral arteries through transverse incisions in the groins.

2 Develop planes around the arteries for proximal and distal control with clamps and elastic slings.

3 Once vessel access has been gained via the Seldinger technique, an infrarenal aortic balloon can be placed over a guidewire to control the aorta proximally if the patient's condition becomes unstable.

4 Using a series of catheters and guidewires a stent-graft prosthesis is placed at the site of the aneurysm under X-ray guidance.

5 A uni-iliac prosthesis (with femoro–femoro crossover graft to facilitate filling of the contralateral limb) is a more practical option than bifurcated modular prosthesis as less stent-graft segments and range of stent-graft sizes are required than with modular bifurcated designs. Exclusion of the opposite CIA with an occluder device is required to prevent iliac backflow and re-filling the aneurysm sac (endoleak).

6 The concentrically folded stent is opened proximal to the neck of aneurysm to ensure that the prosthesis is anchored using various fixing mechanisms to healthy vessel wall.

7 Extension grafts can be utilised for aneurysms extending distal to the aortic bifurcation.

8 A check angiogram is performed to demonstrate aneurysm exclusion (Figure 18.2).

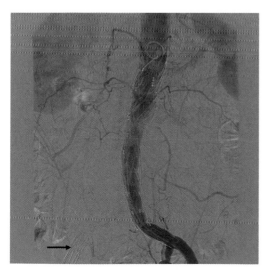

Figure 18.2 Completion angiogram of uni-iliac EVAR, with landing zone in left common iliac artery. Note occluder device to prevent backflow in right common iliac artery (arrow). Distal perfusion of right leg via left to right femoro–femoro crossover graft (not shown).

Complications

The minimally invasive technique leads to fewer complications but most of those associated with open repair still apply albeit at a lower frequency. Complications related specifically to EVAR include:

- Endoleaks – blood continues to flow through the aneurysm as a result of incomplete graft seal (proximally or distally) – type Ia and Ib; backfilling from patent lumbar or inferior mesenteric vessels – type II; modular disconnection – type III; fabric porosity – type IV; continued sac expansion despite no demonstrable endoleak – type V
- Groin wound infection
- Infection of prosthesis
- Displacement of prosthesis

Common pitfalls of emergency EVAR

- Small incisions and little visible blood can allow operating teams to underestimate the severity of the clinical situation.
- Aggressive blood replacement and clotting factor therapy may still be required.
- Angiographic suites are often a long way from the relative 'safety' of the operating theatre department – additional systems must be in place to ensure adequate staffing and availability of essential equipment.

Summary

- Ruptured AAA is a surgical emergency associated with high mortality rates.
- Involve seniors from the outset.
- Rapid diagnosis with ultrasound +/– CT scanning is essential.
- Large bore venous access must be obtained early.
- Cross-match large volumes of blood and clotting products early.
- Open surgical repair remains the mainstay of emergency surgical repair.
- EVAR may be a suitable alternative in non-shocked patients with leaking AAA.

Further reading

http://www.vascularsociety.org.uk/library/aaa-screening.html
http://www.nice.org.uk/nicemedia/pdf/TA167Guidance.pdf
http://www.vascularweb.org/professionals/Podcasts/Abdominal
_Aortic_Aneurysm.html
http://emedicine.medscape.com/article/463354-overview

19

Acute Limb Ischaemia

Matthew Button[1] & Nigel Tai[1,2]

[1]Defence Medical Services, Trauma Clinical Academic Unit, Royal London Hospital, Whitechapel, London, UK
[2]Academic Department of Military Surgery and Trauma, Royal Centre for Defence Medicine, Birmingham, UK

Introduction

An acutely ischaemic limb is one in which symptoms have been present for less than 2 weeks. Beyond this time period, the problem is said to be chronic. This is an arbitrary classification and in reality is of limited clinical relevance. The important clinical decisions to be made are:

• whether the limb is viable or not and
• whether emergency intervention is required

Clinical presentation

Acute presentations of ischaemic limbs (usually legs) have declined over recent years. Childhood sufferers of rheumatic fever have died and there have been improvements in the treatment of atrial fibrillation (the principal causes of embolic ischaemia). Acute deterioration of a chronically ischaemic leg, due to thrombosis within a stenosed arterial segment, is now more common than embolism as a cause of ischaemia.

Other causes of acute ischaemia include graft and aneurysm thrombosis and traumatic arterial damage (Table 19.1).

Clinical assessment

The first and most important decisions to be made are:

1 Is ischaemia responsible for the patient's symptoms?
2 Is the limb viable, threatened or unsalvageable?
3 Is emergency intervention necessary to save the limb?
4 If so, what is the cause of the ischaemic event and what is the safest/quickest treatment option?
5 Is the patient fit enough to withstand planned intervention?

Emergency Surgery, 1st edition. Edited by Adam Brooks, Peter F. Mahoney, Bryan A. Cotton and Nigel Tai. © 2010 Blackwell Publishing.

These decisions can usually be made based entirely on clinical history and examination findings.

The classical signs of acute ischaemia are pallor, coldness, reduced or altered sensation (and later muscle paralysis) and a loss of palpable pulses (hence the easily remembered six P's: Pain, Pallor, Perishing cold, Paraesthesia, Paralysis and Pulselessness). These are useful symptoms and signs in the initial diagnosis of acute ischaemia and will invariably differentiate ischaemic pain from the myriad differential diagnoses for limb pain. They are of less help in deciding viability and need for intervention. Patients with acute limb ischaemia (ALI) present with severe constant disabling pain in the affected tissues. Once tissues have infarcted pain settles. Patients presenting late may complain of pain at the junction between viable and dead tissue. Other symptoms are usually insignificant in comparison to pain.

The most important signs in regard to deciding about viability and the need for intervention are capillary return/skin discolouration, muscle function, nerve function and muscle tenderness (Table 19.2).

Patients with a threatened limb will need urgent intervention if the limb is to be saved. The choice of definitive treatment depends on the likely aetiology. Embolism into a limb with relatively normal arteries usually causes profound ischaemia. Arterial flow must be re-established as rapidly as possible and for this reason surgical embolectomy is preferable to thrombolysis.

The differentiation between embolism and thrombosis can also usually be made clinically. Acute ischaemia due to embolism occurs suddenly with the onset of symptoms occurring over a period of minutes. The patient will give no history of preceding non-critical ischaemia. Contralateral pulses will usually be normal unless multiple emboli have affected both legs or a large embolus lodges at the aortic bifurcation. If palpable the femoral vessels will be soft. These findings contrast with acute thrombosis of atherosclerotic vessels where a pre-existing history of claudication, bilateral disease and hard calcified vessels are the normal findings. The degree of ischaemia is often less in this situation as preceding chronic ischaemia will have stimulated the development of a collateral arterial supply.

Table 19.1 Causes of an acutely ischaemic limb.

Classification	Cause
Thrombotic	Acute thrombosis within atherosclerotic stenosis
	Bypass graft thrombosis
	Thrombosis of popliteal aneurysm
	Luminal thrombosis secondary to thrombophilia
Embolic	From the heart
	Atrial fibrillation 80%
	Mural thrombus 20%
	Valve vegetations
	From proximal aneurysm (luminal thrombus)
	From proximal atherosclerotic plaque
Trauma	Penetrating trauma (arterial transection)
	Blunt trauma (intimal flap)
	Iatrogenic (intimal flap caused by arterial cannulation)
Outside compression	Compartment syndrome
	Popliteal entrapment
Wall Abnormalities	Aortic dissection
	Intra-arterial drug administration

Investigation

The purposes of patient investigation are threefold:
1 To ascertain/confirm the cause of ischaemia.
2 To plan treatment based upon the cause and level of arterial occlusion.
3 To assess patient fitness for surgery/intervention.
Clinical examination should have confirmed presence or absence of atrial fibrillation (AF). An electrocardiogram will confirm this diagnosis. It should be remembered that paradoxical (intermittent) AF is more likely to cause embolisation than persistent fibrillation. Haematological investigation for a thrombophilia is usually not warranted in the acute

setting. There are a number of options available for vascular imaging. The choice of investigation depends upon local expertise as well as patient variables. As always the need for investigation should be questioned. Where diagnosis can be made and treatment planned from clinical findings alone, delay should not be introduced by further investigation. Arterial imaging options include duplex ultrasound, computed tomography (CT) or magnetic resonance (MR) angiography and intra-arterial formal digital subtraction angiography (Table 19.3). Formal digital subtraction angiography is generally reserved for those patients in whom an endovascular treatment is being considered.

Management

The aims of preoperative treatment are to relieve pain, to optimise patient fitness for surgery/intervention and to improve tissue oxygenation in the affected limb prior to definitive intervention.

A checklist of requirements should include:

Analgesia	☐
Intravenous heparin infusion	☐
Intravenous fluids	☐
Facemask oxygen	☐
Nil by mouth	☐
Full blood count	☐
Baseline clotting study	☐
Group and save	☐
Biochemical renal function	☐
Urinary catheter	☐

If, after senior review, surgery is planned then arrangement for on table angiography should be made with both the radiology department and operating theatres.

Table 19.2 Clinical markers of limb viability.

	Capillary return	Sensation	Motor function	Muscle tenderness
Viable tissue (incomplete ischaemia)	Intact	Normal/minimal sensory loss	Normal muscle function	Absent
Threatened tissue (complete ischaemia)	None/markedly delayed	Marked deficiency	Normal or early partial muscle paralysis	Presence suggests emergency revascularisation required to salvage limb
Irreversibly ischaemic tissue	Absent capillary return with fixed skin staining caused by capillary rupture. This forms an irregular pattern over affected skin and will not blanche on pressure (fixed mottling)	Complete sensory loss	Complete paralysis, usually with tensely swollen, exquisitely tender muscle compartments	Present initially, pain and tenderness settle once nerve function ceases

Table 19.3 Special investigations.

	Duplex ultrasound	CT angiography	MR angiography	Intra-arterial digital subtraction angiography (IADSA)
Invasiveness?	Non-invasive	Intravenous contrast required	IV contrast preferable, contraindicated with ferrous implants or metallic foreign bodies and claustrophobia	Arterial puncture carries significant risks but allows therapeutic intervention
Availability	Lengthy investigation by experienced vascular technologist. Not available in all centres and almost never available 'out of hours'	Widely available. Scan duration significantly reduced with recent improvements in scanner technology	Available in most centres but rarely at night and scan duration longer than CT	24 hours service available for emergencies in most large centres
Image quality	Wholly dependent on technologist skill. Increasingly accepted as single modality imaging for operative planning in centres with experienced department	Software allowing vascular reconstructions has extended the role of CT. Good quality images can now be achieved including below the knee	Similar to CT. Choice between these two largely depends on local preferences and any confounding patient factors (renal impairment, metal implants etc.)	Felt by most to be gold standard imaging modality, imaging artefacts around joint replacements can impair views

CT, computed tomography; MR, magnetic resonance.

Patient-specific management

The management options for a patient with an acutely is-chaemic limb are straightforward. There are four broad treatment options: surgical intervention, thrombolysis, amputation or palliation (Figure 19.1).

Acute arterial embolism

An embolus is any solid, liquid or gaseous substance which has travelled within the circulation to lodge at a distant site. In the context of the ischaemic limb, this involves thrombus which has formed in the heart or proximal arterial tree travelling to and occluding one or more large limb arteries. The legs are involved in the majority of patients and the embolus most commonly lodges at the femoral bifurcation. Embolism into an undiseased artery is becoming less common. Most originate in the heart (80% of these being secondary to atrial fibrillation). The other possible sites of origin include thrombus formed within a more proximal arterial aneurysm and (very rarely) thrombus forming in the venous circulation which travels through a right-to-left heart shunt thus passing into the arterial tree. For most patients surgical embolectomy is uncomplicated and is rapidly arranged and performed.

Acute-on-chronic ischaemia

• ALI secondary to a sudden deterioration in flow through an atherosclerotic vessel is now more common than embolic disease in Western populations.
• Chronic ischaemic symptoms often deteriorate in a step-wise manner as atherosclerotic plaques rupture and then expand as bleeding occurs into the plaque. When plaque rupture occurs, luminal blood is exposed to thrombogenic constituents of the plaque core. Blood flow, already reduced by the atherosclerotic process, is prevented.
• Depending upon level of disease and the extent to which a collateral supply to the limb has developed, symptoms may vary from exertional claudication pain to acute limb-threatening ischaemia. The presence of a collateral blood supply usually means that restoration of arterial flow is not as emergent in this situation.
• Intravenous heparin, intravenous fluid resuscitation, analgesia and oxygen should all be administered. If ischaemia is incomplete, definitive treatment can be delayed until arterial imaging has been obtained. In this situation formal arterial angiography not only provides accurate anatomical diagnosis of the disease but also allows treatment by thrombolysis (Figure 19.2).
• Thrombolysis involves the delivery of tissue plasminogen activator directly in to the thrombosed vessel, through a guide-wire directed catheter inserted via a femoral artery sheath by an interventional radiologist. The process usually takes 24–48 hours, depending on the clot burden, and requires several check angiograms to monitor progress and allow re-positioning of the catheter tip as clot is dissolved. Haemorrhagic complications of thrombolysis include stroke, bleeding from the access sheath site and retroperitoneal or gastrointestinal haemorrhage. Thirty-day mortality is around 10%; the technique has declined in popularity and is now generally reserved for clearance of fresh thrombus from occluded synthetic grafts and thrombosed popliteal aneurysms.

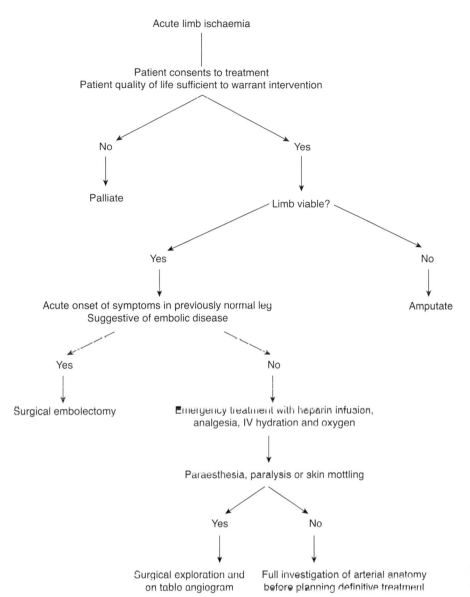

Figure 19.1 Flow diagram for treatment of ALI.

Graft thrombosis

Ischaemia secondary to graft thrombosis is easily diagnosed even when no history is available provided that this diagnosis is remembered and a careful examination is made. The reason for failure of the bypass graft may be more complex. Graft thrombolysis is often possible if the patient has presented promptly. If successful this will reconstitute sufficient flow to allow full investigation of graft anatomy in order to identify the cause of the thrombosis.

Prevention of recurrent thrombosis post-thrombolysis

In the normal arterial system thrombosis is prevented by the functioning endothelium, by the maintenance of brisk laminar blood flow and by a series of anticoagulant factors acting to control the coagulation cascade (Virchow's triad). Throm-

bolysis of either graft or diseased artery alone provides inadequate treatment unless the underlying cause of thrombus formation is identified and steps are taken to prevent recurrence. In atheromatous vessels blood flow is impaired beyond the stenosed segment and endothelial function is reduced over the atheromatous plaque. Treatment is targeted at improving flow or anticoagulation.

Inadequate graft flow rates are due either to anastomotic stenosis or ongoing arterial disease causing deterioration in either inflow to or run off from the graft. Sufficient improvement in flow can be achieved by angioplasty in some cases. Where graft thrombosis is secondary to anastomotic stenosis urgent intervention is needed after thrombolysis. Either intra-arterial balloon or open patch angioplasty of the anastomotic stenosis is essential if recurrent thrombosis is to be prevented.

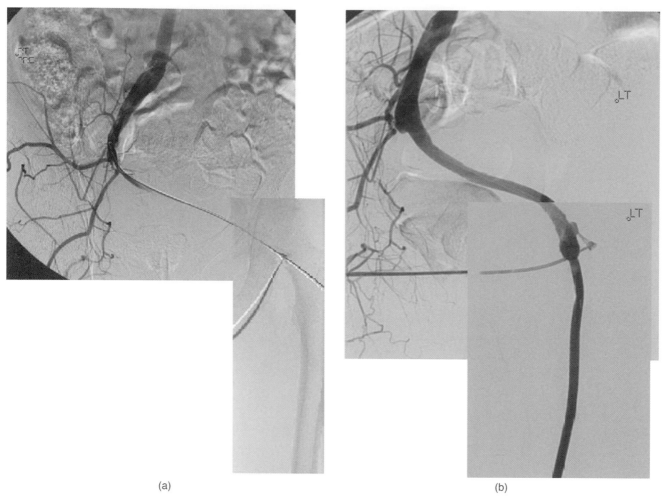

(a)   (b)

Figure 19.2 (a and b) Pre- and post-thrombolysis angiograms of a thrombosed ilio-femoral crossover graft. The patient presented with an acutely ischaemic left leg.

Thrombosis of a popliteal aneurysm

Popliteal aneurysms can present with ALI secondary to either distal embolisation or thrombosis of the aneurysm. Management depends upon the state of crural run off vessels. If one or more vessels remain patent and there is autologous vein available then aneurysm exclusion and distal bypass is the best option. If not and the limb is threatened then thrombolysis may clear the distal arteries sufficiently to allow later urgent planned bypass surgery.

Amputation

Once an acutely ischaemic limb can be seen to be non-viable an amputation should be considered. In the chronic situation indications for amputation include a limb that is a threat to survival of the patient, intractable pain and a useless limb which is inconvenient to the patient. These are less applicable to ALI, here the non-viable, acutely ischaemic limb will always be a threat to patient survival if infarcted

muscle is present. Acidosis and hyperkalaemia secondary to cell death threaten myocardial and renal function. In these cases an amputation should almost always be carried out as an emergency.

Palliation

The majority of patients presenting with ALI are elderly. Amongst this population are a few patients whose severe co-morbidities and/or poor quality of life make treatment to prolong life futile. For this group treatment is aimed at making the end of life as comfortable as possible. This is usually not difficult, principally involving analgesia and avoiding further uncomfortable investigation, intervention or excessive monitoring of observations. The difficulty comes in identifying which patients fall into this category. For patients who fall on the boundary of fitness/life quality, open discussion with the patient, next of kin and family along with further assessment by anaesthetic colleagues will all help to make the decision easier.

Table 19.4 Complications of ALI surgery.

Death
Limb loss
Compartment syndrome
Renal failure
Multi-organ failure
Wound infection
Operative damage to local structures
    Nerve injury
    Lymph leaks

Complications of angiography and thrombolysis
    Bleeding (especially dangerous when retroperitoneal)
    Stroke
    False aneurysm formation
Ischaemic nerve damage
Wound infections
Lymphatic leaks
Nerve injury

ALI, acute limb ischaemia.

Peri-, postoperative and critical care management

Re-perfusion of an ischaemic limb results in the return of acidotic blood with a high potassium concentration to the circulation. This increases the risk of cardiac dysrhythmias if the anaesthetist is not aware or is unable to correct these disturbances.

If a large mass of ischaemic muscle is reperfused, myoglobinaemia will result and renal failure may follow. Adequate intravenous hydration reduces this risk. Urine output must be monitored hourly and renal function checked at least every 24 hours, more frequent measurement of serum potassium may be necessary if levels rise. The indications for renal replacement therapy are a significant and uncontrollable rise in potassium, uncontrollable acidosis and fluid overload. Early advice should be sought from the renal team in any of these circumstances.

Significant limb ischaemia will also trigger a systemic inflammatory response syndrome via neutrophil activation and other inflammatory pathways. There is a potential for this to progress to acute lung injury or multi-organ dysfunction. Treatment is largely supportive with prompt transfer to high dependency/intensive care as required.

As limb reperfusion continues and limb swelling will follow. This is due to both swelling of damaged but viable cells and to rupture of dead cells along with the release of osmotic substances. Acute limb swelling is limited by fascial compartments. This limitation to acute swelling causes compartment pressures to rise with the potential to bring about recurrent limb ischaemia. Where there is any suggestion of muscle compartment swelling/raised compartment pressures, fasciotomies must be completed as quickly as possible. The hallmarks of the syndrome include progressive and severe pain that is worse on passive stretching of the compartmental musculature in the context of a tense, firmly swollen limb. Loss of distal pulses is a late feature. Clinical signs may be obscured in the sedated and ventilated patient. Direct measurement of intra-compartmental pressures may strengthen the diagnosis although the decision to proceed to fasciotomy should not be contingent on the availability of this diagnostic tool. When the duration and severity of acute ischaemia makes post revascularisation compartment syndrome a likelihood, prophylactic fasciotomy should be performed at the time of initial surgery.

Complications

The list of potential complications of ALI is extensive (Table 19.4).

Summary

ALI is most commonly seen in elderly patients. It is a surgical emergency and these patients must be assessed and treated without delay. Senior vascular and radiological input is mandatory if the potential for poor outcome is to be minimised.

4 Soft Tissue Infection

20

Superficial Sepsis, Cutaneous Abscess and Necrotising Fasciitis

Conor D. Marron

The Royal Victoria Hospital, Belfast Trust, Belfast, UK

Introduction

Superficial skin infections, cutaneous abscesses and anorectal abscesses form a large portion of the emergency workload of surgical departments, and indeed many emergency departments. The variety of conditions ranges from minor skin infections, to well localised cutaneous abscesses, to necrotising fasciitis associated with a high morbidity and mortality and severe sepsis. This chapter will discuss the relevant aetiology of a range of conditions affecting skin and subcutaneous tissues, and will aid in the differential diagnosis and discuss differences in surgical management of each condition.

Skin and soft tissue infections are commonplace in many aspects of medical practice and can vary from minor infections and localised abscesses, to systemic conditions that can be life-threatening and require emergency surgical treatment. The major groups of emergency soft tissue infections, and the knowledge and skills required to deal with these can be seen in Table 20.1.

General principles

With all conditions of the skin and subcutaneous tissues, there are several aspects that share many common features that are important to elucidate and understand. Specific variations for each individual condition will be covered later in the chapter.

Bacteriology

The microbiological flora of superficial sepsis and necrotising fasciitis is varied and specific treatment will depend largely on culture-guided sensitivities on an individual case basis. However, there are several groups of organisms that are more common in all skin and soft tissue infections, and this

allows us to use 'best-guess' antibiotic regimens for the initial treatment of skin infections. The microbes that cause surgical infections can be classified into three groups:
- Conventional pathogens, i.e. those which may cause infections in previously healthy individuals.
- Conditional pathogens, i.e. those which cause infections in those with pre-disposing factors.
- Opportunistic pathogens, i.e. those of low threat and virulence but may cause infection in those who are immunocompromised.

In skin and soft tissue infections, it is predominantly bacteria that are of the greatest significance. Bacteria are classified by their shape – bacilli (rods) or cocci (spheres); by their response to gram staining – Gram-positive (pink), or Gram-negative (blue); and their growth requirements – aerobic, anaerobic, or facultative anaerobic.

Of the groups of most importance in skin infections it is the Gram-positive cocci, Staphylococci and Streptococci that predominate.

Staphylococci are arranged into grape-like clusters and may be divided into coagulase-positive and coagulase-negative groups. The coagulase-positive *Staphylococcus aureus* is the predominant organism present in skin and soft tissue infections. Coagulase-negative organisms such as *Staphylococcus epidermidis* are of much lower virulence and rarely cause infections in healthy people. These organisms are skin commensals, but may lead to infections in patients who are otherwise compromised.

Streptococci occur in chains and are further sub-classified depending on their ability to lyse red blood cells that are within blood containing culture media. Furthermore, polysaccharide chains present on the surface of the organisms allow them to be categorised into Lancefield groups. Of the species of Streptococci, it is the *beta-haemolytic group* that are predominantly responsible for severe infections and sepsis. These colonies completely lyse the blood cells on a culture plate resulting in a clear, colourless and sharply defined zone. Within the Lancefield groups, it is the group A organisms, such as *Streptococcus pyogenes*, that cause most problems in relation to skin and soft tissue infections. Other infections related to wounds can arise from Lancefield group

Emergency Surgery, 1st edition. Edited by Adam Brooks, Peter F. Mahoney, Bryan A. Cotton and Nigel Tai. © 2010 Blackwell Publishing.

Table 20.1 Intercollegiate Surgical Curriculum Project (ISCP) syllabus requirements for early years of surgical training.

	Knowledge	Clinical skills	Technical skills
Level 1 Trainee			
Superficial abscess	Aetiology Natural history Bacteriology	History and examination	Abscess drainage
Infected sebaceous cyst/carbuncle	Natural history	History and examination	Abscess drainage
	Bacteriology	Medical management of diabetes perioperatively	Benign skin or subcutaneous lesion excision biopsy
	Associated medical conditions		
Cellulitis	Aetiology Associated medical conditions Immunocompromised patients Bacteriology Antibiotic therapy	History and examination IV therapy	
Infected ingrown toenail	Aetiology	History and examination	Ingrown toenail avulsion/wedge resection /phenolisation
	Bacteriology Atherosclerosis Diabetes		
Level 2 Trainee			
Anorectal abscess and fistula	The origin of cryptoglandular fistula and abscess	Differentiate cryptoglandular abscess and fistula from other causes	Abscess drainage through perineal incision
	Classification of anorectal cryptoglandular abscess based on anatomical spaces	Assessment of abscess/fistula and understanding of Goodsall's rule and digital rectal examination	
	The natural history of surgically treated anal abscess	Management of anorectal abscess	
	Parks classification of anal fistula	Assess rectovaginal fistula	
	Operative strategy for anal fistulas		
	Complications resulting from abscess/fistula surgery		
Gas gangrene and necrotising fasciitis	Natural history of condition	History and examination	Fourniers gangrene /necrotising faciitis debridement
	Vulnerable individuals	Recognition of the early warning signs	
	Physiology of associated conditions	Radical excisional surgery	
	Bacteriology and toxins involved		
	Mechanisms of septic shock		
	Massive blood transfusion complication		
	Knowledge of appropriate antibiotic therapy		
	Knowledge of necrotising fasciitis		

Table 20.2 Risk factors for developing soft tissue infections and necrotising fasciitis.

Aetiological	Patient-related factors
Trauma	Diabetes mellitus
IV drug abuse	Drugs, e.g. steroids
Burns	Immunosuppression
Surgery	Malnutrition
	Age >60
	Chronic disease
	Renal failure
	Obesity
	Malignancy
	Peripheral vascular disease

D organisms such as *Strep. Faecalis*, which is from the enterococci family.

Other clinically important organisms in skin and soft tissue infections are the anaerobic Gram-positive rods, *Clostridium perfringens*, the Gram-negative bacilli, *Pseudomonas aeruginosa*, and the facultative anaerobes (coliforms) *Escherichia coli* and *Proteus*.

Associated medical conditions

Patients presenting with infections of the skin and subcutaneous tissues should be fully assessed in order to elicit an underlying cause for the infection. Often, a simple skin infection or abscess can be the presenting feature for conditions such as diabetes mellitus, and therefore it is important not to overlook the full history and assessment of the patient in order that their condition can be effectively treated, and that the risk of recurrence or further deterioration is reduced. Associated conditions and risk factors for developing infections of the skin, and necrotising fasciitis are divided

into aetiological factors, and patient-related factors, and are summarised in Table 20.2.

Clinical presentation

Frequently during history taking for areas of superficial sepsis, the area is offered for inspection by the patient, which gives the assessing clinician the opportunity to direct questioning in order to ascertain particular relevant details. Critical features that must be ascertained during history taking relate to:

- Chronicity
- Site of lesion
- Other lesions present
- Associated symptoms of redness, heat, pain, tenderness and loss of function
- Predisposing factors and past medical history (outlined in Table 20.2)
- Previous history of similar problems
- Systemic symptoms
- Anaesthetic history
- Time of last food/drink

The clinical features suggestive of an inflammatory process in the skin relate predominantly to the features of acute inflammation; rubor (redness), dolor (pain), calor (heat), tumour (swelling) and loss of function. The clinical features of the various conditions are highlighted in Table 20.3.

The examination of the affected area will depend largely on the symptoms described and whether any lump or swelling is present. Features of lumps that can help define the nature of the problem relate to the size, site, depth within the skin, character of the margin, consistency, fluctuance and temperature. The presence of fluctuance suggests

Table 20.3 Differentiating clinical features of superficial sepsis and necrotising fasciitis.

	Infected sebaceous cyst	Abscess	Cellulitis	Necrotising fasciitis
Symptoms	Pre-existing lump and presence of other similar lumps	New lump	Diffuse	Rapid onset
	Slow onset	Acute onset	Pre-existing trauma	Pain
	Pain	Pain	Pain	Fever/rigors
	Recurrent	Yellowish discharge	Fever	Systemic symptoms
			Systemic symptoms	Multi-organ failure
			Pain on movement	
Signs	Well localised	Well localised	Red	Rapidly progressing beyond marked boundaries
	Tender	Hot	Hot	Purple/black discolouration
	Other lumps	Tender	Swollen	Haemorrhagic bullae
	Firm lump	Fluctuant	Tender	Crepitus
	Punctum visible		No fluctuance	

the presence of fluid within the lesion, which with other features such as tenderness, erythema and heat, would suggest the presence of inflammation and abscess formation. Lesions that are contained within the skin are assessed by feeling for the superficial and deep attachment of the lump, and this helps determine the layer that the lesion has arisen from.

The features of an infected sebaceous cyst, compared with cutaneous abscesses, cellulitis and necrotising fasciitis may initially appear similar; however, subtle differences can allow these to be differentiated clinically from history and examination (Table 20.3).

Within affected areas, it is important to fully assess for evidence of localised collections of fluid/pus in order that these can be adequately treated. Failure to find residual collections could delay healing, or result in deterioration of the condition.

Antibiotic therapy

The antibiotic therapy for most superficial sepsis relates to the underlying condition and the microbiology as discussed above. When considering antibiotic therapy consideration should be given to:

- What are the likely organisms involved?
- Which antibiotic to use?
- Are a combination of antibiotics required?
- What route of administration will be used?
- What duration of therapy is required?
- What is the tissue penetration?
- What dose will be used?

The choice of antibiotic will largely be determined on 'best guess' from experience of the condition, and knowledge of the common microorganisms that give rise to the condition, and to which antibiotics these are commonly sensitive. Samples of the infected material should be sent whenever possible in order to gain accurate culture-guided sensitivities; however, frequently the problem will be treated and settled prior to the samples returning. Based on the previous discussions of the bacteriology, the commonest groups of bacteria giving rise to superficial sepsis are the Staphylococcus and Streptococcus families that are sensitive to flucloxacillin and penicillin respectively. Therefore, there may be a case for utilisation of a combination of antibiotics to achieve a synergistic effect.

The route of administration depends largely on the ability of the patient to absorb the antibiotic, the ability of the antibiotic to be absorbed in large enough dosages to reach therapeutic levels, and the severity of the infection and condition. It is widely accepted that use of intravenous antibiotics is appropriate for those patients with severe soft tissue sepsis, or signs of systemic upset, whilst more minor conditions may be treatable with oral antibiotics, providing that the drug is available in an oral preparation.

The duration of therapy and dose will depend on the patient's response to treatment, but a typical duration for superficial sepsis would be in the region of 5–7 days, in order to avoid problems with antibiotic resistance. The dosage of drugs may need to be altered in patients with renal impairment.

It is also important to consider the relative properties of the antibiotics when considering which to use, as several have good availability in skin and subcutaneous tissue, whilst others do not.

Langer's lines

Within the structure of the skin, the dermis has dense, tough bundles of collagen fibres that interlace and align to create lines of natural resting skin tension. These lines of resting skin tension are called Langer's lines, and are important when carrying out surgical procedures as incisions made parallel to Langer's lines generally heal better and produce less scarring. When treating any lesion by incision and drainage, we should try to ensure that the incisions correspond, as best as possible, to Langer's lines.

Incision and drainage of an abscess/infected collection

The process for effectively treating an infected collection remains the adequate drainage of the infected material in order to allow satisfactory resolution. The main principle is to maintain the wound open in order to allow free drainage and removal of all necrotic material, with healing by secondary intention. The procedure is performed in a sequence of steps that should be followed at all times:

1 *Indications* – ensure that the patient has a collection amenable to drainage and the diagnosis is correct. If the diagnosis is unclear, an attempt at percutaneous aspiration using a needle and syringe can guide you to the collection.

2 *Consent* – as with any procedure, consent should be obtained for the procedure and the patient advised of the indications, complications and alternatives to treatment. Consent should be fully documented in the patient records. This applies regardless of whether performing under local or general anaesthetic.

3 *Anaesthetic* – the choice of using local anaesthetic or general anaesthetic will depend on the local institution policies, the patient's condition, the location of the abscess, the degree of inflammation and the size of the abscess. Local anaesthetic works poorly in inflamed tissues as all local anaesthetics are weak bases. In order that they can effectively block the sodium channel they must diffuse across the cell membrane in their unionised form before becoming ionised in the cytoplasm. However, acidic environments, such as in inflamed tissue, favour the ionised form of the agent, and therefore the anaesthetic is unable to diffuse across the lipid bilayer of the neurones and consequently is far less effective. If local anaesthetic techniques are to be used, this should be via a regional or field block rather than direct infiltration of the abscess. Depending on the site, a general anaesthetic should be used in order to allow satisfactory removal of all necrotic tissue as this may be poorly tolerated in deeper seated abscesses or those in difficult positions such as the perineum. Furthermore, a general anaesthetic will allow adequate inspection and evaluation for potential underlying causes.

4 *Equipment* – the necessary equipment, including the dressing material required should be made available before starting the procedure, and as a minimum will include, a scalpel blade, forceps, artery forcep, curette, swab for microbiology, gauze swabs, saline, skin preparation solution and dressing material.

5 *Incision* – the incision should be made with consideration given to Langer's lines in order that resulting wounds heal as best possible. The incision should be made over the point of maximal fluctuance with an initial stab incision, which is then extended in the direction of Langer's lines. After release of the pus/fluid, the skin opening may then be enlarged by performing a cruciate incision, with small perpendicular incisions at the mid portion of the incision, with the 'corners' of skin then excised to produce a diamond shaped opening. In some situations a cruciate incision is less favourable as it may be deemed to have poorer cosmetic results, and in these settings an individual incision over the abscess, of sufficient size to allow free drainage, will be appropriate.

6 *Dressings* – Using wound dressings, such as fibrous sodium alginate dressings, the cavity edges should be maintained open in order to allow healing to take place from the base of the cavity. Care should be taken not to tightly 'pack' the cavity as this can exert pressure on the cavity wall and cause ischaemia of the surrounding tissues, thereby inhibiting healing. This will allow the wound to heal by secondary intention and to allow further drainage of infected debris, reducing the risk of recurrent abscesses.

7 *Aftercare* – The dressings should be changed regularly, with the interval varying on a case-by-case basis, in order to allow healing to take place, and allow regular inspection of the wound and general patient condition. Whilst there is significant evidence to support the incision and drainage for the treatment of abscesses, there exists little evidence beyond expert opinion to support the post-drainage care for the wound. Antibiotic therapy is rarely required after successful incision and drainage procedures in healthy patients, unless there is evidence of extensive cellulitis beyond the abscess limits, or in the presence of significant co-morbidities. Community acquired methicillin-resistant *S. aureus* (CA-MRSA) has become more prevalent and the focus of media attention. There are reported incidences of up to 74% in cutaneous abscesses in some communities, although there is no evidence to suggest that these require empirical treatment with antibiotics per se.

Cutaneous abscesses

The incidence of skin and soft tissue abscesses is thought to be high, although is not well reported with incidences varying from 2.5% at university clinics to 21% in intravenous drug users. There is no clear aetiology for the development of cutaneous abscesses; however, co-morbid conditions such as diabetes mellitus can pre-dispose the patient to having a lower threshold for development of an abscess. Infection of hair follicles, or trauma and invasion by foreign bodies can allow infection with *S. aureus*, which remains the most common organism resulting in abscess formation.

An abscess is a local collection of pus contained within a barrier of inflammatory reaction, referred to as a pyogenic membrane. Initial bacterial infection leads to cytokine production with a resulting acute inflammatory response and infiltration with neutrophils and polymorphs. Within the abscess cavity, local death of soft tissue results in the production of a solid area of infected dead tissue, along with the liquefaction of tissues and products of infection, which are predominantly neutrophils and polymorphs. Fibrosis then occurs leading to encapsulation of the abscess.

Within the skin and soft tissues, abscesses are common and these tend to 'point' to the nearest epithelial surface, which is predominantly the skin. Within the abscess cavity, local death of soft tissue results in the production of a solid area of infected dead tissue, along with the liquefaction of tissues and products of infection, which are predominantly neutrophils and polymorphs.

The bacteriology of simple cutaneous abscesses largely follows the pattern outlined earlier in the chapter, although perineal abscesses can have a different primary organism responsible due to the proximity of the gastrointestinal tract as will be discussed later.

The clinical assessment of an abscess include accurate evaluation of an underlying cause, and the clinical findings of a localised swelling and the presence of fluctuance on examination as outlined in Table 20.3.

The mainstay of treatment of cutaneous abscesses remains the adequate drainage of the infected and inflammatory material as previously described. Areas of controversy that exist with regards to the treatment of cutaneous abscesses relate to primary closure versus secondary intention, the choice of anaesthetic, routine assessment of microbiology of the abscess and perioperative antibiotic therapy.

Conflicting evidence on primary closure of abscesses evolves from some studies that have shown that there are no detrimental effects of treatment of abscesses using secondary intention versus curettage and antibiotics, and curettage alone in controlled trials. However, further randomised controlled trials found that primary closure led to a failure to heal in 35% of cases, along with a longer median number of days to closure for those primarily closed. Furthermore, there is an increased incidence of pain in those closed primarily. Currently there is a lack of high quality evidence to support primary closure of abscesses, particularly if performed under local anaesthetic.

The evidence suggests that routine culture does not change the management of the patient, or the outcome of the patient presenting with an abscess. Indeed, studies have also shown that most patients improve, even when the identified organism is resistant to the empirically prescribed antibiotics.

The empirical use of antibiotics again is an area of conflict; however, there is a paucity of well-constructed randomised controlled trials in this area. Research dating back to the 1970s fails to support the use of empirical 'best-guess' antibiotics with no difference in outcome from those treated with antibiotics versus placebo. Indeed, the recent emergence of CA-MRSA has led to increasing need for rationalisation of antibiotic prescribing, and even in those patients colonised with CA-MRSA in abscesses, there is no significant difference in the outcome of those treated with antibiotics versus placebo. The Cochrane Library has identified over 60 trials comparing antibiotic therapy for treatment of soft tissue infections including abscesses and has found no significant difference in outcomes. The current recommendations would therefore be to avoid antibiotic prescribing in the management of uncomplicated abscessed which have been adequately drained.

Infected sebaceous cyst and carbuncles

Sebaceous (pilar or epidermal) cysts are common lesions that consist of a stratified squamous epithelium-lined cavity filled with a keratinous debris, and not sebum as the name might suggest. The finding of keratinous debris is consistent with its derivation from a hair follicle. This debris is often 'toothpaste like' and foul smelling. These lesions are commonplace on the scalp, neck, trunk, scrotum and face, but can occur anywhere on the body. These are smooth and rounded and covered by normal epidermis in which a blocked duct (punctum) may be visible.

Trauma to sebaceous cysts can often go unnoticed and this can lead to some of the cyst contents extruding into the surrounding tissue leading to an intense foreign-body inflammatory response. This gives rise to the classical inflammatory symptoms and signs of redness, heat, pain and swelling. This is often described as being an 'infected' sebaceous cyst; however, this is rarely the case, and the liquefied material that may discharge, or be released is, in fact, sterile. Antibiotics are frequently prescribed for the treatment of 'infected' sebaceous cysts, but in reality serve little functional purpose as the condition is more inflammatory than infective; how-

ever, infection can occur as a secondary event in which case surgical drainage is usually required.

A furuncle is a staphylococcal abscess arising in the hair follicles within the dermis leading to the formation of an abscess, which rapidly enlarges and 'points' on the skin and spontaneously discharges pus. Carbuncles are also of staphylococcal origin and are larger than furuncles, being predominantly on the back of the neck due to the structure of the skin in this area being tightly interlaced with fibrous tissue bands. This structure gives rise to a 'honeycomb of abscesses', which often drain (inadequately) through multiple sinuses to the skin. Failure to promptly treat the staphylococcal infections can lead to skin loss, which will ultimately delay healing. Treatment with anti-staphylococcal antibiotics such as flucloxacillin can minimise the pus formation and hence avoid tissue necrosis. Carbuncles and furuncles are more common in diabetic patients, and may even bring this diagnosis to light.

The commonest organisms involved in infected skin lesions and collections are staphylococci, and predominantly *S. aureus*. Occasionally synergistic organisms can be present in the infection, and these are predominantly, although not exclusively, of the Streptococcus species and therefore occasionally a dual antibiotic therapy may be required. Treatment by antibiotics is usually, in the first instance, using flucloxacillin, with or without a penicillin. This obviously depends on patient sensitivities and allergy status.

The presence of infected skin lesions, and in particular carbuncles, should raise awareness of associated medical conditions that may render the patient at risk of developing infections. Carbuncles may be an initial presenting symptom of diabetes, and therefore patients presenting with a carbuncle should have a fasting blood sugar and investigations to exclude diabetes.

The clinical features of an infected sebaceous cyst can be difficult to differentiate from those of an abscess, but critically a history of a pre-existing lump, or presence of other lesions in keeping with sebaceous cysts should raise suspicion.

The treatment of infected sebaceous cysts frequently involves drainage of any infected material if there has been a failure to respond to conservative management, or if there is evidence of significant cellulitis. The drainage of the cyst will leave the cyst wall in place, and effort should be taken to try and destroy this by curetting. Patients with infected sebaceous cysts should be reviewed as they will frequently require further procedures to formally excise the cyst remnant at some stage in the future.

Cellulitis

Cellulitis is an infection of the dermis and subcutaneous tissues, characterised by erythema, pain and swelling of the affected portion. It has well demarcated borders, which often advance as the infection worsens. The commonest cause of cellulitis is trauma, including surgical incisions, although ulceration, tinea infections and co-morbid disease such as venous insufficiency, peripheral vascular disease, or diabetes mellitus, can also lead to cellulitis. In otherwise healthy adults, the isolation of the underlying aetiological factors is often difficult. However, patients with no obvious cause should be investigated for evidence of diabetes. Patients with evidence of lymphoedema or impairment of venous flow can have more extensive problems with cellulitis. Those patients at risk are summarised in Table 20.2.

The commonest organisms involved in cellulitis are the group A beta-haemolytic streptococci, with *S. pyogenes* being the most common, with members of the staphylococci group also prevalent. Rarely Gram-negative organisms, anaerobes and fungi can cause cellulitis, but these are usually in patients with diabetes or who are immunocompromised. The presence of gas associated with cellulitis should raise the suspicion of the presence of *C. perfringens.*

Antibiotic therapy for treatment of cellulitis is based on the 'best guess' of the potential microorganisms, and usually involves treatment in the initial stages with flucloxacillin and penicillin. In patients who are otherwise healthy, not systemically unwell, and with limited signs and symptoms, treatment with oral antibiotics is appropriate. In diabetic patients, or those with systemic symptoms, or more extensive infection, parenteral antibiotics may be required.

The assessment of cellulitis can be aided by marking the boundaries of the limit of the erythema, and monitoring this for evidence of progression. Failure to respond to antibiotic therapy, or rapid advancement of the extent of disease should raise suspicion of necrotising fasciitis and the possible need for urgent surgical intervention, or alteration of antibiotics.

Anorectal abscess and fistula

Anorectal abscesses are variable in nature and classification but arise in the perianal area, and are often associated with a fistulous tract. They arise from the cryptoglandular epithelium in the anal canal which becomes infected and extends through the anal lining to the sphincter muscle layers. Each anal crypt drains four to ten anal glands, which lubricate the anal canal, and when these become obstructed results in stasis of the glandular secretions, which subsequently become infected leading to suppuration and abscess formation. When the abscess breaches the internal sphincter through the crypts of Morgagni, to the intersphincteric space it can penetrate the potential perirectal spaces and result in the presence of a perianal abscess (60%), ischiorectal abscess (20%), intersphincteric abscess (5%), supralevator abscess (4%) or a submucosal abscess (1%).

The peak incidence of anorectal abscesses is in the third and fourth decades of life, with a male predominance of 2:1 to 3:1. Approximately, 30% of patients presenting with an anorectal abscess will have noted a previous abscess which either resolved spontaneously or required surgical intervention.

The commonest organisms involved in anorectal abscesses differ from other cutaneous abscesses, with *E. coli*, *Enterococcus* and *Bacteroides* species being the most prevalent from the normal gut flora. Anorectal abscesses that culture only *S. aureus* rarely have a fistulous connection; however, the presence of coliforms or *Bacteroides* within an abscess should raise suspicion of an underlying fistula (40%).

In patients presenting with anorectal abscesses it is important to consider the perirectal anatomy and the potential spaces that exist, and which therefore need to be assessed in the course of treatment of an anorectal abscess. Anorectal abscesses invariably require adequate drainage to achieve healing and antibiotics have a very limited role and are usually only prescribed for those with extensive cellulitis or necrosis.

Anorectal fistulas occur in 30–60% of those presenting with anorectal abscesses. In patients presenting with fistulating disease, other pathologies such as Crohn's disease should also be considered. The prevalence of cases is 8.6 per 100,000 of the population with a 2:1 male:female preponderance. Fistula-in-ano are hollow tracts lined with granulation tissue connecting an internal opening to the skin.

Anatomy of anorectal fistulas again follows that of the abscesses that tend to cause them. A clear understanding of the anatomy of the pelvic floor muscles is important in determining the fistula location, course and ultimately deciding the treatment. The internal sphincter is a smooth muscle under autonomic control, whilst the external sphincter is a striated muscle with three components (submucosal, superficial and puborectalis) which are under voluntary control. Goodsall's rule can help predict the course of the fistulous tract, stating that fistulae with an external opening anterior to a plane passing transversely through the centre of the anus will follow a straight line to the dentate line, whereas those with openings posterior to the plane will follow a curved course to the posterior midline of the anal canal. An exception to this rule is those with external openings more than 3 cm from the anal verge.

The Parks classification system outlines four categories of fistula-in-ano based on anatomical location, and these can be seen in Table 20.4. The operative strategies are largely based around the preservation of the sphincter muscle complex in order to retain continence, but also paying close attention to draining collections and relieving local sepsis.

Laying open of fistula-in-ano is successful in 85–95% of primary fistulae that are submucosal, intersphincteric and low trans-sphincteric. If there is any doubt about the amount of muscle available within the sphincter complex, a seton suture is placed in order to allow drainage and easy identification of the tract.

Clinical assessment of anorectal abscesses should focus on ensuring that there are no underlying symptoms suggestive

Table 20.4 Parks classification of fistula-in-ano.

Classification	Common course	Percentage	Operative strategy
Intersphincteric	Via internal sphincter to the intersphincteric space and then to the perineum	70%	Usually little muscle involvement and can be treated by laying open
Transsphincteric	Low via internal and external sphincters into the ischiorectal fossa and then to the perineum	25%	An assessment needs to be made of the amount of external sphincter involved in the fistula, and judgement as to whether this can be divided whilst retaining continence
Suprasphincteric	Via the intersphincteric space superiorly to above puborectalis into the ischiorectal fossa and then to the perineum	4%	Usually require placement of a seton suture and more complex fistula surgery
Extrasphincteric	From perianal skin through levator ani muscles to the rectal wall completely outside sphincter	1%	May require defunctioning procedure in order to attain healing

of an underlying cause of the abscess. Furthermore, a full clinical evaluation is usually not possible unless the patient is under anaesthetic as the area is frequently too painful to fully examine. Intersphincteric abscesses often have no external signs; however, patients complain of severe perianal pain, and pain on defecation, and they will be exquisitely tender on digital rectal examination. When the patient is under anaesthetic, a full evaluation of the anorectum by digital rectal examination and rigid sigmoidoscopy should be performed in order to exclude underlying pathology, and to see if there is any obvious fistula-in-ano present.

The surgical drainage of the abscess should be performed as previously described; however, cruciate incisions should be avoided in the perianal area in order to minimise the chance of sphincter injury. A radial incision parallel to the sphincter muscles is usually sufficient. Once the abscess has been drained, excessive curetting and probing of the wound should not be performed due to the risk of creating false passages or fistulae. Care should be taken when examining by digital rectal examination or rigid sigmoidoscopy, also to avoid inadvertent injury and creation of fistulae.

If an obvious fistula is seen at the time of the initial drainage, then it is reasonable practice to insert a seton into the tract at that time. However, excessive searching for a fistulous tract or repeated attempts should not take place for risk of developing multiple fistulae or false passages. A safe practice is to follow the patient up electively with a repeat examination under anaesthetic if there is a strong clinical suspicion of a fistula. Setons can either be used for drainage purposes, or to slowly cut through the sphincter muscles in order to allow the fistulous tract to heal.

Intersphincteric abscesses are treated by draining into the anal canal using a transverse incision at the level of the dentate line and inserting a catheter into the cavity for flushing and in order to keep it open.

Necrotising fasciitis

Necrotising soft tissue infections have been recognised and reported for centuries the earliest dating back to Hippocrates in the fifth century BC.

Necrotising fasciitis is rare within the UK with an estimated 500 new cases each year; however, this is difficult to confirm, as different eponyms are given to describe the same condition. It is associated with a mortality of 70%, with the mean age of survivors being 35 years, and non-survivors 49 years. There is a male:female ratio of 3:1 in all cases of necrotising soft tissue infection, which relates predominantly to the incidence of Fournier's gangrene of the perineum.

The aetiology of necrotising fasciitis is not fully understood, with patients often having a history of trauma, including insect bites, scratches or abrasions. However, in some cases no primary cause can be found. Patients that have pre-existing conditions which increase susceptibility to infection seem to be at an increased risk of developing necrotising fasciitis; these conditions include diabetes mellitus, peripheral vascular disease, chronic renal failure, drug misuse and advanced age.

The microbiology of necrotising fasciitis frequently has a group A beta-haemolytic streptococcus, with or without a staphylococcus as the initiating bacteria; however, the cultures are frequently multi-organism, and usually have a mixed flora with anaerobes and facultative aerobes being present within the culture. *C. perfringens* and *Bacteroides* species are frequently found along with enterococci and coliforms.

The anaerobic bacteria flourish in the hypoxic wounds allowing the facultative organisms to take advantage of the polymorphonucleocytes (PMNs) having decreased function due to the tissue hypoxia. Aerobic metabolism produces carbon dioxide and water, while hydrogen, nitrogen, hydrogen sulphide and methane are produced from the combination of aerobic and anaerobic bacteria within a soft tissue

Table 20.5 Symptoms and signs of necrotising fasciitis.

	Early	Late
Symptoms	Pain	Severe pain
	Skin anaesthesia	
Signs	Cellulitis	Skin discolouration (purple or black)
	Pyrexia	Blistering
	Tachycardia	Haemorrhagic bullae
	Swelling	Crepitus
	Induration	Discharge of 'dishwater' fluid
	Hyponatraemia	Severe sepsis or systemic inflammatory response syndrome
		Multi-organ failure

infection. Accumulation of these gases, except carbon dioxide, within the tissue occurs due to reduced water solubility.

Necrotising fasciitis is associated with a massive systemic inflammatory response characterised by circulating cytokines and increased PMN activity in the systemic circulation leading to end-organ injury; however, the PMNs are decreased in activity at the affected site due to the action of *Bacteroides fragilis* in reducing interferon activity and hence phagocytosis.

The clinical features of necrotising soft tissue infections are characterised in Table 20.5 and can be divided into early and late findings. A high index of suspicion must be held by all clinicians, particularly in the setting of rapidly progressive cellulitis associated with severe pain.

The management of necrotising fasciitis is emergency surgical debridement without delay. Whilst there are several adjuncts such as plain radiographs to look for subcutaneous gas, or computed tomography scanning to evaluate an underlying cause that may require treated, debridement should not be unnecessarily delayed in order to obtain these. Risk factors for death included increased age, female gender, ex-

tent of infection, delay in first debridement, elevated creatinine, elevated lactate level and degree of organ dysfunction.

Urgent radical surgical debridement of all affected tissue is required. The finding of grey subcutaneous tissue should stimulate the surgeon to debride the tissue back to healthy bleeding margins. Tissue hypoxia and ischaemia occur due to thrombosis of the blood vessels within the subcutaneous tissue, potentiating the infective problems. The extent of the disease often exceeds what is apparent on the skin, in keeping with the description of 'undermining synergistic gangrene'. Therefore, debridement may have to be much more extensive than what appears healthy on the skin.

Patients will need regular inspection of the wounds, with a low threshold for re-operation if there is any concern about tissue viability. Support in a critical care unit will be required for management of severe sepsis and pain control. The extent of surgical debridement should not initially be limited in view of the extent of tissue cover required as plastic surgical techniques can cover very large defects.

Further reading

Brook I. Microbiology and management of soft tissue and muscle infections. *Int J Surg* 2008;**6**(4):328–338.

Elliott DC, Kufera JA, Myers RA. Necrotizing soft tissue infections. Risk factors for mortality and strategies for management. *Ann Surg* 1996;**224**(5):672–683.

Hasham S, Matteucci P, Stanley PR, Hart NB. Necrotising fasciitis. *BMJ* 20059;**330**(7495):830–833.

Majeski J, Majeski E. Necrotizing fasciitis: improved survival with early recognition by tissue biopsy and aggressive surgical treatment. *South Med J* 1997;**90**(11):1065–1068.

Parks AG, Gordon PH, Hardcastle JD. A classification of fistula-in-ano. *Br J Surg* 1976;**63**(1):1–12.

Parks AG, Stitz RW. The treatment of high fistula-in-ano. *Dis Colon Rectum* 1976;**19**(6):487–499.

5 Urology

21 Emergency Urology

Thomas J. Walton[1] & Gurminder S. Mann[2]

[1]Leicester General Hospital, Leicester, UK
[2]Nottingham City Hospital, Nottingham, UK

Introduction

Urological emergencies are common, yet increasingly their initial management is provided by trainees for whom urology is often an unfamiliar speciality. This chapter aims to provide the reader with an up-to-date guide to the presentation and primary management of a spectrum of urological disorders, including acute ureteric colic, urinary retention and genitourinary trauma.

Ureteric colic

Urolithiasis represents the commonest cause of acute ureteric colic, with calcium stones accounting for approximately 80% of cases (Table 21.1). Ureteric calculi have a prevalence of approximately 2–3% in Caucasian populations, with a lifetime risk of 10–12% in males and 5–6% in females. They are more common in developed countries, in men, in those with a positive family history, and in those with inadequate daily water intake.

Ureteric colic typically presents with acute severe loin pain – which patients often describe as unrelenting despite a number of postural changes – and haematuria. Vomiting is often a feature of severe uncontrolled pain. Most patients with renal colic present because of severe uncontrolled pain and do not have signs of overt sepsis. Opiates are commonly given, although diclofenac sodium has been shown to be at least as effective for pain relief, particularly via rectal administration. Despite initial concerns, diclofenac sodium therapy has not been associated with renal toxicity in patients with pre-existing normal renal function. Fever, tachycardia, tachypnoea and hypotension suggest sepsis secondary to an infected, obstructed kidney, which represents a life-threatening condition. Immediate management comprises prompt resuscitation, establishment of intravenous

(IV) antibiotics, rapid diagnosis and decompression of the obstructed renal system, usually by ultrasound-guided percutaneous nephrostomy. Early involvement of urology and critical care services is essential in such patients.

Urinalysis should be performed in all patients to assess for urinary pH and the presence of haematuria. Dipstick haematuria is present in 84–90% of patients with stones with a positive predictive value of 60–70%. All urine should be sieved and any retrieved stones sent for biochemical analysis.

Unenhanced spiral CT is the investigation of choice for patients with suspected renal calculi, with a sensitivity and specificity greater than 90%. It avoids problems due to IV contrast reactions, and allows for diagnosis of non-urological pathology. It does however involve significant exposure to ionising radiation (2.5 cGy) and as such should be avoided if possible for follow-up.

The management of ureteric calculi depends upon factors relating to the stone and the patient. Pre-eminent stone factors are size and site. It has been shown that 71–98% of stones <5 mm will pass spontaneously, whereas rates of spontaneous passage for stones >7 mm are low. Stone passage is also related to location in the ureter; 25% of proximal, 45% of mid and 75% of distal ureteric stones will pass spontaneously. In patients in whom stone passage is deemed likely, a trial of conservative management should be employed. Exceptions include patients with a functional or anatomical solitary kidney, bilateral ureteric obstruction, uncontrolled pain, or the presence of infection. Patients without contraindications should receive diclofenac sodium 50 mg tds, which has been shown to reduce the frequency of recurrent renal colic episodes. Recent evidence suggests that additional treatment with smooth muscle relaxants is associated with increased rates of stone passage over analgesics alone. A recent meta-analysis of studies using either nifedipine or tamsulosin, showed an approximate 65% greater chance of stone passage when such agents were used compared with equivalent controls. Intervention is generally reserved for large stones (>7 mm), conservative treatment failures and those with contraindications to a watchful waiting approach. Options include extracorporeal shock-wave lithotripsy and retrograde ureteroscopic stone

Emergency Surgery, 1st edition. Edited by Adam Brooks, Peter F. Mahoney, Bryan A. Cotton and Nigel Tai. © 2010 Blackwell Publishing.

Table 21.1 Causes of acute ureteric colic.

Cause	Frequency	Plain X-ray appearance
Urinary calculi	Common	
Calcium oxalate	60%	Radio-opaque
Calcium phosphate	20%	Radio-opaque
Uric acid	10%	Radiolucent
Cystine	3%	Slightly radio-opaque
Struvite	7%	Radio-opaque
Blood clot	Occasional	Radiolucent
Sloughed renal papilla	Rare	Radiolucent

fragmentation. Whilst a discussion of the relative merits of the two procedures is beyond the scope of this chapter, it is generally accepted that for these strategies equivalent stone-free rates are seen for proximal ureteric stones, whereas ureteroscopic stone fragmentation is thought to be superior for mid and distal ureteric calculi, albeit with a higher complication rate.

Acute urinary retention

Acute urinary retention (AUR) is a common male urological emergency characterised by an inability to pass urine. Although a number of precipitants are associated with the development of AUR (see Table 21.2), the majority of cases are caused by benign prostatic hyperplasia (BPH). The initial management of AUR comprises immediate bladder decompression by either urethral or suprapubic catheterisation. Primary urethral catheterisation is favoured by 98% of urologists in the United Kingdom. Difficulties performing urethral catheterisation are often encountered by the inexperienced surgeon due to inadequate lubrication or by us-

Table 21.2 Causes of acute urinary retention in men.

Cause
Benign prostate hyperplasia (spontaneous AUR)
Postoperative
Excess fluid intake (commonly alcohol)
Drugs
Opiates
Anticholinergics
Antipsychotics
Ephedine/pseudoephedrine
UTI
Haematuria with clot retention
Neurological (MS, cauda equina syndrome etc.)
Pelvic trauma

AUR, acute urinary retention; UTI, urinary tract infection; MS, multiple sclerosis.

ing a catheter which is too thin and flexible. The normal male urethra has a maximum calibre of 30F (approximately 10 mm in diameter), therefore an initial Foley catheter size of 16F which has the requisite rigidity to negotiate an enlarged prostate. Suprapubic catheterisation should be reserved for patients in whom urethral catheterisation is not possible. Absolute contraindications to suprapubic catheterisation comprise therapeutic anticoagulation, a history of bladder carcinoma and an impalpable bladder. Relative contraindications include previous abdominal/pelvic surgery via a lower midline approach, which increases the likelihood of adherent small bowel to the underlying scar.

The significant majority of patients with AUR in the United Kingdom are managed by short duration bladder decompression (1–3 days), followed by a trial without catheter (TWOC). TWOC is successful in up to 23–48% of patients in such cases. Factors predicting an increased likelihood of successful TWOC are lower age (<65 years), a drained volume of <1 L at catheterisation, and an identifiable precipitating factor. Recently the Alf-AUR study has shown that treatment with the α_1-adrenergic blocker alfuzosin improves the likelihood of successful TWOC for all patients compared with placebo (62% versus 48%). Furthermore, continued treatment was associated with a reduced risk of recurrent AUR and the need for BPH surgery among the groups (17.1% versus 24.1%). Patients failing an initial TWOC with alpha-blocker should be re-catheterised with a long-term catheter and referred for consideration of operative urological intervention.

Urinary tract infection

Adult urinary tract infection (UTI) is a large topic; however, a number of infective conditions considered urological emergencies are worthy of review. These include pyelonephritis, pyonephrosis, acute bacterial prostatitis (ABP) and Fournier's gangrene. The management of pyonephrosis, or an infected obstructed kidney, is discussed above. Fournier's gangrene is covered elsewhere in this text. Pyelonephritis and acute prostatitis are discussed below.

Acute pyelonephritis

Acute pyelonephritis is defined as acute inflammation of the renal parenchyma and renal pelvis. It is distinguished from simple uncomplicated cystitis by the presence of flank pain, nausea and vomiting, fever (>38°C) and costo-vertebral angle tenderness, which may or may not occur in association with cystitis symptoms. The clinical presentation ranges from the uncomplicated case suitable for outpatient management, to severe life-threatening sepsis with multi-organ failure. The pathogens responsible for pyelonephritis are the same as for cystitis, denoting a primary ascending aetiology in a majority of cases. Gram-negative bacilli are therefore usually responsible, although Gram-positive organisms, typically *E. faecalis*, are implicated in a minority. A subgroup of *E. coli* which expresses P pili – a surface adherence factor specific for epithelial cells – is responsible for approximately 80% of cases.

The diagnosis of acute pyelonephritis is usually apparent on history and examination alone. Tenderness on percussion over the renal angle is a useful clinical sign associated with a high specificity for pyelonephritis. Urinalysis is usually positive for leucocytes, nitrites and blood, with 80–95% of subsequent cultures positive for values of $>10^5$ CFU uropathogen/mL. Routine imaging is not required in uncomplicated mild cases. However, elderly patients, diabetics, men, children, patients with suspected obstruction, or those failing to respond to appropriate therapy should undergo ultrasonography to exclude upper tract obstruction. In cases of severe sepsis or where abnormalities are identified on ultrasound, contrast-enhanced computed tomography (CT) should be performed as it provides superior information about focal scarring/inflammation, obstruction, stone disease, or the presence of abscess or gas formation.

The management of pyelonephritis hinges on the classification of cases into complicated or uncomplicated, and mild/moderate or severe categories. Factors increasing the likelihood of complicated UTI are shown in Table 21.3. The development of an SIRS response, combined with nausea and vomiting, is believed to distinguish severe cases from mild/moderate disease. Acute uncomplicated pyelonephritis in women may be treated with oral antibiotics alone; recent evidence suggests a 7-day course of ciprofloxacin 500 mg bd has greater efficacy and fewer side effects than the traditional 14-day course of trimethoprim-sulphamethoxazole. The duration of oral ciprofloxacin should be extended to 10–14 days in mild/moderate complicated cases. For severe cases, appropriate resuscitation and establishment of IV antibiotics is required. Choices of antibiotic include ampicillin and gentamicin, ciprofloxacin, or a third generation cephalosporin, dependent upon local microbiological guidelines. Once fever has subsided an oral quinolone is recommended for a total duration of 14–21 days. Because of a reported relapse rate of 10–30%, repeat urine culture is recommended after 4 days on and 10 days off therapy.

Emphysematous pyelonephritis

Emphysematous pyelonephritis describes a severe life-threatening necrosis of the kidney caused by gas-forming organisms. About 70–90% of cases occur in diabetics, who commonly present with severe sepsis. A palpable flank mass is present in 50%. Gas is identified overlying the kidney on plain radiography in 85% of cases, but is commonly missed. Management comprises resuscitation, correction of hyperglycaemia, IV antibiotics and expeditious nephrectomy; surgical removal of the kidney reduces the mortality rate from 60 to 80% to approximately 20%.

Perinephric abscess

A perinephric abscess develops in Gerota's fascia adjacent to the kidney, usually secondary to ipsilateral pyelonephritis. Occasionally haematogenous seeding following a UTI, dental work or skin infection may be responsible. Patients typically present with flank pain and fever, although rigors and nightsweats may be a feature. A palpable flank mass is seen in almost half of all patients. Common pathogens include *E. coli*, *Proteus* spp., *Klebsiella* spp. and *Pseudomonas* spp., although Gram-positive cocci are occasionally seen in those with skin infections and in IV drug abusers. The mortality rate for conservatively managed patients is over 75%, falling to 20–50% for those receiving adequate percutaneous or formal surgical drainage.

Acute bacterial prostatitis

ABP is a rare, occasionally severe infection of the prostate. Patients typically present with fever, pelvic and low back pain, frequency, urgency and occasionally urinary retention. Digital rectal examination reveals an exquisitely tender, hot swollen prostate which is pathognomic. *E. coli* is responsible in 80% of cases, although mixed infections with Gram-negative rods are common. Enterococci are seen in 5–10% of cases. Treatment is by IV antibiotic therapy. Fluoroquinolones are regarded as the oral agent of choice due to broad activity, excellent prostate penetration and a favourable side-effect profile. Treatment duration is 14–28 days.

Table 21.3 Factors increasing the likelihood of complicated UTI.

Factors increasing the likelihood of complicated UTI
Male sex
Elderly
Functional of structural urinary tract abnormality
History of nephrolithiasis
Concurrent pregnancy, diabetes or immunosuppression

UTI, urinary tract infection.

Penoscrotal emergencies

Testicular torsion

Testicular torsion affects one in 4000 males under 25 years. It results from a congenital abnormality of the processus vaginalis which produces a high investment of the tunica around the spermatic cord, leading to the so-called 'bell-clapper' deformity. Contraction of the cremaster muscle thus allows free rotation of the testis, leading initially to venous obstruction, followed by arterial ischaemia and ultimately necrosis. A majority of cases occur spontaneously without an obvious precipitant, although trauma is cited as a cause in 4–8% of cases. Other associated factors are testicular tumour, increased pubertal testicular volume and cryptorchidism.

Patients typically present with an acute onset of severe unremitting scrotal pain. The testis is often swollen and usually exquisitely tender to palpation. It may assume a horizontal lie and, due to shortening of the cord with rotation, may be elevated. This latter finding is quite specific and, where present in a patient with a convincing history, is highly suggestive of torsion. The most sensitive finding, however, is absence of the ipsilateral cremasteric reflex. The reflex, considered to be positive if the testis moves more than 0.5 cm following stroking of the ipsilateral upper inner thigh, is universally present in boys older than 30 months. Two studies have shown that loss of the cremasteric reflex occurs in 100% of cases of acute torsion. Unfortunately, an absent cremasteric reflex is also associated with other causes of an acute scrotum, and thus its specificity is lower at approximately 66% (Rabinowitz Melekos).

The development of testicular ischaemia can occur as rapidly as 4 hours after torsion. Testicular salvage rates of 90% are reported for operative detorsion within 6 hours, falling to 50 and 10% at 12 and 24 hours respectively. Prompt diagnosis and intervention are thus essential in cases of suspected torsion. Imaging should only be performed in cases where clinical suspicion is low or presentation is delayed (>24 hours). Doppler ultrasonography of the scrotum is the modality of choice, but is associated with relatively high false-negative rates (due to early venous occlusion with persistent arterial flow), giving a sensitivity of only 76–78%, with an associated specificity of approximately 90%. Radionucleotide scanning is reportedly associated with sensitivities approaching 100% but is typically unavailable and not commonly performed. Recently a large multicentre trial has shown a sensitivity of 96% and specificity of 97% for high-resolution ultrasound in detecting torsion in 919 children with an acute scrotum.

Successful management of testicular torsion requires prompt restoration of blood supply to the affected testis. Manual detorsion – performed by laterally rotating the affected testis around its natural axis – has been advocated as a rapid non-invasive treatment, but is associated with a success rate of approximately 25% and does not obviate the need for subsequent testicular fixation. As such it cannot be recommended as first-line management. For those undergoing surgery the affected hemiscrotum should be explored to establish a diagnosis. Cases of epididymitis are usually associated with a reactive hydrocele, fluid from which should be sent for microscopy, culture and sensitivity, and chlamydia assay if appropriate. The scrotum should be closed and the

patient placed on antibiotics in lieu of a positive microbiology result. In cases of torsion, the testis should be derotated and placed in warm swabs for at least 5 minutes to assess viability. Non-viable testes should be removed. Viable or dusky testes should be fixed, along with the contralateral testis, using a non-absorbable suture, as there have been a number of reported cases of recurrent torsion following fixation with an absorbable suture. There is no convincing evidence that testicular fixation directly contributes to subsequent male infertility.

Paraphimosis

A paraphimosis occurs when a tight foreskin (phimosis) is retracted over the glans penis and not replaced. The phimotic foreskin acts as a constriction band at the level of the coronal sulcus, obstructing venous outflow from the glans, causing oedema and in rare cases ischaemia and necrosis (Figure 21.1). Treatment consists of prompt manual reduction of the foreskin. This is commonly painful and requires adequate systemic analgaesia, often a penile local anaesthetic block, and occasionally a general anaesthetic. For manual reduction the most reliable technique is a two-handed approach; both thumbs apply firm pressure to the glans penis, with all four fingers arrayed behind the constriction band on each side. Gentle traction is then employed on the foreskin whilst simultaneously compressing the glans penis, in a manner akin to expelling a large tablet from a blister pack. Puncturing of the oedematous foreskin using a sterile 18G needle may be performed as an adjunct in an attempt to accelerate reduction. For cases refractory to manual

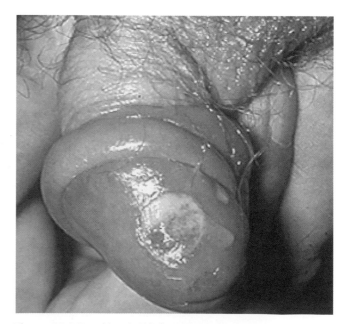

Figure 21.1 Paraphimosis. This figure shows the characteristic appearance of a swollen oedematous foreskin seen in paraphimosis. In addition, an area of superficial ulceration of the glans penis is clearly identifiable.

reduction, a dorsal slit can be performed under local anaesthesia. A formal elective circumcision can then be performed once the swelling has subsided.

Priapism

Priapism is defined as a persistent unwanted penile erection. Typically only the corpora cavernosa are involved. There are two main types: ischaemic (veno-occlusive and low-flow) and non-ischaemic (arterial and high-flow). Ischaemic priapism describes a compartment syndrome of the penis resulting from a failure of detumescence, leading to ischaemia and ultimately fibrosis. The condition is idiopathic in over half of all patients; the remainder are associated with diseases (e.g. sickle cell, leukaemia, spinal cord tumour and malignancy) drugs (e.g. antipsychotics and anticoagulants) and intracavernosal therapy for erectile dysfunction. Patients usually present late with a painful erection and often a history of an antecedent cause or recurrent episodes. Examination reveals hard corpora cavernosa with a soft glans penis, indicating non-involvement of the corpus spongiosum. Non-ischaemic priapism is secondary to penile or perineal trauma and results when injury creates an arterial–sinusoidal shunt within the corpus cavernosum. The erection also involves only the corpora cavernosum with sparing of the corpus spongiosum, but is softer than is seen with ischaemic cases and is characteristically painless. Because the corpora are filled with oxygenated blood, no compartment syndrome exists, and thus non-ischaemic priapism is not considered an emergency.

Whilst it is usually relatively straightforward to distinguish between the two types of priapism on history and examination alone, occasionally difficulties arise, and it is for this reason that blood gas determination of corporeal blood is considered mandatory in all patients. Corporeal aspiration is performed by inserting a 19-gauge butterfly needle into the lateral edge of one corpus cavernosum (two needles are unnecessary as the septum between each corporeal body is incomplete) and aspirating blood for analysis. A PO_2 less than 30 mm Hg or any degree of acidosis requires immediate attempts at detumescence. Conservative measures such as ice-packs, physical exertion and masturbation occasionally have been advocated in the past but are generally ineffective. Therapeutic aspiration is considered to be the first manoeuvre following diagnostic aspiration, achieving detumescence in approximately 30% of cases. Typically, 10–15 mL of blood is aspirated and replaced with an equal volume of normal saline. The procedure is repeated until the aspirate is bright red. The next step if therapeutic aspiration fails is direct corporeal administration of a sympathomimetic agent. Although a number of vasoactive agents have been used, phenylephrine, a selective alpha-1 adrenergic agonist, has the best cardiovascular side-effect profile, and is thus recommended. It can be expected to induce resolution in 65% of cases. A 10 mg of phenylephrine is diluted in normal saline to a concentration of 100 mcg/mL. Under strict pulse and blood pressure monitoring 3–5 mL of solution is injected into the corpora every 5 minutes for up to 1 hour before declaring treatment failure. For refractory cases prompt surgical intervention is required to establish a shunt between the erect corpora cavernosa and either the glans penis (Winter, Ebbehøj or Al-Ghorab techniques), corpus spongiosum (Quackels) or saphenous vein (Grayhack procedure). Shunt procedures have combined resolution rates of 66–77%; more proximal procedures are associated with the highest resolution rates but increased complications, particularly erectile dysfunction. Indeed erectile dysfunction is a major complication of prolonged priapism: 90% of men with a priapism lasting more than 24 hours do not regain the ability to have intercourse. It is for this reason that immediate penile prosthesis insertion is often considered for failed shunting and late presentation (>24 hours) of priapism.

Genitourinary trauma

Renal trauma

Damage to the kidney represents the most common type of urinary tract injury. Even so renal trauma is relatively uncommon, accounting for only 1.4–3.25% of trauma cases. Over 90% are due to blunt injury, of which approximately 90% may be managed conservatively. Initial management of the patient with renal injury follows established ATLS principles, particularly as many patients have associated injuries. Haematuria is present in 80–94% of cases, but its presence or absence gives little indication of the severity of injury. In fact, 18–36% of patients with a major pedicle injury have no evidence of microscopic or gross haematuria. In those with evidence of haematuria and persistent life threatening haemodynamic instability, immediate renal exploration is warranted. For the remainder investigation and subsequent management depends upon mechanism of injury, and the presence of gross haematuria or systemic hypotension.

Blunt trauma

In blunt trauma, gross or microscopic haematuria and a (lowest recorded) systolic BP of <90 mm Hg is associated with a 12.5% incidence of major renal injury. This figure falls to 0.2% in patients with microscopic haematuria only and no recorded evidence of shock. Thus, patients with blunt trauma require radiological imaging if they have gross haematuria, or microhaematuria and a systolic BP < 90 mm Hg. Exceptions include patients with major deceleration injury and children, in whom any evidence of haematuria mandates radiographic assessment. Contrast-enhanced helical CT with delayed (10 minutes) imaging is the gold

Table 21.4 AAST renal injury grading scale.

Grade	Description of injury
1	Contusion or non-expanding subcapsular haematoma
	No laceration
2	Non-expanding perirenal haematoma
	Cortical laceration <1 cm deep without extravasation
3	Cortical laceration >1 cm without urinary extravasation
4	Laceration: through corticomedullary junction into collecting system or
	Vascular: segmental renal artery or vein injury with contained haematoma, or partial vessel laceration or vessel thrombosis
5	Laceration: shattered kidney or
	Vascular: renal pedicle or avulsion

standard, allowing accurate classification of renal injury (see Table 21.4). In general, the only absolute indications for surgery are life-threatening haemodynamic instability believed to arise from a renal injury, renal pedicle avulsion (grade 5 injury), or the finding of an expanding, pulsatile retroperitoneal haematoma at laparotomy. All other renal injuries may be managed conservatively initially, although a small proportion of patients with grade 3/4 injuries develop secondary haemorrhage, which can usually be managed by angiographic embolisation. Urinary extravasation (grade 4 injuries) resolves spontaneously in 76–87% of cases; persistent cases may be treated by percutaneous perinephric drainage with or without ureteric stenting. Occasionally, a non-expanding retroperitoneal haematoma may be encountered during a trauma laparotomy performed for other reasons. In this situation a one-shot IVU (2 mL/kg iodinated contrast, single film at 10 minutes) should be performed to exclude a renovascular (grade 5) injury and to confirm the presence of a functioning contralateral kidney. The presence of contrast in the renal collecting system implies adequate renal perfusion, obviating the need for renal exploration in approximately 30% of cases.

Penetrating trauma

In haemodynamically stable patients with penetrating flank trauma, any degree of haematuria mandates radiological imaging. Exploration of all penetrating renal injuries has been advocated by some, based on a higher reported incidence of secondary haemorrhage, although others have reported the safe implementation of a selective approach in haemodynamically stable patients. In general, surgery is advised for haemodynamic instability, grade 4/5 injuries and when laparotomy is performed for other reasons.

Follow-up after renal trauma

Repeat urinalysis is recommended in all patients with trauma and haematuria, irrespective of severity, to iden-

tify persistent haematuria requiring further evaluation. The incidence of renovascular hypertension and renal insufficiency following renal injury is not well-characterised, nor is the time course for development of such complications. One multi-institutional study of 89 patients with grade 4/5 injuries reported rates of 22.4 and 4.5% for renal insufficiency and hypertension respectively, and it is therefore recommended that such indices are monitored indefinitely following major renal injury.

Ureteric trauma

Ureteric trauma is rare, accounting for only 1% of all cases of genitourinary trauma. Approximately, 75% of cases are iatrogenic, with over half occurring to the distal third of the ureter during gynaecological surgery. The remainder occur during general, urological and vascular surgery. In Europe, blunt abdominal trauma accounts for the majority of remaining ureteric injuries, whereas in the United States gunshot injuries are the most common cause.

Damage is identified intraoperatively in approximately one third of cases, whereupon urological specialist input should be immediately sought. Simple ligation injury can usually be managed by immediate de-ligation and ureteric stenting. Where ureteric integrity is questionable the affected segment should be resected followed by reconstruction. Satisfactory results are obtained by establishing a tension-free, spatulated anastomosis. Often this may be achieved by simple ureteric mobilisation and ureteroureterostomy, followed by prophylactic ureteric stenting. Where this is not feasible, a number of alternative approaches are possible, dependent on location of injury (see Table 21.5).

Delayed diagnosis of iatrogenic ureteric injury occurs in approximately two-thirds of patients; patients may present with postoperative loin pain, ileus, fever, and occasionally

Table 21.5 Site-specific options for repair of complete ureteric injuries.

Location of injury	Surgical option
Upper third	Uretero-ureterostomy
	Transuretero-ureterostomy
	Ureterocalycostomy
Middle third	Uretero-ureterostomy
	Transuretero-ureterostomy
	Boari flap and re-implantation
Lower third	Direct re-implantation
	Psoas hitch
	Blandy cystoplasty
Complete ureteric loss	Ileal interposition
	Autotransplantation

with a urinary leak, where elevated fluid creatinine is diagnostic of a urinary tract fistula. IVU and contrast-enhanced CT are the most appropriate first-line diagnostic modalities; where they are equivocal, retrograde pyelography (RPG) should be performed as it has been shown to be the most accurate imaging modality for establishing the presence and degree of ureteric injury. Retrograde ureteric stenting is usually unsuccessful in cases of delayed ureteric injury; therefore, in cases where the diagnosis is established on IVU or CT, percutaneous nephrostomy is advocated to provide temporary urinary diversion prior to definitive urinary reconstruction, as outlined in Table 21.5.

Bladder trauma

Bladder injuries may be categorised as blunt, penetrating or iatrogenic. Injury to the bladder is identified in 1.6% of blunt abdominal trauma cases, of which 80% have an associated pelvic fracture. Up to 30% will have a concomitant urethral injury. Bladder rupture is conventionally classified as intraperitoneal or extraperitoneal. Intraperitoneal rupture accounts for approximately 40% of cases. It occurs when there is a sudden rise in intravesical pressure, usually experienced following a blow to the pelvis or lower abdomen. The weakest part of the bladder is the dome, which ruptures into the abdominal cavity, leading to extravasation of urine. Extraperitoneal ruptures due to blunt trauma account for approximately 60% of cases, and are seen almost exclusively in the context of pelvic fractures. Injury is either due to a bony spicule piercing the bladder, or more commonly a tear of the bladder wall, typically on the anterolateral bladder wall. External penetrating trauma to the bladder is rare. Iatrogenic bladder trauma is more frequent, most commonly complicating hysterectomy, caesarean section and transurethral resection of bladder tumour.

The hallmark of bladder injury is gross haematuria, which is seen in 82–95% of cases. Additional features include an inability to void, suprapubic pain and suprapubic tenderness. The development of ileus, abdominal distension, urinary ascites/fistula, and unexplained elevations in serum urea and creatinine, suggest intraperitoneal bladder rupture. Multiple studies have shown that passive filling of the bladder by catheter clamping following the administration of IV contrast is inadequate for the diagnosis of bladder injury: a cystogram is thus the investigation of choice. It is performed by gravity-filling the bladder to capacity with dilute contrast before performing either CT or antero-posterior, oblique and post-drainage films. Filling of the retrovesical space, paracolic gutters and outlining of intra-abdominal viscera is indicative of intraperitoneal rupture (Figure 21.2a). Extraperitoneal rupture is associated with characteristic 'flame-shaped' areas of extravasation confined to the perivesical tissue (Figure 21.2b), and occasionally a so-called 'teardrop deformity' caused by a large pelvic haematoma.

Patients presenting with haematuria, an isolated pelvic fracture and a normal cystogram usually have a bladder haematoma, which is self-limiting and requires observation and catheter drainage alone. A similar management strategy is employed for a majority of patients with extraperitoneal bladder ruptures. Exceptions include patients with bladder neck or associated vaginal/rectal injuries, those undergoing open repair and internal fixation of pelvic fracture, and those in whom the indwelling catheter fails to provide adequate drainage. External penetrating injuries and blunt intraperitoneal bladder ruptures require formal surgical exploration and open repair. Small iatrogenic intraperitoneal bladder ruptures may be repaired laparoscopically where expertise is available, or alternatively may be managed by urethral catheter drainage alone, with prompt operative repair in patients who deteriorate under observation. In patients who require operative repair, absorbable sutures are

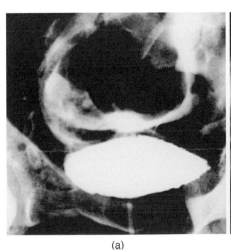
(a)

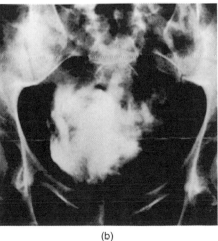
(b)

Figure 21.2 Cystographic appearances of bladder rupture. (a) Intraperitoneal bladder perforation is demonstrated on stress cystography by filling of the retrovesical space, paracolic gutters and outlining of intra-abdominal viscera. (b) Extravesical bladder rupture is signified by the presence of characteristic 'flame-shaped' extravasation, occasionally in association with a 'tear-drop deformity', indicating compression of the bladder by surrounding pelvic haematoma.

mandatory to prevent the formation of subsequent bladder stones. A follow-up stress cystogram, performed at 10 days, is generally performed prior to catheter removal.

Urethral trauma

Damage to the urethra represents the second commonest form of urinary tract injury after renal trauma. It is commoner in men, where it is associated with blunt external trauma in approximately 90% of cases. The male urethra is divided into anterior and posterior segments by the urogenital diaphragm. The anterior urethra, subdivided into penile and bulbar parts at the peno-scrotal junction, is relatively exposed and thus at higher risk of blunt and penetrating external trauma. Anterior urethral damage typically occurs following a blow to the perineum such as experienced during 'fall-astride' injuries. Stab wounds, gunshots, dog bites and blast injuries account for most cases of external penetrating trauma, whereas urethral instrumentation and catheterisation are common forms of iatrogenic internal trauma. Penile fracture, a rare cause of anterior urethral trauma, is separately discussed below. The posterior urethra consists of membranous and prostatic components and is almost exclusively injured in the context of a concomitant pelvic fracture. Overall the male urethra is injured in 3.5–19% of pelvic fractures and the female urethra in 0–6% of pelvic fractures. The risk of urethral injury is related to the type of pelvic fracture; unstable diametric pelvic fractures and bilateral ischiopubic rami fractures carry the highest likelihood of posterior urethral injury.

Blood at the urinary meatus is considered to be the hallmark of urethral injury. It is present in 37–93% of posterior and at least 75% of anterior urethral injuries. Blood at the vaginal introitus is seen in 80% of female urethral injuries. Other features are an inability to void, penile/perineal haematoma and a high-riding prostate. This latter feature is often difficult to assess in the acute setting, where pelvic haematoma often precludes adequate palpation of the prostate. The presence of blood at the urinary meatus mandates formal urethral imaging prior to any attempts at urethral catheterisation. Retrograde urethrography is easily performed using a 14F Foley catheter inserted into the distal urethra, with the balloon inflated using 1–2 mL of water. About 20–30 mL of undiluted contrast is injected and radiographs taken in a 30° oblique position. In the absence of a significant urethral injury the urinary bladder may be catheterised. Whilst relatively easy to perform, retrograde urethrography is time-consuming and thus inappropriate for unstable patients; for these patients a supra-pubic catheter should be inserted when the bladder becomes palpable and a retrograde urethrogram performed when practicable.

The management of urethral injuries is controversial. Most surgeons believe that immediate open exploration is required for stable patients who have sustained either penetrating urethral trauma or blunt posterior urethral trauma involving the bladder neck or rectum, due to the high rate of fistula, incontinence and infection. For the remaining majority of blunt urethral injuries, there is also a consensus advocating immediate urinary diversion, primarily via the suprapubic route, to limit urinary extravasation and its associated infective complications. For patients with partial urethral injuries, retrograde urethrography is then usually performed at intervals until satisfactory healing is demonstrated. The management of the diverted patient with a complete posterior urethral disruption secondary to blunt trauma is where much of the controversy rests, centred on the option of establishing early or delayed urethral continuity. The early establishment of urethral continuity, or primary realignment, takes place within 2 weeks of injury and typically involves a combined suprapubic/urethral endoscopic approach to realign the disrupted urethral ends over a stenting urethral catheter. The associated stricture rate is approximately 60%, meaning that at least 40% of patients require no further surgery, and in those that do, further stricture surgery is simplified due to reasonable urethral apposition. Ultimately, however, urethroplasty can be expected in up to one third of patients. Delayed urethroplasty involves prolonged suprapubic urinary diversion, usually for 3 months, during which time a urethral stricture forms at the site of injury in almost all patients, necessitating primary anastomotic urethroplasty. Proponents of this technique argue that although suprapubic catheterisation is necessary for at least 3 months, re-stricture rates are much lower (<10%) with this technique than with primary re-alignment.

External genital trauma

Blunt scrotal trauma

Eighty-five per cent of scrotal injuries result from blunt trauma, usually associated with athletic activity. Injuries range from simple bruising of the scrotum, through haematocoele to overt testicular rupture. Testicular torsion and dislocation are rare but well-described complications of blunt scrotal trauma. In testicular rupture the tunica albuginea is torn with evisceration of testicular tubules, mandating urgent surgical repair. Diagnosis may be made clinically by palpation or radiologically by ultrasound. Scrotal ultrasonography is considered the most sensitive modality for detecting tunica albuginea rupture, with a reported accuracy of up to 94%. Even in the absence of testicular rupture, a number of studies have shown increased rates of delayed intervention (>3 days) and subsequent orchidectomy in patients treated conservatively for haematocoele. Current guidelines

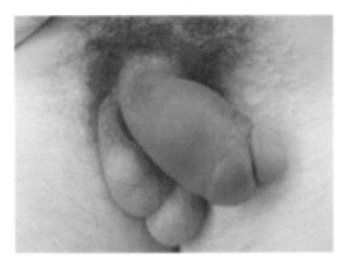

Figure 21.3 Penile fracture. This figure shows the typical appearance of the penis following penile fracture. Often likened to an aubergine (or egg-plant), a large haematoma confined to the penile shaft is seen, indicating that Buck's fascia has not been ruptured.

therefore recommend early scrotal exploration in all cases of testicular rupture, torsion and dislocation, and in patients with large symptomatic haematoceles.

Penile fracture

Penile fracture is uncommon (Figure 21.3). It occurs due to excessive bending of the erect penis, usually during vaginal intercourse. A tear of the tunica albuginea of the corpus cavernosum occurs, leading to immediate penile pain and rapid detumescence. Often an audible crack or popping sound is heard. Penile examination reveals swelling and bruising confined to the penile shaft, often described as an aubergine, or egg-plant, deformity. If Buck's fascia is torn, blood may extravasate along fascial planes into the scrotum, perineum and occasionally into the suprapubic areas. Associated urethral injury occurs in approximately 20% of cases. In most cases penile fracture may be diagnosed on history and clinical examination alone. Magnetic resonance imaging is the most sensitive modality for determining tunica albuginea rupture in equivocal cases. Once diagnosed, management comprises prompt surgical repair. Because of the possibility of occult and partial urethral injuries, some proponents advocate routine preoperative retrograde urethrography, whereas others believe an adequate assessment of urethral

integrity may be made at operation. Surgery typically involves a distal circumferential penile incision with degloving of the penile skin to the location of injury, followed by primary repair of the tunica albuginea defect.

Further reading

Brandes S, Coburn M, Armenakas N, et al. Diagnosis and management of ureteric injury: an evidence-based analysis. *BJU Int* 2004; **94**(3):277 289.

Gomez RG, Ceballos L, Coburn M, et al. Consensus statement on bladder injuries. *BJU Int* 2004;**94**(1):27–32.

Kalfa N, Veyrac C, Lopez M, et al. Multicenter assessment of ultrasound of the spermatic cord in children with acute scrotum. *J Urol* 2007;**177**(1):297–301; discussion 301.

Knudson MM, Harrison PB, Hoyt DB, et al. Outcome after major renovascular injuries: a Western trauma association multicenter report. *J Trauma* 2000;**49**(6):1116 1122.

Manikandan R, Srirangam SJ, O'Reilly PH, et al. Management of acute urinary retention secondary to benign prostatic hyperplasia in the UK: a national survey. *BJU Int* 2004;**93**(1):84–88.

McNeill SA, Hargreave TB, Roehrborn CG. Alfuzosin 10 mg once daily in the management of acute urinary retention: results of a double-blind placebo-controlled study. *Urology* 2005; **65**(1):83–89; discussion 89–90.

Montague DK, Jarow J, Broderick GA, et al. American Urological Association guideline on the management of priapism. *J Urol* 2003; **170**(4, Pt 1):1318–1324.

Morey AF, Iverson AJ, Swan A, et al. Bladder rupture after blunt trauma: guidelines for diagnostic imaging. *J Trauma* 2001; **51**(4):683–686.

Morey AF, Metro MJ, Carney KJ, et al. Consensus on genitourinary trauma: external genitalia. *BJU Int* 2004; **94**(4):507–515.

Naber KG, Bergman B, Bishop MC, et al., for Urinary Tract Infection (UTI) Working Group of the Health Care Office (HCO) of the European Association of Urology (EAU). EAU guidelines for the management of urinary and male genital tract infections. *Eur Urol* 2001;**40**(5):576–588.

Santucci RA, Wessells H, Bartsch G, et al. Evaluation and management of renal injuries: consensus statement of the renal trauma subcommittee. *BJU Int* 2004;**93**(7):937–954.

Talan DA, Stamm WE, Hooton TM, et al. Comparison of ciprofloxacin (7 days) and trimethoprim-sulfamethoxazole (14 days) for acute uncomplicated pyelonephritis in women: a randomized trial. *JAMA* 2000;**283**(12):1583–1590.

Tiselius HG. Epidemiology and medical management of stone disease. *BJU Int* 2003;**91**(8):758–767.

6   Trauma

22

Abdominal Trauma: Evaluation and Decision Making

Lesly A. Dossett[1] & Bryan A. Cotton[2]

[1]Department of Surgery, Vanderbilt University Medical Center, Nashville, TN, USA
[2]Department of Surgery and The Center for Translational Injury Research, The University of Texas Health Science Center at Houston, Houston, TX, USA,,

Introduction

Abdominal injuries are divided into blunt and penetrating categories based on the mechanism of injury. Blunt mechanism intra-abdominal injuries result from one of several mechanisms: (1) compression causing a crush injury, (2) an abrupt shearing force causing tears or (3) a sudden rise in intra-abdominal pressures causing a rupture of abdominal viscera. Motor vehicle crashes account for 75% of blunt abdominal injuries. Penetrating mechanism injuries result from lacerations or blast effect.

The abdomen includes three basic regions: (1) the peritoneal cavity with its intrathoracic component, (2) the retroperitoneum and (3) the pelvic portion. Because the diaphragm may rise as high as the fourth intercostal space, blunt and penetrating injuries to the lower chest may involve abdominal organs.

The evaluation of the patient with abdominal trauma begins with a focused history and physical examination, as time and the critical nature of the injury permits, and continues with adjuncts to the physical examination including laboratory investigations and abdominal sonography. As with the evaluation of all multi-trauma patients, the basic principles of the advanced trauma life support (ATLS®) course hold in the evaluation of patients with abdominal trauma.

The primary goals of the abdominal evaluation in the setting of trauma are (1) to identify whether or not an intra-abdominal injury is present and (2) to determine if the injury requires operative repair.

Blunt abdominal trauma

History

In the abdominal trauma patient who is able to provide a reliable history, the character and duration of any abdominal complaints is of particular importance. Worsening abdominal pain or tenderness may signal progression of a solid organ injury or a hollow viscus injury towards peritoneal irritation (from succus, bile or blood). Many patients, however, are unable to provide a history secondary to hypotension/haemorrhage, head injury, intoxication and endotracheal intubation. Therefore, it is important to obtain information from prehospital personnel regarding the time of injury, mechanism and use of restraint devices. A brief medical history including current medications, drug allergies and a history of prior abdominal surgery may be particularly helpful when available.

Physical examination

The physical examination begins with inspection of the front and back of the abdomen, the perineum and the lower chest. Visual inspection for bruising or abdominal distension and palpation for abdominal tenderness are key elements of the examination. Auscultation of the abdomen is rarely helpful. Palpation may detect localised or generalised tenderness, guarding or other signs of peritoneal irritation. A digital rectal examination can be performed to assess rectal tone and the presence of gross blood. A substantial proportion of trauma patients will have unreliable physical examinations because of associated head injuries, spinal cord injuries or intoxication. In these patients, a careful inspection for scars from previous surgery should be noted during the physical examination.

> The primary objective of the physical examination in abdominal trauma is to rapidly identify the patient who needs a laparotomy.

Laboratory evaluation

The majority of laboratory values obtained in the acute setting will provide little guidance to the work-up and management of the patient with blunt abdominal trauma. In patients who are to undergo computed tomography (CT) scan (regardless of the laboratory results) the only laboratory

Emergency Surgery, 1st edition. Edited by Adam Brooks, Peter F. Mahoney, Bryan A. Cotton and Nigel Tai. © 2010 Blackwell Publishing.

values likely to be of any benefit are a group and save (or cross-match).

In those patients that one wishes to avoid a CT scan, a handful of laboratory values may help to safely eliminate the possibility of intra-abdominal injury. Used in conjunction with a reliable, *completely* benign and atraumatic torso examination, a normal urinalysis and normal serum hepatic transaminases are likely to identify those patients that may be spared CT scan of the abdomen. The utility of other laboratory values, such as haemoglobin-haematocrit and amylase-lipase, lies in their being followed in a serial manner (e.g. – every six to eight hours) in patients with established intra-abdominal injuries who are being being managed non-operatively.

Plain radiography

Chest radiograph (CXR) is likely to be the only plain film of value in the evaluation of blunt abdominal trauma. A CXR, especially with a nasogastric tube in place, may help to identify an elevated or disrupted hemidiaphragm. Pelvic plain films are of benefit as a triage tool in those patients who arrive with haemodynamic abnormalities. They may help in identifying a fracture pattern with potential for haemodynamically significant blood loss.

Computed tomography

In the haemodynamically stable patient who sustains blunt abdominal trauma, CT of the abdomen and pelvis remains the preferred method of evaluation (Figure 22.1). CT scan can reliably identify solid organ injuries (including the presence of active extravasation) and free intraperitoneal fluid or air.

> Critical limitations of CT scan in abdominal trauma include identification of hollow viscus and diaphragmatic injuries.

Abdominal CT is very accurate in assessment of the liver, kidney and spleen. CT has limited value in identifying intra-abdominal injury to hollow viscus and the diaphragm. Findings suggestive of these injuries may include thickened bowel wall, asymmetric bowel wall enhancement, interloop fluid and free fluid not explained by other injuries. Free intra-abdominal fluid in the absence of solid organ injuries should prompt further evaluation for a hollow viscus injury. Women of childbearing age may have a small amount of physiologic free fluid in their pelvis ($\approx$50 cc). Patients greater than 24 hours from their injury who have been vigorously resuscitated may have ascites and interloop fluid due to a capillary leak syndrome.

Diagnostic peritoneal lavage

The open technique for diagnostic peritoneal lavage (DPL) consists of a small (2–5 cm) incision below the umbilicus and dissection of the subcutaneous tissue to the fascia. The fascia and peritoneum are opened sharply under direct

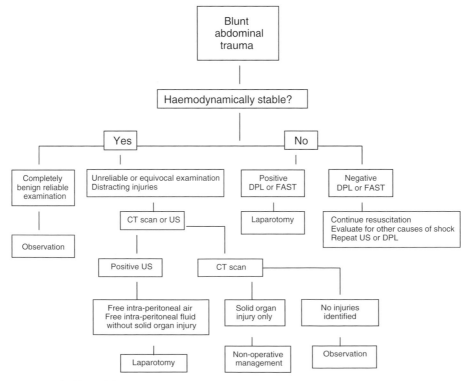

Figure 22.1 Evaluation algorithm for blunt abdominal trauma.

visualisation. A catheter is inserted through the opening and directed towards the pelvis. The percutaneous technique is performed in a Seldinger fashion by making a small (0.5 cm) incision below the umbilicus. A needle is inserted through the fascia until a 'give' is felt after penetration of the peritoneum. A syringe containing fluid may be used to confirm intraperitoneal placement. The syringe is disconnected and a guidewire is inserted through the needle. After serial dilation, a catheter is inserted and directed towards the pelvis.

If aspiration of the DPL catheter does not reveal gross blood, 1 L of warm saline is infused. The fluid is then siphoned back into the empty saline bag by lowering the bag below the level of the patient. A specimen of the recovered fluid is then examined macroscopically, microscopically and biochemically.

The major advantage of DPL is that it is very sensitive (>95%) for identifying intraperitoneal haemorrhage. However, because the technique is invasive and fails to identify the source of bleeding it is used with decreasing frequency. Additionally, because most solid organ injuries are now managed non-operatively, the specificity of DPL for identifying *operative* intra-abdominal injuries is quite low.

DPL currently has limited application in the initial evaluation of the patient with abdominal trauma. Indications for DPL in blunt trauma include the (1) unconscious patient with question of potential abdominal injury where CT is not available or they are unstable and the source is not readily identifiable and (2) the patient with high-energy injury, suspected intra-abdominal injury and an equivocal examination.

Focused assessment with sonography for trauma

Focused assessment with sonography for trauma (FAST) has largely replaced DPL as a rapid technique to evaluate for the presence of intra-abdominal free fluid. It is highly operator-dependent, and even in the best hands has relatively low specificity.

> Patients who remain hypotensive or labile in the presence of (+) FAST or DPL findings should undergo immediate laparotomy.

Four areas of the thoraco-abdomen are examined: the pericardial/subxiphoid region, the right upper quadrant (Morrison's pouch), the left upper quadrant and the pelvis/bladder.

In the hands of most operators, FAST will detect a minimum of 200 mL of fluid. Massive subcutaneous emphysema or morbid obesity can prevent a satisfactory examination. In addition, FAST is not a reliable method for excluding hollow viscus injury, or reliably grading solid organ injuries; therefore, FAST should be followed by a CT scan in patients who are haemodynamically stable and not proceeding directly to the operating theatre.

Rigid sigmoidoscopy

Rigid sigmoidoscopy is useful when evaluating the extraperitoneal rectum. Injuries to this part of the intestinal tract may not produce symptoms until septic complications prompt further investigation. In patients with suspected extraperitoneal rectal injuries, the digital rectal examination is often unreliable. Rigid sigmoidoscopy can be performed in the emergency department or operating room. Gross blood or other signs of injuries should prompt further evaluation and treatment.

Diagnostic laparoscopy

Diagnostic laparoscopy has a limited role in the evaluation of the blunt abdominal trauma patient. The major limitations of laparoscopy in this setting include the technical difficulty in 'running' the bowel, the inability to diagnose retroperitoneal injuries and the difficultly of adequately exposing deep lying organs such as the spleen.

Evaluation of the urogenital tract

Patients who sustain blunt intra-abdominal injury are also at risk for injury to the urogenital tract. The injuries can have a delayed presentation and a high index of suspicion is necessary to promptly identify these injuries. Gross blood at the urethral meatus, or gross haematuria should prompt further evaluation. Microscopic haematuria in the setting for haemodynamic instability is also an indication for evaluation of the urogenital tract.

Gross blood at the urethral meatus may signal an injury to the urethra, and a urinary catheter should not be placed blindly until this injury has been ruled out by a retrograde urethrogram. In the absence of gross blood, difficulty in placing a urinary catheter should also prompt either urologic consultation or a urethrogram. Injury to the female urethra is rare but should be suspected in the setting of vaginal bleeding or external genitalia injury.

Injury to the bladder is particularly common in patients with severe pelvic fractures. Gross haematuria is an indication for a cystogram which can be performed at the bedside or in the radiology suite. Plain radiographs after the injection of contrast through a urinary catheter and after evacuation of the contrast should be obtained. Free spillage of contrast in the abdomen (often visualised along the para-colic gutters) signals an intraperitoneal bladder rupture. Extravasation of contrast lateral to the bladder is often the result of an extraperitoneal bladder rupture. CT cystography is as accurate as conventional cystography and may be used interchangeably for the evaluation of bladder trauma.

The ureters are rarely injured from a blunt mechanism. Their integrity can be assessed with an intravenous pyelogram (IVP) or a delayed CT scan, but both tests have unacceptable high false-negative rates. A high index of suspicion must be maintained in order to detect these injuries. CT scan has the highest sensitivity and specificity for the evaluation of renal injuries and is the imaging modality of choice in patients suspected to have renal injuries.

Blood at the urethral meatus, gross haematuria or difficulty placing a urinary catheter may signal an injury to the urogenital tract.

Penetrating abdominal trauma

History

For penetrating injuries an attempt should be made to identify the weapon used.

A brief medical history including current medications, drug allergies and a history of prior abdominal surgery may be particularly helpful when available.

Physical examination

For penetrating injuries, determining trajectory is the single most important function of a physical examination or radiograph prior to laparotomy. The physical examination should involve a quick and focused survey for all skin wounds. Patients should be log rolled to provide a thorough inspection with careful attention to the axilla and perineum. All skin wounds should be marked with flat small radio-opaque objects (e.g. paperclips taped over the wound) if radiographs are to be performed. The addition of these markers can assist in approximating the trajectory of a missile, and therefore assist in the identification of likely injuries (Figure 22.2). Wounds located on the anterior abdomen have the highest likelihood of intra-abdominal injury, but flank and back wounds may also penetrate the peritoneum.

Uncontrolled haemorrhage or evisceration from penetrating wounds warrants immediate operative exploration.

Laboratory evaluation

The majority of laboratory values obtained in the acute setting will provide little guidance to the work-up and management of the patient with penetrating abdominal trauma. The only initial laboratory specimen likely to provide any benefit to the patient or physician is a group and save and cross-match.

Plain radiography

Chest and pelvic radiographs can be useful to identify retained ballistic fragments and estimating a trajectory of gun-

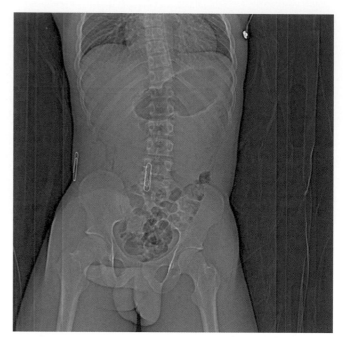

Figure 22.2 Application of radio-opaque markers to penetrating wounds to assist in trajectory, and hence injury, identification.

shot wounds to the abdomen. All wounds should be marked with paperclips prior to the radiographs. Adequate films should include both diaphragms and the pelvis in the case of penetrating abdominal trauma. Given the nature of ballistic fragments not respecting the boundaries of the chest and abdomen (not to mention the potential lethality of a missed intra-thoracic injury), patients who sustain ballistic injuries to the abdomen and pelvis should have a chest radiograph obtained immediately upon arrival. Patients who sustain penetrating knife injuries to the upper abdomen should also undergo chest radiography to rule out intra-thoracic injury.

Computed tomography

In addition to its role in blunt abdominal trauma, CT can be of use in the evaluation of the patient with penetrating abdominal trauma. High-resolution CT scans can often accurately identify missile tracts and in some cases, identify patients who do not need operative exploration. This is especially helpful for wounds in the pelvic, gluteal, thoracoabdominal (right diaphragm) and flank areas (Figure 22.3a and b).

Local wound exploration

A local wound exploration (LWE) can be performed when physical examination and/or imaging studies are inconclusive as to whether or not a stab wound has violated the anterior abdominal fascia. LWE can be performed at the bedside with a local anaesthetic and basic instrument

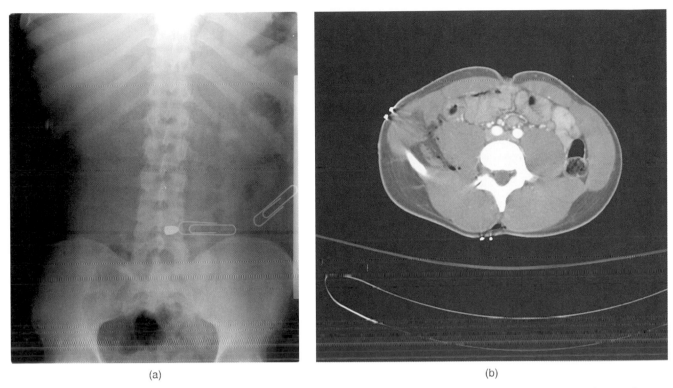

(a)   (b)

Figure 22.3 (a) Radio-opaque markers (paper clips) provide two-dimensional trajectory of the ballistic fragment and allow for the identification of 'one-hole, one-bullet'. (b) CT scan demonstrating retroperitoneal trajectory of the ballistic fragment; thereby excluding the need for operative management of intra-abdominal injury.

tray. An incision should be made and carried down to the level of the fascia to determine whether or not there is a violation of the anterior fascia. If the anterior fascia has been violated, a laparoscopy may be performed to assess for peritoneal violation, in which case or when posterior fascial penetration cannot be ruled out a full exploratory laparotomy should be performed in the operating room. LWE can be difficult in obese or uncooperative patients.

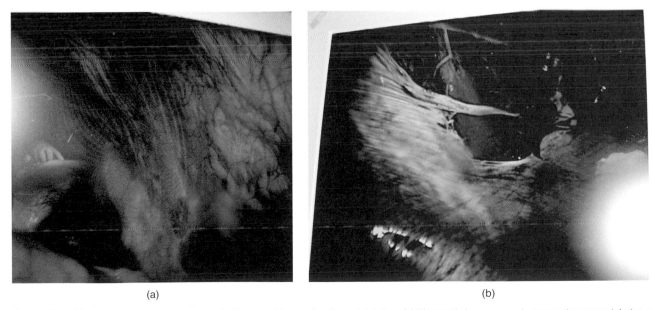

(a)   (b)

Figure 22.4 (a) Diagnostic laparoscopy demonstrating no evidence of peritoneal violation. (b) Diagnostic laparoscopy demonstrating gross violation of the peritoneum.

Laparoscopy

For stable patients with penetrating abdominal trauma, laparoscopy can have a role in evaluation, particularly when there is suspicion that the wound is tangential. In these cases, laparoscopy may avoid an unnecessary laparotomy and significantly shorten hospital length of stay for patients without peritoneal penetration (Figure 22.4a). Findings of peritoneal penetration at laparoscopy warrant full abdominal exploration (Figure 22.4b). This can be performed either via laparoscopy or via conversion to a laparotomy. Accurate exploration of the abdomen using a laparoscope is highly operator-dependent and carries a higher risk of missed injuries.

Rigid sigmoidoscopy

Penetrating injuries with trajectories near the rectum should be evaluated with rigid sigmoidoscopy. Gross blood or other signs of injuries should prompt further evaluation and treatment.

Evaluation of the urogenital tract

Patients who sustain penetrating intra-abdominal injury are also at risk for injury to the urogenital tract. Suspected trajectories that may involve the kidney, ureter, bladder or urethra should prompt further evaluation.

Penetrating injury to the bladder is typically discovered at laparotomy. Patients who are otherwise candidates for non-operative management, but are at risk for a bladder injury should undergo conventional or CT cystography.

Most ureteral injuries are the result of gunshot wounds. Both IVP and CT are unreliable in excluding these injuries since they have high false-negative rates. Patients with colonic injuries are at high risk for concurrent ureteral injury and the ureters should be inspected at the time of operation.

Unnecessary laparotomies versus missed abdominal injuries

The incidence of unnecessary (non-therapeutic) laparotomies for trauma varies from 2 to 38% and depends on the experience and policies of individual trauma centres. Morbidities directly related to a non-therapeutic laparotomy or the associated anaesthesia can be as high as 25%. The reported incidence of delayed diagnosis in patients with penetrating abdominal injuries selected for non-operative management is about 3.5%.

Further reading

Brooks AJ, Civil I, Braslow B, Schwab CW. Abdomen and pelvis. In: Mahoney PF, Ryan J, Brooks AJ, Schwab CW, eds. *Ballistic Trauma: A Practical Guide*, 2nd edn. Springer-Verlag, London, 2005.

Cotton BA. Blunt abdominal trauma. In: Brooks AJ, Mahoney PF, Hodgetts TJ, et al., eds. *Churchill's Pocketbook of Major Trauma*. Elsevier, Edinburgh, UK, 2007.

Simeone AA, Frankel H, Velmahos G. Abdominal injury. In: Peitzman AB, Rhodes M, Schwab CW, Yealy DM, Fabian TC, et al., eds. *The Trauma Manual: Trauma and Acute Care Surgery*, 3rd edn. Lippincott Williams & Wilkins, Philadelphia, PA, 2008.

23

Thoracic Trauma: Evaluation and Decision Making

Stella R. Smith[1], Thomas König[2] & Nigel Tai[2,3]

[1] Department of Surgery, The Royal London Hospital, London, UK
[2] Defence Medical Services, Trauma Clinical Academic Unit, Royal London Hospital, Whitechapel, London, UK
[3] Academic Department of Military Surgery and Trauma, Royal Centre for Defence Medicine, Birmingham, UK

Introduction

Thoracic trauma accounts for 25% of all trauma fatalities in the UK. Only 10% of patients with thoracic trauma require surgical intervention and the majority can be managed conservatively with supportive therapy (oxygen and pain relief) and a chest drain where necessary. The key task in thoracic trauma is to rapidly identify the sickest subset of patients who merit urgent surgical or critical care interventions (Table 23.1).

Anatomy

Mechanisms and patterns of injury

Blunt mechanisms

Blunt chest trauma is predominantly due to road traffic accidents and falls from height. Fractures of the first and second ribs, sternum and scapulae are particularly indicative of a high-energy mechanism. Fractures of the first rib may be associated with injury to the brachial plexus, sympathetic chain and subclavian artery. Sternal fractures may be with blunt cardiac injury and traumatic aortic disruption. Fractures of the scapulae frequently coexist with underlying pulmonary contusion in 50% of cases.

Penetrating mechanisms

Penetrating injuries are caused by gunshots and stabbing implements, e.g. knives and machetes. Ballistic wounds are classified by the energy transferred to the tissue with those missiles with greater kinetic energy having the most potential to cause extensive tissue destruction. However, the relative elasticity of aerated lung parenchyma rarely retards the passage of such missiles sufficiently to allow for high-energy exchange, meaning that lung may be spared from the more

devastating consequences observed when rounds encounter denser tissues such as bone or liver.

Blast injury

Damage to the delicate alveolar structures can occur from exposure to the peak overpressure associated with the initial blast wave and result in alveolar haemorrhages, oedema and an exudative response manifested as bilateral pulmonary infiltrates on chest X-ray (CXR) – 'blast lung'. This condition is a marker of poor outcome and is an early cause of death in patients exposed to 'contained' explosions initiated in a building or semi-closed structure such as a bus.

Initial assessment and resuscitation

Primary survey

The initial in-patient assessment of all trauma patients should follow Advanced Trauma Life Support (ATLS®) guidelines to identify and treat life-threatening conditions. Rapid evaluation by a well coordinated and resourced team practising 'horizontal' resuscitation is ideal.

- The standard mantra of 'ABC' should be supplemented by a preliminary check for massive haemorrhage with swift control of any bleeding wounds as the primary survey progresses (C-ABC).
- A full but rapid examination of the thorax (inspection, palpation/percussion, auscultation – Tables 23.2 and 23.3) to rapidly assess for the presence of the 'lethal six' and intervene as appropriate.
  - Airway obstruction
  - Tension pneumothorax
  - Massive haemothorax
  - Open pneumothorax
  - Cardiac tamponade
  - Flail chest
- During this phase, IV access is established or refined, blood is drawn for cross-matching and arterial blood gas analysis, echocardiography (ECG) and oxygen saturation monitoring equipment is placed and a CXR and focused

Emergency Surgery, 1st edition. Edited by Adam Brooks, Peter F. Mahoney, Bryan A. Cotton and Nigel Tai. © 2010 Blackwell Publishing.

Table 23.1 Decision making in major thoracic trauma.

Key questions:
- Is patient stable?
  - Pulse, blood pressure, respiratory rate, saturations and mentation
  - Blood gas analysis
- Is the chest injury the cause of instability?
  - Injury mechanism, pattern of injuries, signs and symptoms
  - Triage of body cavities: CXR, PXR, FAST scan
- What adjuncts to stabilisation does the patient need?
  - Oxygen therapy
  - Intravenous fluid resuscitation, blood product transfusion
  - Needle thoracentesis
  - Pain relief
- What stabilisation manoeuvres does the patient need?
  - Intubation, ventilation and surgical airway
  - Tube thoracostomy +/− suction for airway leak
  - Thoracotomy and relief of tamponade, hilar clamp or aortic compression
- What definitive investigations does the patient need?
  - CT
  - CTA
  - Bronchoscopy
  - Oesophagoscopy
  - Angography
  - Echocardiogram
- What definitive surgical repairs does the patient need?
  - Repair of arch vessels (stent and open)
  - Repair of aorta (stent and open)
  - Repair of myocardial injury
  - Repair/resection for major airway leak
  - Repair of oesphageal injury
  - Repair of diaphragmatic injury
- What are the *patient* complicating factors?
  - Elderly patient, pre-existing COAD and IHD
  - Polytrauma: head, pelvic and limb injuries
- What are the *logistical* complicating factors?
  - Hospital facilities (interventional radiology and cardiothoracic support)
  - ICU/HDU bed availability
  - Blood requirement

Table 23.2 Thoracic examination in trauma patients.

Exposure	Neck to waist
Observation	Any obvious injuries? – examine the back early in penetrating trauma
	Distress – ? air hunger
	Respiratory rate and depth
	Breathing pattern – shallow and deep
	Chest wall movement – asymmetrical and flail segment
	Cyanosis – late sign
	Distended neck veins
Palpation	Trachea – central or deviated (late sign)
	Subcutaneous emphysema
	Expansion – equal or reduced on one side
	Tenderness or obvious bony disruption
Percussion	Dull, resonant or hyper-resonant
Auscultation	Breath sounds – listen in axillae, apices and posteriorly – normal or reduced, one or both sides
	Heart sounds – normal or muffled

Investigations

Chest X-ray (see Skill Box 23.1)
- Supine films are less sensitive for detecting haemopneumothoraces and diaphragmatic injuries.
- Heart size and mediastinum may be artefactually widened by AP projections.
- Fractures of the first and second ribs and scapulae are indicative of a high-force injury and a high index of suspicion should be for great vessel injury, cardiac contusions and severe lung contusions.

Focused Assessment with Sonography in Trauma
- Four areas examined: pelvis, perihepatic, perisplenic and pericardial.
- Extended FAST (eFAST) involves additional examination of pleural movement to check for presence of pneumothorax and pleural cavity to assess for presence of fluid (blood).

Computed tomography
- Computed tomography (CT) scan is established as the most valuable imaging modality in major chest trauma:
  - Evaluation of arch/great vessels (CT angiography)
  - Assessment of vertebral fractures
  - Volume of haemothorax/pneumothorax; position of chest drain
  - Trajectory of cross-torso ballistic injuries and relation to mediastinal structures
  - Concordant assessment of intracranial, intra-abdominal and pelvic injuries
- CT is fast and 64 slice machines can complete a torso scan within 30 seconds; but the movement to and from the CT

assessment with sonography in trauma (FAST) scan is performed – within the resuscitation suite to allow triage of the body cavities for bleeding within a controlled environment.

- In general, the IV fluid management of shocked patients with penetrating thoracic trauma should be undertaken according to the principles of hypotensive resuscitation (target systolic blood pressure of 90 mm Hg) and damage control resuscitation (1:1 transfusion of packed cells to plasma) in order to prevent 'popping the clot' and minimise traumatic coagulopathy. Such techniques are adjuncts to definitive surgical control of haemorrhage and do not lessen the urgency to stop the bleeding.

Table 23.3 Signs of commonly presenting conditions in chest trauma.

Condition	Signs				
	Haemodynamic stability	Chest wall movement	Trachea	Percussion note	Breath sounds
Airway obstruction	Unstable	Reduced, accessory muscle use and intercostal recession	Central or deviated	Normal	Reduced bilaterally
Tension pneumothorax	Unstable	Decreased	Deviated away from side of tension	Hyper-resonant	Decreased or absent
Open pneumothorax (sucking chest wound)	Unstable	Decreased and obvious injury	Central	Hyper-resonant	Decreased
Massive haemothorax	Unstable	Decreased	Central	Dull	Decreased
Cardiac tamponade	Unstable	Normal	Central	Normal	Normal
Flail chest	Stable	Paradoxical	Central	Normal	Normal or decreased
Simple pneumothorax	Stable	Decreased	Central	Hyper-resonant or normal	Normal or decreased
Simple haemothorax	Stable	Decreased	Central	Dull	Normal or decreased

suite, plus time to safely transfer the patient on to the scanner, still makes CT unsafe in the evaluation of hypotensive patients.

Specific thoracic injuries

There are a 'deadly dozen' chest injuries. Six of these should be identified and treated in the primary survey (the lethal six as above). The presence of simple pneumothorax, haemothorax and fractured ribs may be inferred from clinical examination, CXR and e-FAST early on in the resuscitation process. Six other, subtler injuries that may be missed and cause late mortality include pulmonary contusion, blunt cardiac injury, tracheo-bronchial injury, traumatic aortic disruption, traumatic diaphragmatic rupture and oesophageal injury.

Cardiac tamponade
• Usually results from penetrating trauma; but; occasionally as a result of high energy blunt trauma.
• Blood from an injured great vessel, cardiac chamber, coronary or pericardial vessel accumulates in the restrictive, fibrous pericardial sac and restricts diastolic filling – 15–20 mL is sufficient to produce shock.
• The typical clinical picture is of a shocked, very agitated patient who bears a penetrating wound to the 'Box' (bounded by the nipples, the jugular notch and the xiphisternum):

   ○ Beck's triad (hypotension, distended neck veins and muffled heart sounds), pulsus paradoxus (systolic blood pressure falling by more than 10 mm Hg in inspiration) and Kussmaul's sign (raised jugular venous pressure with inspiration) may be observed.
   ○ Neck vein distension may be absent in hypovolaemia, or may be the result of a tension pneumothorax.
   ○ The most helpful investigation is the FAST examination to detect intrapericardial blood. Whilst this test is very specific, sensitivity is reduced and there is a 5–10% false-negative rate, heightened by the presence of associated haemothorax.
   ○ Other features may include a globular heart on CXR and low-voltage ECG complexes.
• Thoracotomy, pericardiotomy and repair of the injury are the definitive treatment.
• This may be required immediately in the resuscitation bay in cases where circulatory collapse has occurred or is imminent (BP < 70 systolic), or may be done in theatre if the patient is sufficiently well to allow transfer.
• There is no place for percardiocentesis in the diagnosis of tamponade (low sensitivity and specificity).

Tension pneumothorax
• Displacement of mediastinal structures secondary to pressurised air within the pleural space ingressing from a breach of the chest wall (penetrating injury) or disruption of an airway structure (blunt injury).

> **Skill Box 23.1 A systematic approach to examining a CXR performed for trauma**
>
> - Identification – check the name, hospital number and date
> - Side – differentiate left from right
> - Quality
>   - Rotation – the spinous process of T4 should be between the heads of the clavicle
>   - Penetration – in a properly penetrated film the vertebral interspaces should be visible behind the central (cardiac) shadow. Penetration can be altered on modern computer X-ray images
>   - Respiration – ideally chest X-rays are performed during full inspiration
> - Soft tissue – look for subcutaneous emphysema, soft tissue swelling and fragments
> - Bone – look for fractures
>   - Ribs – number, side, flail segment, any first or second rib fractures?
>   - Scapulae
>   - Clavicles
>   - Spine – alignment of spinous processes
>   - Humerus
> - Lungs
>   - Pneumothorax
>   - Haemothorax
>   - Contusions
>   - Apical cap – indicates aortic rupture
> - Cardiac shadow
>   - Widened or aneurismal
>   - Borders – an indistinct heart border may indicate lobar collapse
> - Mediastinum
>   - Widened – a wide mediastinum suggests great vessel injury
>   - Midline shift – caused by blood or air
>   - Aortic knuckle – loss of definition in aortic rupture
>   - Air
> - Hila – depression of left main bronchus or loss of space between aorta and pulmonary artery can indicate aortic rupture
> - Abdomen – look for free abdominal air
> - Tubes
>   - Endotracheal – correctly placed just above carina and deviated
>   - Nasogastric tube – in chest or abdomen and deviated

- Air does not escape through the breach due to a 'flap valve' effect with consequent mediastinal shift, kinking of large veins and reduction in cardiac filling.
- Usually associated with positive pressure ventilation; infrequent in spontaneously breathing patients.
- Clinical features include:
  - Sudden drop in saturations in ventilated patient without evidence of tube dislodgement
  - Hyper-resonant percussion note and reduced breath sounds on the affected side
  - Neck vein distension (not if coexistent severe haemorrhage)
  - tachycardia and hypotension
  - tracheal deviation (a very late sign)

- Differentiate from cardiac tamponade (careful elicitation of the percussion note and auscultation may aid discrimination).
- Treatment:
  - CXR is usually not required to make the diagnosis, and action should not be deferred.
  - Immediate large bore needle decompression in the second intercostal space, mid-clavicular line of the affected side.
  - Characteristic 'hiss' of air may or may not be heard on removal of the needle.
  - Failure to achieve immediate improvement in patient condition requires default to thoracostomy followed by chest drain placement.
  - Chest drain placement should also follow the 'successful' needle decompression, as the tension will likely (quickly) recur.

Simple pneumothorax

- Air enters the pleural space and causes the underlying lung to collapse as intrapleural pressure equilibrates with atmospheric pressure.
- CXR features include:
  - Visible lung edge with absent lung markings beyond
  - Deep sulcus sign: this is where the hemidiaphragm on the affected side is deeper in the midline than expected
- Treatment involves chest drainage (see Skill Box 23.2).
- Very small pneumothoraces (<10% of the volume of the affected hemithorax) may be managed conservatively if repeat clinical reassessment and repeat CXRs are satisfactory (positive pressure ventilation and extra-hospital transfer are contraindications to conservative management).
- The key elements of inpatient management include adequate pain relief and early mobilisation to assist lung re-expansion.
- The drain should be removed once it has stopped 'swinging' (movement of fluid meniscus < 2 cm with inspiration), draining (<25 mL/day) and clinical examination is consistent with full lung expansion. A single post-removal CXR is taken to confirm that there is no re-accumulation of pneumothorax prior to discharge.

Open pneumothorax

- Marked reduction of alveolar ventilation due to preferential movement of air through a large chest wall 'sucking' defect (at least 2/3 the diameter of the trachea) instead of via the major airway.
- Associated with large pneumothorax, severe hypoxia and hypercarbia.
- Initial treatment options:
  - Asherman chest seal
  - Occlusive wound dressing taped on three sides (flutter-valve allowing air out on expiration)

Skill Box 23.2 Chest drain insertion (Figure 23.2)

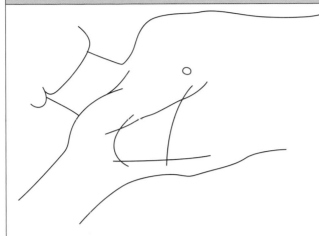

1 Set up the chest drain kit
   a. Pour the sterile water into the bottle up to the correct level and insert the tubing to create an underwater seal.
   b. Open the chest drain kit or suture pack. Place a gown and sterile gloves onto the pack. Open the drain, 2/0 nylon suture (or similar) and scalpel.
2 If the patient is conscious, infiltrate local anaesthetic (1% lidocaine), along the upper border of the 6th rib and down between the intercostals to the parietal pleura.
3 Prepare the area with antiseptic solution and drape.
4 Make a 2-cm incision, through skin and fat, along the upper border of the 6th rib within the 'triangle of safety': anterior to the mid axillary line, posterior to the lateral border of the pectoralis muscle and superior to the 6th rib. – Figure 23.2.
5 Bluntly dissect through intercostal muscles with arterial forceps down to pleura.
6 Open the pleura by perforating the membrane with the forceps in a controlled manner.
7 Digitally explore the pleural cavity; confirm entry and assess state of underlying lung (inflated and collapsed), presence of adhesions.
8 Replace digit with a large (36 French) drain directed with the assistance of arterial forceps (upwards and anteriorly for a suspected pneumothorax, downwards and posteriorly for a suspected haemothorax) ensuring at least 10 cm of tubing is intrapleural.
9 Connect the drain to the underwater seal.
10 Secure the drain with a robust skin suture.
11 Check the drain is bubbling or draining. Do not clamp.

   ○ Ipsilateral chest drain placed remotely from the wound on the affected side with occlusive dressing
• Definitive treatment:
   ○ Surgical closure of defect (muscle transposition and flap coverage)
   ○ Diaphragmatic transposition to exclude defect from pleural cavity

Flail chest

• Two or more adjacent rib fractures in two or more places results in isolation of a segment of the chest wall that has lost bony continuity with the rest of the thoracic cage. Hypoxia is common and due to:
   ○ Underlying pulmonary contusion (usually severe)
   ○ Ventilatory mechanical inefficiency of flail segment
   ○ Associated pain causing inhibition of ventilation, coughing and deep breathing
• Clinical features include:
   ○ Asymmetrical 'paradoxical' chest movement (segment moves outwards on expiration, inwards on inspiration) – not observed if patient ventilated or if 'splinting' chest wall due to pain
   ○ Crepitus of rib fractures, reduced expansion and abnormal chest wall movement on palpation
   ○ Reduced air entry on affected side
   ○ Hypoxia on arterial blood gas; reduced saturations on pulse oximetry
• Treatment consists of:
   ○ Transfer to high dependency unit/intensive care unit
   ○ Humidified high flow oxygen to maintain saturations >95%
   ○ Aggressive analgesia and pain control. A thoracic epidural should be used assuming that the patient is haemodynamically stable. Patient-controlled infusion of opiates is an alternative although ventilatory effort may be prejudiced due to narcosis
   ○ Early involvement of anaesthetic expertise in order to plan for subsequent respiratory failure (arterial $pO_2 < 8$ kPA; respiratory rate of >30; rising pCO_2 on serial venous gases)
   ○ Intubation and ventilation may be avoided by early application of continuous positive pressure ventilation therapy in deteriorating patients
   ○ Chest physiotherapy in order to maximise clearance of bronchial secretions
   ○ Scrupulous monitoring of fluid balance and careful titration of IV fluids   the injured lung will rapidly become oedematous if overloaded
   ○ Rarely, surgical fixation of flail segments is indicated in patients with gross mechanical instability in order to assist efforts to wean the patient from mechanical ventilation

Rib fractures

• Patients with fractures of ribs 8–12 should be suspected of having sustained injury to liver, spleen or kidney.
• First or second rib fractures require further investigation by CT to rule out injuries such as great vessel trauma and severe pulmonary contusions.
• Clinical features:
   ○ Localised tenderness with crepitus or subcutaneous emphysema

  ◦ Pleuritic pain
• Balanced analgesia (paracetamol, NSAID and oral opiate) is the key to managing these injuries.

Pulmonary contusion
• Pulmonary contusion represents the damage to lung parenchyma caused by the transmission of a high energy blunt force to the thorax.
• A potentially lethal condition in which respiratory failure develops over hours to days.
• Often associated with overlying fractures to ribs, sternum or scapula, although less so in children due to flexibility of the young bony skeleton.
• May accompany haemothorax, flail chest, lobar collapse/atlectasis or occur in isolation with significant shunt.
• Key diagnostic task is to differentiate evolving contusion from other causes of respiratory failure in the trauma patient (ventilator-associated pneumonia, acute lung injury/ARDS).
• The CXR demonstrates patchy interstitial shadowing, although these changes may be delayed for 48 hours. CT thorax (pulmonary windows) can determine volume of contusion and aid prognosis.
• Treatment priorities as per flail chest, with lung-protective ventilation strategies (low-tidal volumes) to prevent baro- and volutrauma in vulnerable pulmonary parenchyma.

Massive haemothorax (Figure 23.1)
• Defined as the rapid accumulation of more than 1500 mL (or one third of the circulating blood volume) in a pleural cavity, as measured on subsequent chest drainage.
• Results in both respiratory and cardiovascular compromise so the clinical picture is one of shock with hypoxia.
• Frequently associated with the requirement to definitively control haemorrhage via thoracotomy.
• Clinical features include:
  ◦ Shock
  ◦ Dullness to percussion and absent/reduced breath sounds on affected side (anterior chest exam may be normal due to fluid dependency)
• Treatment:
  ◦ Chest drainage
  ◦ Ongoing resuscitation with blood product
  ◦ Thoracotomy (urgent)
• Chest drain output may be misleading if the drain becomes blocked; ongoing shock despite cessation of output mandates a further CXR to appraise the thoracic cavity as part of a strategy to re-triage the body cavities for sources of haemorrhage.
• In the context of less acute presentations of haemothorax, the continued loss of more than 200 mL per hour or more of blood from a chest tube over a 4-hour period is traditionally used as an indication for thoracotomy.

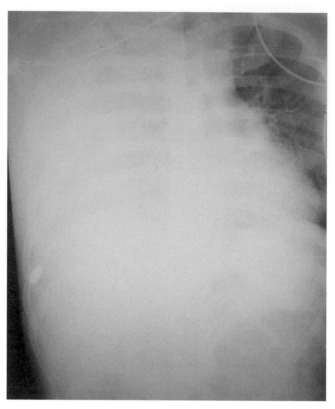

Figure 23.1 Massive haemothorax secondary to a thoracic gunshot wound – note bullet in right thoracoabdominal junctional zone.

Haemothorax
• These bleeds are usually self-limiting (15% require operative intervention) but must be drained in order to encourage lung expansion and optimal ventilation, and to reduce the risk of infection (empyema) or the development of a fibrous 'cortex'.

Tracheobronchial tree injury
• These injuries are the result of penetrating or blunt (deceleration) mechanisms that injure the major intrathoracic airways (distal trachea and large bronchi).
• Signs and symptoms are dependent upon the site of the airway breach with respect to the pleural reflection: i.e. extrapleural (proximal) or intrapleural (distal) injury.
• Extrapleural injuries (proximal airway) are associated with stridor and massive subcutaneous emphysema.
• Intrapleural injuries are associated with large pneumothorax, low saturations even on very high FiO_2, severe difficulties in mechanical ventilation, persistent air leak from a chest drain manifested as excessive bubbling throughout the respiratory cycle.
• Early involvement of critical care staff is mandatory. Other steps:

○ Passage of the endotracheal tube beyond the site of injury for extrapleural injuries followed by in-theatre fibre-optic inspection of the injury and definitive repair
○ Intrapleural injury:
 – Insertion of a second chest drain with application of high volume, low pressure suction
 – Intubation with a double lumen tube and selective ventilation
 – Thoracotomy: repair of bronchus, resection or lobectomy as required

Blunt cardiac injury

• Blunt injury to the heart can result in chamber rupture, valvular disruption or cardiac contusion. Rib or sternal fractures may be present, although blunt cardiac injury is present in less than 20% of sternal fractures.
• The classic presentation is one of sinus tachycardia (following blunt chest injury) that is refractory to generous pain medication and adequate volume expansion.
• Chamber rupture typically presents as a tamponade, which may be slow to develop if the atria are ruptured.
• Serious cardiac contusion presents with hypotension, tachycardia +/− arrhythmias (multiple premature ventricular ectopics, bundle branch block (right) in a casualty with no other explanation for shock.
• The mainstay of diagnosis is a standard 12-lead ECG. Troponin measurements do not confer any additional benefit. ECG is useful in excluding valvular injury.

• The risk of significant dysrhythmias is high within the first 24 hours and at-risk patients should remain on continuous cardiac monitoring in a monitored bed for this period.
• Arrhythmia is treated according to standard ACLS guidelines.

Traumatic aortic disruption

• Usually fatal: of those who present to hospital the majority have a contained tear at the aortic isthmus (segment between the left subclavian artery and ligamentum arteriosum) resulting in a false aneurysm.
• Specific signs of traumatic aortic disruption are usually absent and a CXR can be helpful but is not very sensitive, especially in a supine view. CT angiography scanning should be used liberally in patients with a wide mediastinum, high-energy injury or fractured 1st rib, 2nd rib, sternum or scapula. CXR signs include:
 ○ Widened mediastinum
 ○ Obliteration of the aortic knuckle
 ○ Tracheal deviation to the right
 ○ Obliteration of space between pulmonary artery and aorta (obscured AP window)
 ○ Depressed left main bronchus
 ○ Deviation of oesophagus (nasogastric tube) to right
 ○ Widened paratracheal tissues or paraspinal interfaces
 ○ Pleural or apical cap
 ○ Left haemothorax
• Endovascular stenting has gained increased popularity and may soon become the mainstay of treatment, as it appears to

Table 23.4 Complications of chest drain insertion.

Complication	Notes
Haemothorax	This occurs when the intercostal vessels are lacerated on insertion of the drain. To avoid this, the tract should always be made over the top of the 6th rib, rather than directly under the 5th rib.
Lung laceration	This occurs when the lung underneath is inadvertently damaged as the chest drain is inserted. Care must be employed when using forceps to penetrate the pleura. Adhesions can result from lung lacerations. These reduce lung expansion and predispose to infection.
Inappropriately placed drain	Selection of an inappropriately low intercostal space or failure to recognise visceral herniation via a ruptured diaphragm can result in injury to abdominal organs. Unguarded and over forceful puncture of the pleura or a "plunging" trochar can result in catastrophic damage to the mediastinum.
Pain	This is usually due a drain placed in too far; it should be pulled back.
Subcutaneous emphysema	This occurs when the drain is not in far enough or has slipped; it should be advanced or replaced.
Ineffective drain	The drain has either been placed subcutaneously or has slipped out of the pleural cavity. Sometimes drains can be become blocked with clot or lung (particularly when sitting in a fissure). These should be re-sited.
Retained haemothorax	Clotted blood will not drain. Requires video-assisted thoracoscopy, wash-out and drainage. Can occasionally be managed with intra-pleural instillation of thrombolytic agents and ultrasound guided drainage.
Empyema	Pleural collection (pus) secondary to infection of a retained haemothorax. May be avoided by proper aseptic technique during chest drain insertion and adequate drainage of intra-pleural blood. Treated with directed antibiotic therapy, ultrasound guided drainage +/− video-assisted thoracoscopy and washout. Occasionally requires formal thoracotomy, washout and rib resection/decortication procedure.
Persistent pneumothorax	Removing a chest drain too early when air is continuing to leak from damaged lung will result in re-accumulation of a pneumothorax. A further drain is required. If pneumothorax still persists an airway(tracheo-bronchial tree) injury should be suspected.

carry significantly less morbidity than standard open repair while achieving equivalent short and medium-term outcomes.

• In shocked patients stenting can be deferred until incompressible haemorrhage from other sources (abdomen and pelvis) has been addressed.

Traumatic diaphragmatic rupture

• Occurs more commonly on the left than right where the liver protects the diaphragm or obliterates the defect.

• Blunt trauma produces large radial tears through which the stomach and bowel can herniate acutely into the chest. Penetrating trauma results in smaller lesions and the hernia can take years to develop.

• Clinical features include:
  ○ Reduced air-entry and presence of bowel sounds on side of rupture
  ○ Palpation of bowel loops/stomach during chest drain insertion (Table 23.4)

• Features on CXR include:
  ○ Stomach or air-filled loops of bowel in the chest
  ○ A nasogastric tube in the chest
  ○ May be confused with an elevated diaphragm or loculated haemopneumothorax

• A CT scan or gastrograffin swallow can aid the diagnosis and should be used where these injuries are suspected although a small diaphragmatic breach may well be missed without accompanying herniation.

• Thoracoscopy/laparoscopy is the required step if the diagnosis is equivocal.

• Surgical repair is always needed. This may occasionally be accomplished at laparoscopy, although the need to evaluate and repair accompanying visceral trauma necessitates formal laparotomy in most cases.

Oesophageal trauma

• Oesophageal trauma usually observed in penetrating injury; occasionally seen in blunt trauma.

• In blunt trauma, the distal oesophagus usually ruptures and spills gastrointestinal contents into the left chest.

• Should be suspected in patients who have evidence of torso subcutaneous emphysema, mediastinal air on CXR and a left-sided pleural effusion.

• Gastric content in a chest drain is confirmatory. CT scanning, gastrograffin swallow and/or oesophagoscopy are the appropriate investigations.

• Urgent surgical repair is needed. Delayed diagnosis is associated with a much poorer outcome.

Summary

The vast majority of patients with thoracic trauma can be managed safely with chest drainage, analgesia and oxygen supplementation. A high index of suspension, vigilant observation and aggressive investigation are effective strategies in identifying the minority who require expeditious surgical intervention.

24 Vascular Trauma

Nigel Tai[1,2] & Nora Brennan[3]

[1]Defence Medical Services, Trauma Clinical Academic Unit, Royal London Hospital, Whitechapel, London, UK
[2]Academic Department of Military Surgery and Trauma, Royal Centre for Defence Medicine, Birmingham, UK
[3]The Royal London Hospital, Whitechapel, London, UK

Introduction

Vascular trauma can constitute an urgent threat to life and limb. Surgeons managing such patients have to gain rapid haemorrhage control, often in the setting of profound physiological disturbance, whilst planning for re-establishment of tissue perfusion. These factors, combined with the relative infrequency of vascular trauma and the poor tolerance of vascular structures to sub-optimal surgical technique, pose marked challenges to the on-call surgeon.

As with all major trauma, management of these patients begins around the primary survey of airway, breathing and circulation. This is especially important in the context of a mangled limb as the appearance can be shocking to the rest of the team and lead to an inappropriate prioritising of the limb injury over immediately life-threatening but less obvious injuries. However, this well-accepted paradigm of trauma care should not prevent the rapid control of exsanguinating extremity haemorrhage by concurrent application of directed pressure or tourniquet as the primary survey is initiated.

Mechanisms, injury patterns and sequelae

Penetrating injury to vessels from blades, cutting weapons and low-energy handgun bullets may result in vessel puncture, laceration or transection. Arterial transection facilitates vessel spasm and retraction, which in the shocked patient may lead to cessation of haemorrhage. Adaptive vessel spasm is less effective at reducing bleeding when axial continuity is maintained in simple lacerations, and bleeding is less likely to stop in this situation.

Blunt crushing or de-gloving mechanisms, with exposure and disruption of vasculature, may result in segmental con-

tusion or loss of vessel. Fracture dislocations, resulting from falls from height or motor vehicle accidents, may threaten vascular integrity through disruption of the intimal layer, with consequent peeling forwards of the delicate intima and the creation of a dissection flap with subsequent thrombosis. The popliteal artery and brachial artery are especially threatened by fracture-dislocations to the knee and elbow joints respectively.

Similar dissection flaps may be produced by the passage of a high energy military round, adjacent to a vessel, or by the transit of an explosive blast wave through the vessel wall, or by the damage caused by intraluminal instrumentation as a result of endovascular, radiological or cardiological misadventure. Miscellaneous causes of vascular injury include external compression from splints and plaster casts, extremes of temperature or injection of noxious agents. Trauma that results in perforation to adjacent segments of vein and artery may result in the establishment of an arteriovenous fistula.

The early consequences of vascular trauma include haemorrhage and/or ischaemia. Bleeding may be obvious due to external manifestation along a wound track – or concealed, with haemorrhage either restrained by surrounding soft tissues or unconstrained when bleeding occurs into a neighbouring body cavity. Haemorrhage that is constrained by the overlying soft tissue may eventually result in the development of a pseudo-aneurysm that either thromboses spontaneously or continues to grow, resulting in compression of adjacent tissues and eventual rupture with exsanguinating haemorrhage. The degree of limb ischaemia and tissue compromise will be dependent upon the proximity and site of injury and the extent of potential collateral circulation.

Emergency department assessment and management

Although vascular trauma may present dramatically, the clinical picture is often subtle and can easily be overlooked when attention is directed at competing injuries. A high degree of suspicion combined with careful and thorough

Emergency Surgery, 1st edition. Edited by Adam Brooks, Peter F. Mahoney, Bryan A. Cotton and Nigel Tai. © 2010 Blackwell Publishing.

evaluation is essential. This should include a careful debrief of the attending pre-hospital medical technicians to ensure that the mechanism of injury is completely understood and that the elapsed time of injury, time of any tourniquet application and witnessed arterial bleeding are recorded. The diagnosis of vascular trauma is essentially a clinical exercise with special investigations used to evaluate the site rather than confirm the presence of a significant injury. Senior vascular expertise should be sought at the earliest time once the diagnosis is suspected.

Initial key steps in extremity vascular trauma

1 If there is obvious and ongoing heavy bleeding, then this needs to be stemmed in the emergency department (ED) – even as other trauma team members are concurrently addressing the patient's airway and breathing. Evidence of ongoing haemorrhage includes obvious arterial bleeding, rapid soaking through of in situ dressings or pooling of blood on to the trauma trolley mattress or floor.

  ○ Tighten or reposition an ineffective in situ tourniquet if already applied by pre-hospital medical technicians to gain control whilst addressing other life-threatening injuries.
  ○ If no tourniquet is in situ, remove any ineffective dressings and evaluate wound.
  ○ Apply firm manual pressure over the bleeding point and maintain pressure.
  ○ Evaluate if bleeding is high or low pressure. Venous bleeding may be controlled with additional gauze and compressive bandaging. Arterial bleeding may be controlled by continued and direct manual pressure pending rapid transport to theatre or, if pressure cannot be maintained, the application of a pneumatic tourniquet above the bleeding point (documenting the time and site of application).
  ○ Application of surgical haemostats to bleeding vascular structures in the ED is not recommended unless lighting, suction, equipment, exposure, assistance and expertise is favourable. Better results are obtained in theatre!

2 If there is no obvious and heavy external haemorrhage, or if the above steps have succeeded in controlling the bleeding, further patient management consists of:
  ○ Appropriate primary survey
  ○ High flow oxygen
  ○ Establishment of large bore venous access (not in injured limb)
  ○ Drawing of blood for trauma panel and cross-match (four units packed cells per mangled limb with equivalent plasma volumes)
  ○ Full clinical survey of limb, documenting presence of HARD or SOFT vascular signs (Table 24.1) and alteration of motor or sensory function. The absence of hard signs effectively 'rules out' a significant vascular injury. Soft signs merely point towards the possibility of arterial injury and confirmatory investigations will be required.

Table 24.1 Hard and soft signs in vascular trauma.

Vascular trauma	Notes
Hard signs	
Active arterial bleeding	
Expanding haematoma	
Signs of end organ ischaemia	'6 P's: paralysis, paraesthesia, pallor, pain, pulselessness and poikilothermia Stroke or hemispheric signs in neck trauma
Bruit/thrill	Indicates AV fistula ('machinery murmur')
Expansile swelling	Indicates false aneurysm
Soft signs	
History of arterial bleeding	Check with pre-hospital staff
Wound close to major vascular structure	
Non-expanding haematoma	
Neurological deficit	

  ○ Assessment of external wounds, skin breaches and possible trajectory of penetration in penetrating mechanisms
  ○ Assessment of limb angulation and shortening if blunt mechanism, with reduction of fractures
  ○ There is little point in removing dressings to evaluate a compound extremity fracture in the ED when this diagnosis has already been established by pre-hospital medical staff. This is better done in theatre – which is where definitive care will be undertaken – in order to avoid further disturbance and contamination of tenuous soft tissues.

3 Pulses in an injured patient may be difficult to palpate if there is ongoing shock; the same caveat applies to the diagnostic value of assessing skin temperature and capillary refill in a cold, exposed trauma patient. However, isolated pulse abnormalities and significant asymmetry in pulse quality are strong indicators of underlying proximal vascular injury. Similarly, the presence of a distal pulse does not guarantee that there is not a vascular injury since collateralisation may compensate for proximal arterial trauma. The presence of pulses will be affected by any proximal tourniquet and, in older patients, by co-existent peripheral vascular disease.

4 Resuscitation room investigations:
  ○ Mobile plain X-ray of the affected limb (two views, two joints) is essential in gunshot wounds, blast fragmentation wounds and blunt trauma to gauge the presence of retained fragments and to assess skeletal integrity. Entry and exit wounds should be marked with a paper clip so that trajectory can be ascertained.
  ○ Hand-held Doppler (HHD) is a valuable adjunct to physical examination and can be used to assess the presence and quality of distal pulses. The Doppler probe should be held at 45–60° to the skin overlying the vessel. An acoustic gel should be used to obliterate air from the probe–skin

Table 24.2 Zones of the neck in vascular trauma.

Zone	Description	Notes
Zone I	From jugular notch to cricoid cartilage	Root of neck structures may be involved (subclavian and arch vessels). Proximal control may require median sternotomy
Zone II	From cricoid cartilage to angle of jaw	Carotid sheath structures may be involved. Proximal and distal control may be readily obtained via a standard full-length neck incision, anterior to sternocleidomastoid muscle
Zone III	Superior to angle of jaw	Distal internal carotid artery structures may be involved Gaining distal control and repair may require special manoeuvres (subluxation of the jaw and division of digastric, styloglossus muscles) or placement of an endovascular balloon/stent

interface and improve sound wave transmission. Used to generate an ankle-brachial pressure index (ABPI), the tool can rule out significant arterial injury if

- ABPI is >0.9
- ABPI does not differ from the contralateral limb by more than 20 mm Hg.

Initial key steps in cervical vascular trauma

1 The first step is to recognise the patient who requires early rapid sequence induction (RSI) and endotracheal intubation because of impending loss of airway. There is usually no doubt that the patient has a vascular injury. RSI is required when

- The patient presents with a rapidly swelling cervical haematoma
- The patient is coughing blood
- Signs of airway obstruction are present
- Manual compression is required to stem ongoing cervical bleeding

2 RSI for penetrating cervical vascular trauma may be very challenging due to inability to visualise the vocal cords on indirect laryngoscopy because of blood or displacement from haematoma and swelling. Such patients require.

- Expert anaesthetic input
- Presence of intubation adjuncts (bougie, difficult airway kit, flexible laryngoscope etc.)
- Availability of surgical tracheostomy kit, lighting and suction as a salvage option.

3 Haemorrhage should be concurrently stemmed by appropriate digital pressure of the bleeding tract.

4 Once airway control is achieved, or if it is not required, attention can be directed at characterising the physiological status of the patient, the site of the cervical injury and the likelihood that a major vascular structure has been injured (Table 24.1). Although the site of skin breach does not always tally with the location of the vascular injury, the 'zone' of the injury should be determined (see Table 24.3) as this will guide the preoperative planning.

5 A chest X-ray should be undertaken to rule out associated pneumo- or haemothorax and to assess trajectory in gunshot wounds.

ED decision making: investigate or operate?

Unstable patients with clear evidence of a vascular injury to the neck or extremity (i.e. the presence of hard signs) require definitive haemorrhage control and should be triaged to the operating theatre. In extremity trauma, if there is doubt around the exact site of the vascular injury (e.g. in those who have sustained multiple fragment or pellet injuries, or several bony fractures, related to the axial course of an artery along a limb) on-table angiography can assist the incision planning. In cervical trauma incisions should be planned around the zone of the injury. In junctional regions (root of the neck – zone I; para-inguinal injuries) the adjacent body cavity may need to be rapidly opened to gain proximal vascular control. Theatre and scrub staff should be briefed, thoracotomy/median sternotomy or laparotomy instruments should be ready and the patient must be prepped and towelled in accordance with the 'worst case scenario' principle (Table 24.2).

In stable patients, the assessing surgeon should now be in a position to triage the patient as either (1) vascular injury present and site identified, (2) vascular injury present but site obscure, (3) vascular injury possibly present and (4) vascular injury not present. Patients falling into either groups 2 or 3 require further vascular imaging – typically taking the patient away from the resuscitation area – whereas patients in groups 1 and 4 do not. Patients in group 1 may proceed to definitive vascular reconstruction – once prioritisation of management for other injuries is agreed – whereas patients in group 4 do not need further vascular imaging or treatment.

Further investigation

Computed tomography angiography

Modern multi-detector computed tomography angiography (CTA) has displaced formal contrast angiography as the primary mode of vascular imaging in many institutes (Figure 24.1). It is particularly useful in scrutinising cervicothoracic vascular injury. Whilst images can be gained rapidly, the modality involves transport of a potentially unstable patient

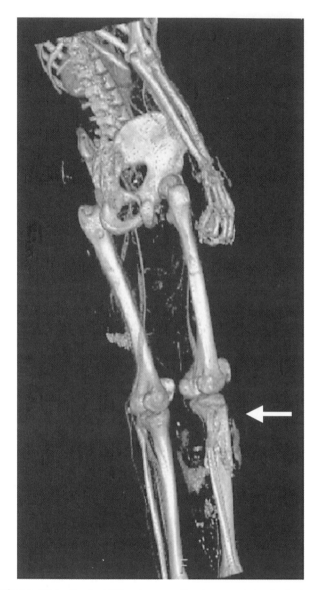

Figure 24.1 Contrast CT angiogram with volume rendering to display course of infrainguinal arterial tree in victim of left lower limb fragmentation injury. Image rotated to view popliteal vasculature from posterior viewpoint. Note lack of filling of popliteal artery and crural vessels on right (arrow).

to a hazardous area, exposure to a large radiation dose and nephrotoxic dye. The patient should be accompanied by the full trauma team who should discuss the suspected injury burden with the radiographer/radiologist in order that the best imaging protocol be selected. Logistic challenges include the integration and timing of vascular CTA protocols into an acquisition sequence that may also need to interrogate for the presence of other injuries to brain (uncontrasted scan) and abdominal viscera (porto-venous phase scan), and correct loading of the patient into the scanner (feet-first in lower limb CTA acquisition as opposed to head-first arrangement for standard trauma CT).

Intra-arterial digital subtraction angiography

The role of invasive contrast angiography for diagnosis alone has diminished, although the modality has superior utility in blast and gunshot injuries when the presence of retained metallic foreign bodies can significantly degrade the image quality of CTA. Apart from this indication, DSA is indicated prior to deployment of endovascular techniques to either control haemorrhage (balloon, coil and gelfoam) or to restore vessel continuity (covered stent).

Duplex ultrasonography

This non-invasive modality combines pulsed Doppler and B-mode (brightness) ultrasound imaging to yield information about vascular anatomy. In M (motion) mode blood flow and velocity can be measured. The technique requires skilled technicians, is highly operator-dependent and is rarely available out of office hours – curtailing utility for trauma patients.

Operative management

The decision-making process now proceeds to a choice between operative or endovascular management using either a definitive or a damage control approach.

Endovascular techniques

Compared to the marked shift towards endovascular procedures over open surgery in non-traumatic vascular disease, interventional radiology techniques have yet to find widespread applicability in trauma patients. Endovascular approaches remain favourable when vessel exposure may be technically difficult or highly morbid – such as in the subclavian and vertebral arteries – or when standard surgery is complex and physiologically demanding – such as in repair of traumatic disruption of the thoracic aorta. Covered stents may be used to bridge vessel disruptions and intraluminal balloons can be placed to provide distal vascular control in difficult access areas such as the distal internal carotid artery. Whilst such techniques are less morbid and impose a reduced surgical insult, there are potential disadvantages. Timely, 24-hour availability of a dedicated angiography suite and interventional radiologist is not a universal feature in trauma and non-trauma hospitals. Time lost in opening the suite and summoning personnel may put the patient at an undue risk. Stents may be malpositioned, embolise, thrombose, undergo structural failure or become infected, with potentially catastrophic consequences.

Damage control

In patients who have suffered massive trauma with gross physiological derangement, operative interventions should be limited to those required to restore physiological be expedited following skeletal stabilisation. In combined arteriovenous injuries both vessels should be shunted, as venous patency benefits arterial patency.

In cases of severe arterial injury and haemorrhage where the patient will not tolerate a definitive repair, vessel ligation may be undertaken. The clinical consequence of ligation depends upon the degree of collateral circulation that the dependent end organ enjoys and the nature of the end organ in question. The external carotid and subclavian arteries (in their second part) may be safely ligated whereas ligation of the popliteal artery is likely to cause significant limb-threatening ischaemia. Ligation of the internal carotid artery is associated with a 25–40% chance of major stroke. Single vessel injuries to the calf or forearm can usually be ligated without notable sequelae.

In the unstable patient with extremity vascular trauma the surgeon should balance the desire to save the limb with that of preserving the patient's life. In these circumstances – particularly when there has been significant trauma to bone, soft tissue and nerve in addition to vascular injury – amputation remains a life-saving intervention. Whilst scoring systems such as the mangled extremity syndrome index, mangled extremity severity score and predictive salvage index have been developed to assist the decision making in these circumstances, none has been shown to be superior to mature clinical judgement. In borderline cases amputation is best decided by two consultant surgeons in concert. There should be no attempt to form flaps at the first surgery as lines of demarcation are difficult to judge in shocked, poorly perfused patients. Instead, the limb should be taken at the lower boundary of the viable soft tissue envelope, with appropriate ligation of major vessels, debridement of residual dead tissue, washout and dressing with gauze and crepe. There should be no attempt to close the stump at this point as this will encourage infection of contaminated stump tissues and rapid sepsis. Instead, the stump should be debrided and washed at subsequent surgeries until formal flap formation and closure can be expedited when the patient has recovered physiological stability.

Definitive repair

The key operative steps and points of considerations to be undertaken in any vascular repair are given in Tables 24.3 and 24.4 respectively. Of paramount importance is to plan surgical incisions that allow proximal and distal control of blood vessels prior to exploration of the injury site.
• Simple lacerations that do not involve more than a third to a half of the vessels' circumference may be closed with interrupted transverse sutures.
• Patch angioplasty with autologous vein may be more appropriate in long ragged tears where tissue loss is evident. Prosthetic material should not be used routinely in heavily contaminated or military wounds due to the risk of graft infection.

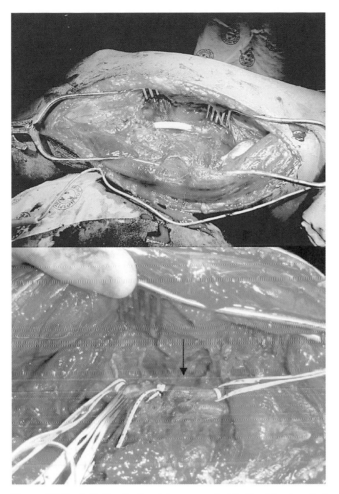

Figure 24.2 Definitive (top) and damage control (bottom) treatment of distal superficial artery injuries in different patients using PTFE end-to-end graft and an improvised shunt (arrow) respectively. The shunt – a piece of sterile-sized intravenous drip tubing – is being held in place with vascular slings. Proximal vascular clamps are applied prior to distal control, removal of the shunt and repair with reversed saphenous vein.

normality. A lower burden of surgical insult will offset the likelihood that traumatic coagulopathy will result and allow earlier transfer to the intensive care unit. This strategy – damage control surgery – should be combined with haemostatic resuscitation (1:1 use of packed cells to plasma; early use of platelets and cryoprecipitate) and effective casualty re-warming in an over-arching strategy of 'damage control resuscitation'. Damage control vascular surgery refers to the use of measures such as shunting and ligation to this end.

Shunting (Figure 24.2, bottom) consists of the temporary insertion of a hollow, sterile tube into the proximal and distal ends of the interrupted vessel in order to restore distal perfusion in the unstable casualty, deferring the need to embark on a definitive repair. Shunts can also be used as an interim measure to revascularise a limb prior to a prolonged orthopaedic procedure. Definitive reconstruction can then

Table 24.3 Key principles in any vascular repair.

Long, extensile axial incisions

Proximal and distal control gained *prior to* exploration of the haematoma/site of injury

Resection/debridement of injured segment of vessel

Inspection of intimal integrity and 'tacking down' of intimal flaps

Check of inflow and backflow, with Fogarty sweep if reduced and heparinised saline flush downstream

Assessment of surgery required and the patient's physiology

Definitive surgery/damage control as appropriate and restoration of perfusion if possible

Quality control

Coverage of repair with viable tissue

Consider fasciotomy

• In near or complete transection without segmental tissue loss, end-to-end anastomosis may be used to restore continuity. A sufficient length of the vessel is mobilised and an end-to-end anastomosis carried out without undue tension. The vessel ends should be cut obliquely (spatulated) to reduce the risk of stenosis. Stay sutures should be placed at equal intervals to prevent purse-stringing and luminal narrowing.
• An interposition graft of reversed long saphenous vein or polytetrafluoroethylene (PTFE) should be used if a segment of vessel is damaged or missing (Figure 24.2, top). Vein should not be taken from a leg with a concomitant venous injury as it may provide important collateral venous drainage in situ.

Table 24.4 Checklist for operative vascular repair.

Preoperative:	Consent (including possibility of limb loss)
	Marking of limb
Images:	Results from relevant studies available
Equipment:	X-ray compatible operating table and image intensifier
	Vascular set, Fogarty catheters
	Chest set for zone I injury
	Abdominal set for groin injury
	Shunts (commercial or improvised)
Expertise:	Orthopaedic and plastic surgeons for mangled extremity
	Radiographer
Preparation:	Include chest in zone I injury and abdomen in zone II injury
	Prep entire limb in extremity trauma
	Prep contralateral groin and thigh for access to long saphenous vein
Postoperative:	Mark distal pulse; regular review of at-risk compartments
	Book return to theatre (if fasciotomy inspection/closure required)

• In complex vascular injuries, bypass procedures should be considered. In severely contaminated wounds or wounds with large areas of soft tissue loss an extra-anatomic route should be chosen to enable graft coverage with uncompromised tissue to reduce the chance of graft infection.
• The anaesthetist should be forewarned prior to clamp removal and restoration of perfusion in order to mitigate the prospect of reperfusion injury.
• Assessment of the quality of repair is best done using post-reconstruction on-table angiography or, as a less accurate substitute, HHD insonation of the vessel immediately distal to the repair.
• Compartment syndrome is common after major vascular injury to the limbs and difficult to diagnose in the intubated, sedated trauma patient. For that reason, the default position is to perform full-length fasciotomies of the vulnerable limb segment following repair, ensuring all relevant compartments have been decompressed. Fasciotomies may be performed at the start of the surgery if a prolonged time to revascularisation is anticipated.
• Veins should be repaired in the stable patient and either shunted or ligated in the unstable patient.

Postoperative management

The patient should be cared for in a high dependency or intensive care environment with frequent monitoring and vascular observation (presence and quality of pulse, capillary refill) for the first 24–48 hours. Consideration of anticoagulation and anti-platelet agents should be balanced with the risk of haemorrhage from other injuries (e.g. head and chest injuries) and in general, patients are not systemically heparinised. Adequate hydration is essential, especially after administration of contrast dye, after episodes of hypotension and in the presence of concomitant renal injury.

Management of late presentations of vascular trauma

False aneurysm

A false aneurysm occurs when a haematoma caused by a lacerated vessel is surrounded by fibrous tissue forming a sac, and the sac remains in continuity with the vessel. The cavity of the sac is increased by the continued arterial pulsation eroding the wall of the false aneurysm. False aneurysms are more common in penetrating and iatrogenic trauma, and present as a swollen, expansile mass overlying the course of an artery, associated with a skin laceration or breach and a degree of bruising. There may be signs of soft tissue infection – typically in intravenous drug users where the aneurysm has arisen through mistaken injection into an adjacent artery. The natural course of false aneurysms is to

Table 24.5 Early complications of operative repair of vascular trauma.

Time scale	Complication	Notes	Prevention
Acute	Compartment syndrome (see Chapter 19)	Triggered by ischaemia/reperfusion, fractures, soft tissue injury causing tissue oedema within constrained fascial envelope. Compartment pressure defeats perfusion pressure and flow to tissue bed ceases	Minimisation of time-to-reperfusion Prophylactic fasciotomy if prolonged periods of hypotension or ischaemia, combined arterial and venous injury, vein ligation, severe crush injury or high-energy transfer trauma Early fasciotomy if compartment syndrome established
	Reperfusion injury	Tissue damage caused by free radicles, activated white cells, potassium and lactate from ischaemic limb following reperfusion May result in cardiac depression, arrhythmia, acute kidney injury/failure, adult lung injury/respiratory distress syndrome, intestinal oedema/abdominal compartment syndrome	Minimisation of time-to-reperfusion; careful intravenous fluid therapy
Sub-acute	Thrombosis of repair	Usually due to technical issue and presence of variable degree of end organ ischaemia dependent on injured vessel. Requires early surgical re-exploration and correction of underlying issue (poor inflow, poor graft, poor anastomoses and poor runoff)	Correct selection of appropriate repair tactic, careful tissue handling and strict vascular technique
	Unviable tissue	May be observed in fasciotomy wounds at subsequent re-look surgery with 'die-back' of watershed areas of muscle. Debride using '4C' rule to discriminate between viable and unviable tissue (colour, consistency, contractility and capacity to bleed)	Minimisation of time-to-reperfusion; prophylactic fasciotomy
	Graft infection	Indicated by evolving soft tissue infection and self-limiting but possibly severe 'herald' bleeds from graft of anastomotic suture line. Often requires re-exploration, ligation of proximal vessel, graft removal, debridement and extra-anatomic reconstruction plus protracted antibiotic therapy	Perioperative antibiotic therapy Appropriate choice of graft material Routing grafts away from deep wound bowls (extra-anatomic by-pass) Coverage of graft with viable muscle flap

progressively enlarge and rupture. Management consists of anatomically defining the aneurysm via duplex ultrasound and CTA as a prelude to intervention. Options include open surgery (resection of the aneurysm and repair/ligation of the vessel) or endovascular treatments (ultrasound-guided injection of thrombin into the aneurysm sac and transcatheter embolisation of sac).

Arteriovenous fistulae

Arteriovenous (AV) fistulae may occur with penetrating trauma resulting from simultaneous partial laceration to a neighbouring vein and artery. Blood passes from the high-pressure artery into the low-pressure vein, usually via a common haematoma cavity, causing a palpable thrill or bruit. AV fistulae are typically present for a few days following the injury and are associated with a 'machinery murmur' bruit. The haematoma cavity may become aneurysmal in due course. Management consists of definition of anatomy – usually via duplex or CTA – prior to treatment if it is symptomatic (distal ischaemia or cardiac failure); options include surgical resection or the use of a covered stent to seal the arterial side of the defect.

Summary

Vascular trauma is a demanding condition to manage successfully and early senior vascular specialist input is very important in securing a good outcome. Clinical examination is the cornerstone of accurate diagnosis, with CTA being the preferred investigation for stable patients with equivocal findings, or where there is uncertainty about the site of the vascular injury, or where the zone of injury borders an adjacent body cavity. Endovascular repair is limited to a few key injury patterns. Operative repair should be conducted with the aim of stopping bleeding and restoring perfusion via generous skin incisions that allow proper proximal and distal control. Shunts are increasingly recognised as a mainstay of the damage control approach.

Further reading

Aucar JA, Hirshberg A. Damage control for vascular injuries. *Surg Clin North Am* 1997; **77**: 853–862.

Miranda FE, Dennis JW, Veldenz HC, Dovgan PS, Frykberg ER. Confirmation of the safety and accuracy of physical examination in the evaluation of knee dislocation for injury of the popliteal artery: a prospective study. *J Trauma* 2002; **52**: 247–251.

Rasmussen TE, Clouse WD, Jenkins DH, Peck MA, Eliason JL, Smith DL. The use of temporary vascular shunts as a damage control adjunct in the management of wartime vascular injury. *J Trauma* 2006; **61**: 8–12.

Rozycki G. Blunt vascular trauma in the extremity: diagnosis, management and outcome. *J Trauma* 2003; **55**: 814–824.

Starnes BW, Beekley AC, Sebesta JA, Andersen CA, Rush RM. Extremity vascular injuries on the battlefield: tips for surgeons deploying to war. *J Trauma* 2006; **60**: 432–442.

25 Damage Control Surgery

Timothy C. Nunez[1], Igor V. Voskresensky[1] & Bryan A. Cotton[2]

[1]Department of Surgery, Vanderbilt University Medical Center, Nashville, TN, USA
[2]Department of Surgery and the Center for Translational Injury Research, The University of Texas Health Science Center, Houston, TX, USA

Introduction

Stone and colleagues initially described the concept of *damage control* (DC) *surgery* in 1983 while examining the application of temporary abdominal closure in critically injured patients who developed significant intraoperative coagulopathy. They described a technique of aborting the laparotomy after control of surgical haemorrhage and gross contamination, returning to the operating room once the physiology of the patient had been corrected. In 1993, Rotondo et al. further expanded on the technique, implementing the 'open abdomen' and 'lethal triad' components and coining the actual term of 'damage control laparotomy'.

The DC approach is now well established in both civilian and military trauma practice and is the standard of care for the severely injured patient with disturbed physiology. Though initially limited to patients with abdominal trauma, DC is now applied to vascular, chest and orthopaedic trauma as well as emergency general surgery patients with intra-abdominal catastrophes. The concept has even been central to the evolution of trauma resuscitation and the treatment of trauma-associated coagulopathy; a concept known as *damage control resuscitation*. The lethal triad of hypothermia, acidosis and coagulopathy is often found in the severely injured patient and accounts for the incredibly high mortality seen in this population. DC surgery and resuscitation are intended to try and break this bloody vicious cycle and allow clinicians to restore normal physiology.

Indications

The clinician must use a variety of objective and subjective data to apply damage control techniques to the appropriate patients (Tables 25.1 and 25.2). So far, however, no author or group has been able to identify strict criteria to

guide the clinician. There are injury patterns and mechanisms that should be a red flag for the institution of damage control measures. To achieve maximal benefit, damage control measures should be implemented as early as possible in the patient's course (Figure 25.1). This includes both management of their life-threatening injuries and directly treating the trauma-associated coagulopathy that is present in up to 35% of trauma patients.

The surgeon should strive to stay out of trouble rather than trying to get out of trouble ('keeping up, not catching up'). In order to achieve the objectives of this approach, damage control surgery and resuscitation demands open and effective communication with all members of the team treating the patient. The surgeon must keep the anaesthetist, haematologists, blood bank and nursing staff fully involved and aware of the management of the patient.

Damage control flow and phases

Phase 0

Damage control in reality begins in the field. This is applicable for both civilian and military trauma victims. Prehospital personnel should focus their efforts to decrease time on scene and transport patient as rapidly as possible to definitive care. Medics are instructed to stop bleeding as rapidly as possible with the use of direct pressure, dressings or tourniquets. Most trauma surgeons now advocate that their prehospital personnel resuscitate patients with a minimal amount of crystalloid solution. These saline-based fluids have been shown to increase coagulopathy, acidosis and the incidence of secondary abdominal compartment syndrome.

Since the landmark paper from Houston on the benefits of *hypotensive resuscitation* this has been proposed as the preferred method of managing injured patients prior to obtaining surgical control of haemorrhage. While many argue that its benefit was demonstrated only in penetrating trauma, application of low volume resuscitation with permissive hypotension to blunt trauma has led to similar findings. This method of resuscitation is currently practiced both in the civilian world as well as in ongoing military conflicts.

Emergency Surgery, 1st edition. Edited by Adam Brooks, Peter F. Mahoney, Bryan A. Cotton and Nigel Tai. © 2010 Blackwell Publishing.

Table 25.1 Indications to apply damage control technique.

Hypothermia < 35°C

Coagulopathy defined as non-surgical bleeding or abnormal coagulation studies

Acidosis <7.20

Major injury requiring extensive procedure for definitive repair or inaccessible venous injury

Need to reassess intra-abdominal organs for viability

Peak airway pressure increase of >10 with closure of abdomen

Other life-threatening injuries in other anatomic location

On arrival to the hospital it is essential that the surgical team recognise as early as possible the patients who will require damage control. They can use both subjective and objective data as described previously. There is no ideal trigger or score, the clinician must use all the data available along with their clinical acumen. Just as with the prehospital phase the surgical team will want to spend as little time as possible in the resuscitation area. The goal is to get the patient safely to the operating room as soon as is feasible.

Establishment of intravenous access above the diaphragm and above the suspected injuries is critical. This is often overlooked, but it is important that resuscitative products be infused in a vessel above where the main injuries are located.

Phase 1 – the initial operation

After a rapid evaluation in the trauma bay, the patient is transported to the operating room to obtain control of haemorrhage, limit peritoneal contamination and apply temporary abdominal closure. It is essential that the entire operating room team be prepared for the critically ill patient who requires damage control. The operating room should be warmed to a minimum of 25°C. The anaesthetic team should be prepared and knowledgeable of the 'keeping up' approach to resuscitation. If your facility has a massive transfusion protocol it should already be activated. Once the decision has been made that the patient will require damage control the surgeon should be making plans to terminate the operation as soon as possible (Table 25.2).

Table 25.2 Injury patterns and mechanism identified to indicate need for damage control.

Penetrating thoraco-abdominal injury with severe shock
High energy blunt trauma
Victims of primary blast injury
Two proximal amputations
Major vascular injury with major visceral injury
Severe multi-body cavity injury (major vascular injury with severe TBI or pelvic fracture

Control of haemorrhage

To achieve rapid and adequate haemorrhage control may require a variety of techniques. Initially, the patient should undergo packing of all four quadrants. Be sure to establish and keep open communication with the anaesthetist regarding the patient's ongoing haemorrhage, time to completing the case and temporary closure and what problems (if any) they are facing. In order to locate the source of injury in a sea of blood may require control of the supra-celiac aorta through the gastrohepatic ligament. This can be done with an aortic occlusion device, fingers or an aortic clamp.

Truncal arterial and venous injury will often lead to the patient's demise and rapid repair is essential. Lateral repair is the easiest and typically the quickest method to control these vessels but will have some down sides. It is likely to cause a stenosis. When taking the patient back for the definitive phase of damage control you may have to revise previous repairs to prevent long-term complications.

Ligation of any truncal vessel can be considered. Obviously some arteries and veins will tolerate ligation better than others. The vena cava and portal vein may be ligated with the known postoperative problems of lower extremity limb oedema with the former and extremely low survival with the latter. Shunting is also an option for control of a major vascular injury. It can be done rapidly to control haemorrhage and maintain distal perfusion. This obviates the need for a prolonged operative time trying to do a complex vascular repair.

Control of contamination

Control of contamination is a must, though many argue as to how early in the first operative procedure this has to be done. With respect to stool and succus, one may employ linear stapling devices to resect those limited segments that are the source of contamination. More rapid control can be obtained with proximal and distal placement of heavy suture (ligature fashion) such as 0-silk or umbilical tape. These sutures/ties are passed along the mesenteric border and across the bowel lumen and secured. Alternatively, if faced with non-circumferential 'holes' in bowel, the defect may be quickly repaired with 2- or 3–0 absorbable suture. Large bladder injuries can often be ignored until physiology, haemorrhage and contamination have been addressed. If there is a large bladder injury, a suction device can be placed into the pelvis and a lap pad placed over this and packed. Alternatively, a rapid repair with suture can be performed with revision at a later time.

Temporary abdominal closure

While initial descriptions of DC described fascial closure, most would now agree that the fascia should not be 'disturbed' at the initial procedure. At a minimum, however, primary fascial re-approximation should not be attempted. The most common method employed is the 'vac-pack'

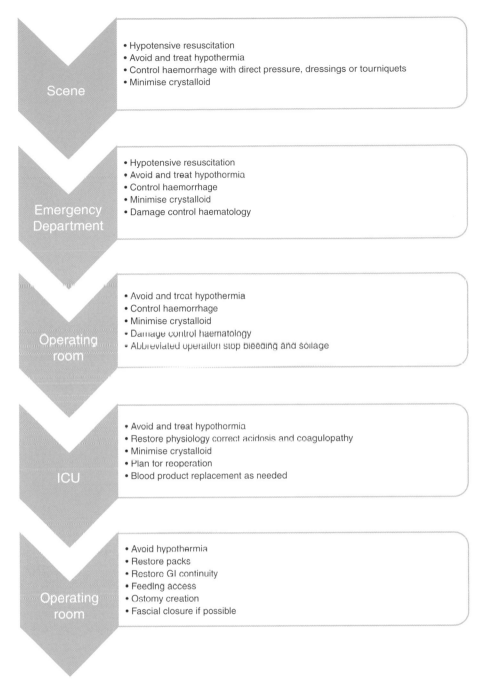

Scene
- Hypotensive resuscitation
- Avoid and treat hypothermia
- Control haemorrhage with direct pressure, dressings or tourniquets
- Minimise crystalloid

Emergency Department
- Hypotensive resuscitation
- Avoid and treat hypothermia
- Control haemorrhage
- Minimise crystalloid
- Damage control haematology

Operating room
- Avoid and treat hypothermia
- Control haemorrhage
- Minimise crystalloid
- Damage control haematology
- Abbreviated operation stop bleeding and soilage

ICU
- Avoid and treat hypothermia
- Restore physiology correct acidosis and coagulopathy
- Minimise crystalloid
- Plan for reoperation
- Blood product replacement as needed

Operating room
- Avoid hypothermia
- Restore packs
- Restore GI continuity
- Feeding access
- Ostomy creation
- Fascial closure if possible

Figure 25.1 The flow of the damage control concept.

technique that employs a self-made vacuum pack dressing. This involves the use of a non-adherent bag placed against the bowel, followed by placement of an Ioban-wrapped towel over the 'bowel-bag,' and finally an additional Ioban covering the abdominal wall and one or two drains (placed into the 'gutters' of the subcutaneous tissue) (Figure 25.2). Commercially available negative pressure devices are also frequently employed to address the open abdomen at the completion of phase 1. In fact, this technique has quickly become the favoured method in light of its simplicity of application and recent data demonstrating superior 'time-to-fascial-closure' compared to the traditional vac-pack. Other institutions utilise towel clip or 'Bogotá bag' closure (suturing plastic bag to the skin, to avoid compromising the fascia). One point to remember is that if the patient's airway pressures increase by more than 10 cm H_2O then your closure is too tight. If this occurs you will need to reassess and change your strategy. While this is less likely with

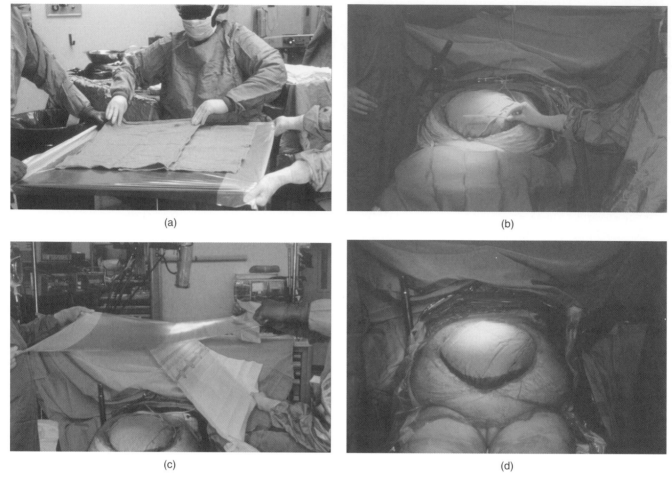

(a)

(b)

(c)

(d)

Figure 25.2 Application of 'vac-pack' dressing. (a) Creation of Ioban-wrapped towel for non-adherence to and protection of underlying bowel. (b) Towel placed Ioban side down into abdomen with drains laid laterally. (c) Application of Ioban seal to anterior and lateral abdominal wall. (d) Drains placed to suction with evidence of adequate seal and successful negative pressure dressing.

temporary closure techniques the development of recurrent abdominal compartment syndrome (compartment syndrome in patients with an open abdomen) is well described.

Phase 2 – physiologic restoration

Restoration of physiology is the goal of the second phase of damage control. The principles of this phase of are to break the bloody vicious cycle of hypothermia, acidosis and coagulopathy. While the correction of these components of the lethal triad is described here in the second phase of DC, the correction should begin on first contact with the patient. Damage control is broken down into steps for the benefit of description, but the concept should be applied in a continuum.

Hypothermia

While hypothermia is generally defined as a core body temperature <35°C, its severity is usually divided into those temperatures <35°C, 32–35°C and <32°C. Severe hypother-

mia (<32°C) is associated with near 100% mortality in the severely injured population. Hypothermia affects coagulation by decreasing platelet activation and adhesion and by slowing down the metabolic rate of coagulation factor enzymes, specifically the serine proteases.

Treatment begins with on scene care, which can include removal of wet clothing and quickly covering the patient after exposure. Warmed intravenous fluids and blood products should be used as soon as the ability to deliver such warming is available. As well, ventilator circuits should be warmed and humidified. Passive external re-warming techniques include wrapping the patient (including the head) in warm blankets. Active external re-warming, such as radiant heat blankets, is also effective early on. Invasive manoeuvres include the use of active internal and extracorporeal methods.

Acidosis

Similar to hypothermia, the other component of the triad negatively impacts the ability to form and maintain clot.

Acidosis disturbs the coagulation system through an inhibition of key enzyme activity. Its effects on coagulation are potentiated in the hypothermic patient. It is vital that the team attempts to not only treat the obvious acidosis that has developed but also to prevent worsening acidosis as well. To this end, aggressive crystalloid resuscitation and hypoventilation (both of which can worsen acidosis and coagulopathy) should be avoided. Following base deficit and lactate levels may provide some evidence that the resuscitation is heading in the right direction but should not be used as end-points 'to be achieved at all costs'. Should the patient's pH demonstrate a severe *metabolic* acidosis (ph < 7.20), sodium bicarbonate can be used to buffer the system until resuscitation efforts have caught up. Alternatively, tris-hydroxymethyl-aminomethane (THAM) may be used without the subsequent excess CO_2 production associated with bicarbonate administration. However, both of these agents must be used in combination with adequate resuscitation.

Coagulopathy

Trauma-associated coagulopathy is present in up to a one-third of trauma patients on admission. The concept of *damage control haematology or haeostatic resuscitation* directly attempts to address this process with a proactive rather than reactive approach to transfusion of blood and blood component therapy. While the optimal ratio of blood products to be transfused is currently being debate, it is now well accepted that the use of fresh frozen plasma and platelets should start earlier and in higher ratios than has been traditionally administered. The transfusion of blood products to the exsanguinating patient should mimic the transfusion of whole blood; component therapy approaches whole blood but has significant differences (Table 25.3).

Early identification of patients who will require damage control haematology is an ongoing area of investigation. Several authors have attempted to identify the ideal scoring system to objectively identify trauma patients who are likely to require a massive transfusion. The ideal scoring system will be easy to use, sensitive, specific and be rapidly available within minutes after arrival to the trauma centre. The ABC (assessment of blood consumption) score provides rapid identification of patients who will require massive transfusion (>10 units PRBC in 24 hours). If any two of the following are identified, the patient has almost a 40% incidence of requiring massive transfusion:

- Heart rate on arrival of ≥120
- Systolic blood pressure ≤90
- Free fluid on FAST examination
- Penetrating mechanism

Phase 3 – completion and definitive surgery

The third phase of damage control surgery was originally described as the definitive surgery or second look. This may take one trip back to the operating room or it may take several trips depending on the severity of the injury. This phase should occur after the patient's physiology has been restored and the bloody viscous cycle has been interrupted. This may occur just a few hours from the original operation or it may take 24 hours or more. However, phase 3 should not be delayed longer than 72 hours. The 'second look' or 'take back' tenets include removal of packing, restoration of intestinal continuity and colostomy formation. Further exploration for injuries not detected during the original operation should be carefully undertaken; it is easy to miss injuries when rapidly exploring and controlling haemorrhage in an unstable patient. At this time, a nasoenteric feeding tube or percutaneous feeding tube should be placed.

Fascial closure may not be possible at the initial take back and one should plan to return to the operating room once significant oedema has resolved. Pay careful attention to airway pressures when attempting primary closure; if an increase of >10 cm H_2O is observed, attempts at primary closure should be aborted and a temporary negative pressure dressing employed. In this situation then percutaneous tubes and stomas should be avoided if possible. One may also need to consider aggressive diuresis upon return to the ICU and another planned trip back to the operating room for primary closure. When failure to achieve primary closure occurs, a comprehensive plan for long-term management of the open abdomen needs to be made. If stomas are required, these should be placed lateral to the rectus muscle.

Damage control outside of the abdomen

Peripheral vascular injuries

Peripheral vascular injuries may need to be temporised because of the deranged physiology of the patient. While these injuries are more likely to cause permanent disability than death, inability to obtain timely control of haemorrhage from these wounds is most often fatal. Principles in

Table 25.3 Comparison of fresh whole blood to one unit of PRBC, FFP and platelets.

	Fresh whole blood	Component therapy (one unit of PRBC, FFP and platelets)
Haematocrit	38–45%	29%
Platelets	150,000–400,000	87,000
Coagulation function	100%	65%
Fibrinogen	1500 mg	750 mg
Volume	500 mL	660 mL

PRBC, packed red blood cells; FFP, fresh frozen plasma.

managing peripheral vascular injuries are the prevention of exsanguinating haemorrhage and preservation of end-organ function. The indications and the flow of damage control for vascular injuries is essentially the same as for damage control in the abdomen.

Haemorrhage control

Cessation of haemorrhage prior to obtaining surgical control centres upon direct pressure. This method has always been advocated by American College of Surgeon's ATLS® course as the primary means of haemorrhage control. This is most often accomplished with a well-placed bandage that applies enough pressure to control haemorrhage. Alternatively, personnel can use their own gloved hand to apply pressure. While historically seen as a technique of last resort, recent data from both the Israeli and US military suggest that tourniquet use is an extremely reliable and safe adjunct for preoperative haemorrhage control. Haemostatic agents have been an area of intense research over the past several years and there are several different commercial types available. None of these meet the exact characteristics which are needed for the ideal haemostatic dressing; these include 'ready-to-use' right out of the package, simple to apply, and durable and stable over time.

Damage control haematology is also essential in the patient who has had large amount of bleeding from the isolated extremity wound, these patients may very well have significant physiologic derangements that warrant damage control. The lethal triad is not limited to the patients with truncal injuries only. The resuscitation practice for this population is the same as previously described, blood products will be given early and often in predefined ratios to attempt to prevent the patient getting to a physiologic point of no return, the bloody viscous cycle.

Shunting

Temporary shunting has recently gained renewed interest on the heels of reports from both the civilian and military settings. Temporary shunting is a valuable option in the cold coagulopathic patient who cannot withstand a long complex vascular repair. This simple technique can provide flow to the distal extremity or end-organs even in patients being transferred to the ICU for the phase 2 of damage control. The decision to shunt is based on the same physiologic parameters that are used to decide using a damage control technique. With aggressive use of shunting there are many patients who can survive injuries with preservation of their extremities. There are many commercially available shunts, but you also may have to improvise (intravenous tubing or paediatric chest tubes). Commercial shunts include the Javid, Argyle and Sundt. Once the shunt is inserted proximally and distally it needs to be secured, using umbilical tape, suture or Rommel tourniquets. While the shunt may stay in for several days (if necessary), it should be evaluated constantly for shunt patency as well as for distal perfusion.

Musculoskeletal issues

Fasciotomy in this patient population is a must. The typical compartments that need to be released are the four muscle compartments of the lower leg or the forearm; these are done through two long incisions. Failure to perform (or perform adequately) can lead to limb loss. The key with compartment syndrome is to prevent or anticipate its development rather than detect it early.

Peripheral vascular injuries that require shunting may be also associated with skeletal injury that will require temporary fixation. In these situations the shunt should take precedence over the skeletal fixation. Once you have established distal flow and the patients' physiology can withstand more time in the operating room you may allow the orthopaedic surgeon the short time that is need to apply external fixation. If this is not possible, the injured extremity will need to be splinted as best that it can. External fixation with shunt in place is safe.

Definitive operative stage

Once the patient's physiology has corrected (they are warm, not coagulopathic and not acidotic) it is safe to return to the operating room for definitive vascular repair. The majority of principles of elective peripheral vascular surgery (proximal and distal control, appropriate anatomic exposure) apply here as well. Two particular (potential) departures are worth noting though. The use of heparin at the time of definitive reconstruction is still a difficult question and is best made on a 'case-by-case' basis. In isolated extremity trauma it is reasonable to heparinise the patient during the definitive repair. In the patient with multisystem trauma (especially with associated intracranial injuries) systemic heparinisation should be used with caution (if at all). Saphenous vein is the preferred conduit in these settings (given the higher likelihood of a contaminated field and potential PTFE graft infection). Finally, wound closure may be extremely difficult in this group and the use of flaps and skin grafts may be needed to achieve adequate coverage.

Thoracic injuries

Thoracic damage control while not a new concept and has not been well described in the literature. The principles, however, are the same: an abbreviated operation with rapid transport to the ICU in an effort to restore the patient to normal (or near-normal) physiology prior to definitive repair.

Emergency department thoracotomy

Emergency department (resuscitative) thoracotomy is a well-established procedure often performed in patients who have had penetrating injuries and are in extremis. This temporising measure allows the surgeon to get the patient expeditiously to the operating room for more secure control of haemorrhage. It can also be used as a diagnostic tool, easily identifying injuries in the left chest or mediastinum. As well, it can identify injuries in the right chest when the anterolateral thoracotomy is extended across midline. Once the chest is opened, several manoeuvres can be employed to quickly address life-threatening issues. These include decompression of a cardiac tamponade, gaining proximal aortic control and packing the chest cavity for general haemorrhage control. If a tamponade is encountered and released, one is faced with immediate control of cardiac/great vessel bleeding. This can be accomplished by applying a finger (or two) over the area with gentle pressure or by rapid suture or staple closure. With large defects, some have described balloon occlusion with the use of a Foley catheter placed into the defect. A pulmonary twist has also been described in cases of significant haemorrhage from the lung and pulmonary vessels. The damaged lung is twisted 180° to provide compression of the main pulmonary artery and vein. In cases where intravenous access is limited or non-existent, a large bore catheter (or simply intravenous tubing) can be placed directly into the right atrium to facilitate resuscitation. This should be quickly but appropriately secured with a purse string suture.

Damage control procedures

An abbreviated thoracic operation is triggered by the same parameters as for abdominal and vascular injuries. If the patient is cold, coagulopathic and/or acidotic, it is imperative that the operating team be thinking immediately as to how they will get the patient out of the operating room and on their way to the ICU for physiologic restoration. The principles of stopping haemorrhage and controlling soilage and in the chest air leak are the same.

Even when the primary surgical concern is in the chest cavity, it is usually not practical to have the patient in ex tremis in any other position other than supine. Placing the arms out at 90° or placing the patient into a 'taxi-hailing' position with a slight 'bump' from a blanket or towel may assist in exposure. However, given the potential for requiring an emergent laparotomy (even in those in whom it is not anticipated preoperatively) the supine position is the safest and most 'forgiving' position. Unlike elective or semielective cases, there is usually insufficient time to place a double lumen endotracheal tube.

Exposure

The extra difficulties of injury to vessels in the chest are that not all of them are accessible through one incision. One missile may have traversed the chest that can injure structures that have to be approached through three different approaches. Anterolateral thoracotomy will give you good exposure and control of the descending aorta, pulmonary artery/vein and proximal left subclavian. Bilateral thoracotomy (clam shell) gives you good control of the descending aorta, proximal left subclavian, bilateral pulmonary artery/vein and atriocaval junction. A sternotomy gives good access to the aortic arch and its proximal branches as well as you can extend this incision up into the neck for control of the carotid vessels. Some authors have also described the division or removal of the clavicle (or portions of it) to get control of the subclavian vessels.

Vascular injuries

Injuries to vascular structures in the chest are approached the same as described for truncal vascular injuries, control of haemorrhage is essential and the same methods of control are available. Ligation is fairly well tolerated in the chest. Lateral repair is simple but may not be technically feasible and may be time consuming.

Cardiac injuries

Cardiac injuries will typically require suture repair (usually with polypropylene). When possible, pledgets should be used, using good horizontal mattress sutures in place with secure knots.

Lung parenchyma injuries

Lung injuries are typically the easiest to deal with from a technical standpoint. These injuries can be addressed in a rapid fashion and there are several options to control lung parenchymal bleeding. The pulmonary twist is simply rotating the lung 180° to control haemorrhage. Placing a clamp across the hilum will also control bleeding. Both of these manoeuvres can be used as a temporary intraoperative adjunct or can be used for an extended period of time while you attempt to restore the physiology of your patient. Devitalised lung should be excised. A surgical stapler (with 'vascular loads') provides simultaneous removal of non-viable tissue, resection of the lung segment and a staple-sealed edge.

Oesophageal injuries

Oesophageal injuries encountered in a patient with severe physiologic disturbances can be challenging. Primary repair would be ideal but is likely to be too time-consuming. If physiology allows repair, most authors would recommend a two-layered closure with wide drainage. As well, many would recommend buttressing the repair with pericardium or intercostal muscle. If primary repair is not feasible these injuries can be managed with wide drainage using at least two large bore chest tubes and with a nasogastric tube placed at the site of injury connected to continuous low wall suction. Distal feeding access as described before will take place when the patient's physiology has been restored and the patient has gone back for their definitive operation.

Tracheal injuries

Most of these injuries are amendable to passing the endotracheal tube past the site of injury. Occasionally, a penetrating injury with an anterior–posterior trajectory will make an anterior defect in the trachea that can be managed by passing a temporary airway through this defect.

Temporary chest wall closure

Temporary chest wall closure may take some creative techniques depending on the incision made as well as how much damage to the chest wall was done by the injury. The key is to have the patient maintain adequate perfusion, oxygenation and control of haemorrhage. Packing the thoracic cavity with towel clip closure is acceptable, but the patient may develop secondary compartment syndrome during phase 2 of damage control because the chest is not allowed the ability to 'swell'. We prefer to employ one of the two techniques discussed above in the abdominal section; either the 'vacpack' or black sponge vacuum assisted closure. Remember to place chest tubes to monitor ongoing blood loss. A bowel bag is placed over the lung (without perforations), acting as pleura. Two chest tubes are then placed and a negative pressure dressing applied over the open wound.

Applying damage control principles to non-trauma settings

Along with surgical critical care and trauma, emergency general surgery has become part of the triad of acute care surgery. While often seen as a 'natural' extension of trauma, not all applications of care of the severely injured patient are easily (or appropriately) translated into the emergency surgery realm. While the widespread adoption of damage control principles is not advisable based on available data, there are clearly clinical situations where the damage control concept can be appropriately applied. In those cases of widespread peritoneal soilage or life-threatening haemorrhage, few would argue that implementation of such principles is warranted. However, once bleeding is medically and surgically controlled, contamination has been cleared, and 'source control' achieved, there is no indication for further planned explorations or peritoneal washouts. At this point, the adage of 'the longer you leave them open, the longer they stay open' applies.

Summary

Damage control surgery, regardless of the body cavity to which it is applied, is a concept that can be stated as staying out of trouble rather than getting out of trouble. The 'bloody viscous cycle', and an exhaustion of your patient's physiology, should be aggressively avoided by restraining oneself from attempts to do a thorough but complex heroic surgical procedure. Damage control resuscitation is an essential component to the survival of these severely injured patients. Not only do we need to warm the patient, stop their bleeding and correct the acidosis that is present, but we must aggressively attack the trauma-associated coagulopathy that they present with. This is done most efficiently with predefined ratios of blood products delivered in a systematic fashion. Trauma surgeons need to be actively involved with blood bank and the transfusion committees in their respective institutions. Finally, damage control is often described as occurring in phases or steps. Describing it this way makes it simpler to understand all the components of damage control. However, the best way to think of damage control is a constant flow from the scene to the emergency department to the operating room, ICU, and back to the operating room.

Further reading

Beekley AC. Damage control resuscitation: a sensible approach to the exsanguinating surgical patient. *Crit Care Med* 2008;**36**(7): S267–S274.

Cotton BA, Gunter OL, Isbell J. Damage control hematology: the impact of a trauma exsanguination protocol on survival and blood product utilization. *J Trauma* 2008;**64**(5):1177–1182; discussion 1182–1183.

Fox CJ, Starnes BW. Vascular surgery on the modern battlefield. *Surg Clin North Am* 2007;**87**(5):1193–1211, xi.

Holcomb JB, Jenkins D, Rhee P, et al. Damage control resuscitation: directly addressing the early coagulopathy of trauma. *J Trauma* 2007;**62**(2):307–310.

Phelan HA, Patterson SG, Hassan MO, Gonzalez RP, Rodning CB. Thoracic damage-control operation: principles, techniques, and definitive repair. *J Am Coll Surg* 2006;**203**(6):933–941.

Rotondo MF, Schwab CW, McGonigal MD. 'Damage control': an approach for improved survival in exsanguinating penetrating abdominal injury. *J Trauma* 1993;**35**(3):375–382; discussion 382–383.

Stone HH, Strom PR, Mullins RJ. Management of the major coagulopathy with onset during laparotomy. *Ann Surg* 1983; **197**(5):532–535.

26 Trauma Laparotomy

Victor Zaydfudim[1] & Bryan A. Cotton[2]

[1]Department of Surgery, Vanderbilt University Medical, Center, Nashville, TN, USA
[2]Department of Surgery and The Center for Translational Injury Research, The University of Texas Health Science Center, Houston, TX, USA

Introduction

The aim of this chapter is to provide a brief practical outline to what every surgical trainee needs to know about the initial laparotomy for trauma so that he or she can understand the procedure and be a useful assistant to a more experienced surgeon. The chapter focuses on basic exposure, vascular and bowel control, and resection/repair strategies. This chapter will not address the details of all the available exposure techniques, operative approaches and intraoperative decision-making. These can be gained through experience, textbook reading and intraoperative learning.

The primary goals of the trauma laparotomy are (1) rapid control of exsanguination, (2) control and minimisation of bowel spillage and (3) avoidance of the lethal triad: hypothermia, coagulopathy and acidosis (Table 26.1). Initial trauma laparotomy cases are unscheduled and usually need to be performed rapidly on patients with markedly disturbed preoperative and intraoperative physiology. As such, there is little tolerance of error, but plenty of opportunities to make mistakes. In light of this, it is best to approach this operation the same way every time.

Preparatory considerations

It is crucial that you accompany your patient from resuscitation bay to the operating room. Upon moving a sick, often unstable, patient to the operating room suite please establish communication with the rest of your team. Ongoing communication with the anaesthesia and nursing teams is essential throughout the operation.

Anaesthesia

At the time of 'hand-off/hand-over', provide a brief account of anticipated injuries and patient's haemodynamics. Brief

Emergency Surgery, 1st edition. Edited by Adam Brooks, Peter F. Mahoney, Bryan A. Cotton and Nigel Tai. © 2010 Blackwell Publishing.

discussion should include: airway, access, injuries expected, potential need for blood products, whether or not the institution's massive transfusion protocol has been activated, and what preoperative antibiotics have been (or are to be) given.

Circulator and scrub nurse

As staff is usually limited during the time of day these cases arrive, identify those instruments or trays you anticipate needing; specifically those not routinely kept in the room. Remember to request blood-salvage systems, fluid warmer/infuser, or special suction devices that may be required. Specify exactly how you would like the patient to be positioned, prepped and draped – always remind the team even if it is the same way every time. Let them know of any procedures you might want to do prior to laparotomy (e.g. chest tubes and lines). Ensure that the room is warm enough for this critically ill trauma patient who needs an emergent operation ($>80°F$ or $>27°C$). Let them know if you think you might do something out of sequence such as open the chest while someone else is opening the abdomen.

You

Carefully place and set up over headlights and always consider placing a headlight on yourself. This may give you a headache but will almost always help you. Make sure you are comfortable with everything in the room before leaving for the scrub sink. Table 26.2 lists few things that might help you.

Patient

For a 'standard' laparotomy, the patient is placed supine with arms out and prepped from the neck to the knees and down to the table on both sides. This will allow access to abdomen, both sides of the chest, mediastinum, zone 1 of the neck and bilateral groins (Figure 26.1). At the same time, the anaesthesia team can access both arms and enough of the neck to establish sufficient vascular access and invasive monitoring.

In setting up the patient, ask yourself whether you suspect thoracoabdominal trauma; if so, the patient should be placed

Table 26.1 Deadly triad.

Acidosis
Coagulopathy
Hypothermia

Table 26.2 Helpful adjuncts.

All circumstances	Selected cases
Headlight	Argon beam coagulator
High-power suction (Neptune™)	Hemostatic agents (Nu-Knit™)
	Blood bank notification
	Another assistant

into a 'taxi-cab hailing' position. This positioning affords better access to the chest while not limiting abdominal exposure and is accomplished by placing the patient up slightly on one side using a 'bump' or rolled blanket.

Beginning the operation

'Getting into' the abdomen and identifying injuries is often perceived as the most exciting part of the operation. However, the concept 'same way, every time' certainly applies here. Unless the patient is crashing and needs an emergent aortic cross-clamp, patient should be prepped and draped in the sterile fashion.

Retractors

The majority of self-retaining retractors will help to free-up your hands. We typically position the post for the retractor between the chest and the abdomen on the left side of the table. This allows for adequate abdominal retraction, as well as leaves open access to the left chest. Remember to have

access to bilateral chest cavities and groins, as well as sternal notch.

A 'big' incision

The incision should be large enough to accommodate rapid and adequate exposure for a thorough exploration. As such, the midline incision is preferred in almost all cases. Some authors suggest a bilateral subcostal incision for patients with previous midline explorations, but remember it might be tough to reach the pelvis from the epigastrium.

While an incision spanning xiphoid to pubis is the mantra of trauma laparotomy, being judicious does not hurt.

Most operative movements can be aided with the help of assistants. Certainly while opening the abdomen, it helps to use the traction/counter-traction principle of surgery.

Classic teaching ascribes to using the knife to cut through the skin, subcutaneous tissues and the fascia in three broad knife strokes. However, not every trauma patient is crashing

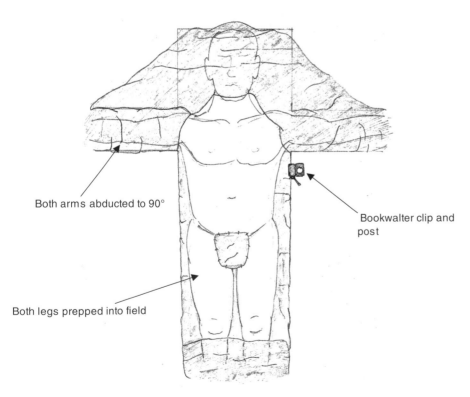

Both arms abducted to 90°

Bookwalter clip and post

Both legs prepped into field

Figure 26.1 Patient positioning, draping and set-up. Indicate positioning of the Bookwalter.

and it is important not to cause injury to either the patient or the scrub team, so care needs to be exercised. Once the preperitoneal fat is exposed, the abdominal cavity is entered with a blunt finger push just above the umbilicus where the peritoneum is the thinnest. The peritoneal cavity is then fully opened with Mayo scissors, taking care to avoid iatrogenic injury to liver, bowel or bladder. In this manner a skilled surgeon should be able to enter the abdomen in seconds.

Inform the anaesthesia team prior to entering the peritoneal cavity and decompressing the intra-abdominal haematoma. Unless the patient is *in extremis* give the anaesthesia team time to get ready prior to diving-in. Once the abdomen is opened divide the *ligamentum teres* between clamps and sharply divide the falciform ligament towards the central tendon to facilitate exposure.

Initial packing

Packing starts in the quadrant with most suspicion for an injury and proceeds towards area of least suspicion for an injury. Use of large handheld Richardson/Morris retractor provides adequate exposure for the operator on the contralateral side of the table to systematically pack off one quadrant at a time. Once the abdomen is adequately packed, the self-retaining retractor, which has already been set up, can be simply dropped into the field.

Blunt versus penetrating

There are many differences between blunt and penetrating trauma. In penetrating trauma, the trajectory of the injury can be ascertained and an injury pattern can be expected. There are a number of potentially different injury patterns and treatment strategies and we will list some of these in this chapter. Knowing whether the injury is blunt or penetrating and expecting a pattern suggested by the trajectory or possible seat-belt sign or abdominal wall haematoma will help you manage your patient during the operation.

Bleeding

Bleeding always needs to be addressed first. Hopefully the packing has temporary quenched rapid haemorrhage and you are now free to explore the abdomen. At this point, check out the zones of the retroperitoneum prior to removing packing. Should these demonstrate large or expanding haematomas, notify the anaesthetist of the increased risk for tremendous blood loss, make sure your institution's massive transfusion protocol is in place, and determine whether proximal and distal control are needed prior to proceeding with exploration.

Next, begin removing the packs. If you recall, the order of packing was from the quadrant with most suspicion for injury to the quadrant with least suspicion for injury. To remove the packs reverse order should be followed. Remove the packs first in the quadrant where you do not expect an injury and proceed to the quadrant with suspicion for an injury.

Vascular injuries

If packing did not help with ongoing haemorrhage chances are you are dealing with active intraperitoneal bleeding from the great vessels or from the porta/retrohepatic area. While the mechanics of injury are different in both blunt and penetrating trauma, intraperitoneal haemorrhage of these largely retroperitoneal structures needs to be addressed first. If the haemorrhage is a contained retroperitoneal haematoma, judicious exposure and control depends on zone of the haematoma and mechanism of injury.

Temporary control

When haemorrhage is resulting in haemodynamic instability, obtain immediate and rapid vascular control either in the abdomen or in the chest. The aorta can be accessed either through a left anterolateral thoracotomy or at the diaphragmatic hiatus with either an aortic occluder or a vascular clamp.

Areas of injury

Active haemorrhage or contained haematoma is usually associated with either great vessel injury in one of the three zones of the retroperitoneum or vascular trauma within the porta/retrohepatic area. Anatomic boundaries of the retroperitoneal zones are delineated in Figure 26.2. While areas of active haemorrhage need to be explored and fixed,

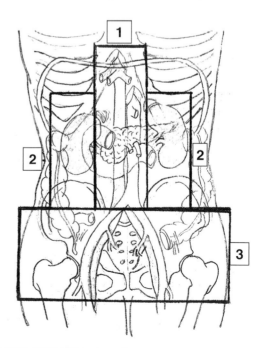

Figure 26.2 Zones of the retroperitoneum.

Table 26.3 Zone of vascular injury and plan of attack.

	Penetrating trauma	Blunt trauma
Zone 1	Explore	Explore
Zone 2	Explore	Explore only if active exsanguination
Zone 3	Explore	Explore only if active exsanguination
Porta	Explore	Explore
Retrohepatic	Do not explore unless active exsanguination	Do not explore unless active exsanguination

not all contained haematomas need exploration. Table 26.3 summarises zones of injury and plan of action.

Zone 1 is centrally located and encompasses aorta with its intra-abdominal branches and the inferior vena cava (IVC). It is further divided into supramesocolic and inframesocolic areas, which not only orients vascular structures with relation to the colon, but also helps distinguish injuries above and below the renal vessels. Zone 2 is located lateral to the IVC and contains the renal vessels and the kidneys. Zone 3 encompasses the pelvis and contains the iliac vessels. Porta/retrohepatic area consists of the portal structures as well as the venous confluence of hepatic veins and the IVC.

Approach

Supramesocolic (zone 1)
Injury to the supramesocolic (zone 1) structures (aorta above the renal vessels) is best approached through left medial visceral rotation (Figure 26.3). The left colon is mobilised medially to expose the aorta. If a very high aortic injury is suspected, such as laceration to the supraceliac aorta, the kidney should be rotated medially as well, and the left crus of the diaphragm should be divided to allow best exposure.

Inframesocolic (zone 1)
Injury to the inframesocolic aorta can be accessed via the left medial visceral rotation as well. However, should an injury to the IVC be suspected, a right medial visceral rotation (Figure 26.4) will help expose all great vessels with the exception of aorta above the superior mesenteric artery (SMA).

Alternative approaches to great vessels without completing a medial visceral rotation are available. For example, injury to the celiac or SMA aorta can be identified and isolated by stapling and dividing the stomach.

Zone 2
Zone 2 injuries can be accessed through medial visceral rotation on the side of the injury. Zone 2 injuries rarely need exploration. As summarised in Table 26.3, non-expanding haematoma in zone 2 does not need exploration unless the patient suffered a penetrating injury and the trajectory suggests injury to the renal vessels.

Zone 3
As with zone 2, non-penetrating injuries to zone 3 do not need exploration unless an expanding haematoma is present. However, penetrating injuries to this area should be explored as injury to major vascular structures of the pelvis, rectum or ureters will have dire consequences unless identified and addressed. One of the tricks in exploring injuries to the common or external iliac arteries is obtaining distal control with a Foley catheter with inflated balloon. While this

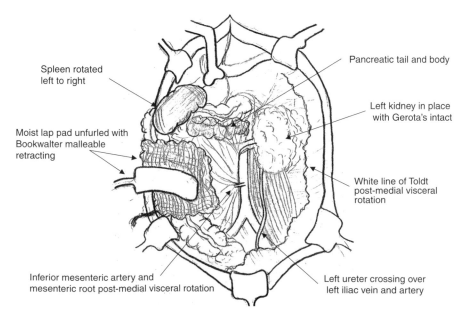

Spleen rotated left to right

Moist lap pad unfurled with Bookwalter malleable retracting

Inferior mesenteric artery and mesenteric root post-medial visceral rotation

Pancreatic tail and body

Left kidney in place with Gerota's intact

White line of Toldt post-medial visceral rotation

Left ureter crossing over left iliac vein and artery

Figure 26.3 Mattox manoeuvre (left medial visceral rotation).

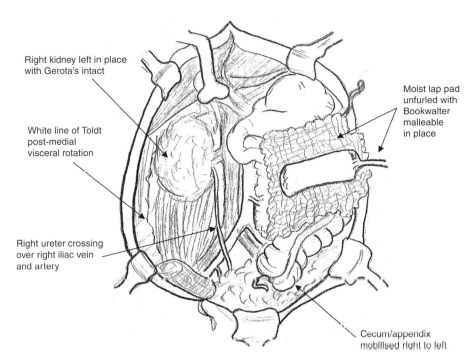

Right kidney left in place with Gerota's intact

White line of Toldt post-medial visceral rotation

Right ureter crossing over right iliac vein and artery

Moist lap pad unfurled with Bookwalter malleable in place

Cecum/appendix mobilised right to left

Figure 26.4 Cattell-Braasch manoeuvre (right medial visceral rotation)

manoeuvre might work in other vessels, the arteries of the pelvis are best suited for this approach.

Porta/retrohepatic

Injuries to the portal structures should be explored regardless of mechanism or appearance of the haematoma. Vascular control can be obtained with a Pringle manoeuvre proximally and individual vascular control distally. Pringle manoeuvre can be rapidly performed by opening the hep-

atoduodenal ligament and occluding all three portal structures with either a vascular clamp or a Rummel tourniquet (Figure 26.5). The retrohepatic area contains the confluence of hepatic veins and retrohepatic IVC and, if at all possible, should not be explored. Unless there is evidence of active 'in-your-face' haemorrhage – avoid opening haematoma in this area. If you must approach this area be prepared to perform total hepatic isolation by controlling the porta, as well as infrahepatic and suprahepatic IVC. Alternatively, control

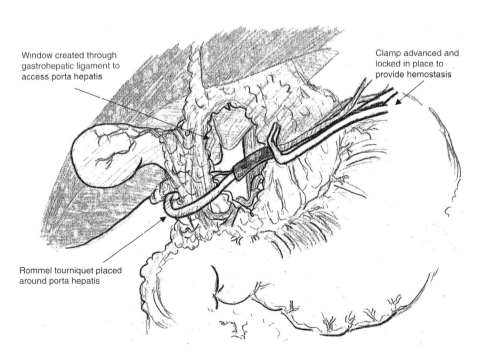

Window created through gastrohepatic ligament to access porta hepatis

Clamp advanced and locked in place to provide hemostasis

Rommel tourniquet placed around porta hepatis

Figure 26.5 Pringle manoeuvre.

Table 26.4 Repair or ligate.

Vascular structure	Plan of action	Potential complications if vascular structure is ligated
Aorta	Repair	
Infrarenal IVC	Repair or ligate	Lower extremity venostasis, oedema, DVT
Suprarenal IVC	Repair or ligate	Same as infrarenal; also renal failure
Celiac	Ligate	
SMA	Repair or ligate	Bowel ischaemia
SMV	Repair or ligate	Bowel ischaemia
Portal vein	Repair or ligate	Bowel ischaemia
Hepatic artery	Repair or ligate	Cholecystectomy if ligated
Common iliac artery	Repair or ligate	Will need extra-anatomic revascularisation of extremity
External iliac artery	Repair or ligate	Will need extra-anatomic revascularisation of extremity
Internal iliac artery	Ligate	
External/internal iliac vein	Ligate	Oedema and DVT
Renal artery	Repair or perform nephrectomy	
Left renal vein	Ligate	
Right renal vein	Repair or perform nephrectomy	

IVC, inferior vena cava; SMA, superior mesenteric artery; SMV, superior mesenteric vein; DVT, deep vein thrombosis.

of massive retrohepatic haemorrhage might necessitate atri-ocaval shunting bypassing IVC flow into the right atrium (this manoeuvre would require a rapid sternotomy).

Control and repair

Some vascular structures should be repaired while other can be ligated (Table 26.4). Options for simple and efficient vascular control differ depending on whether an arterial or venous injury is present and on accessibility of the vessel.

Arterial

Major arterial injuries typically need to be controlled with vascular clamps. If necessary, initial proximal control can always be obtained in the chest or at the diaphragmatic hiatus. Once the area of injury is identified, proximal and distal control should be obtained around the area prior to haematoma 'entry' or repair. Ligation of arterial vessels is more problematic but can be done in selected circumstances with proper flow reconstitution methods. In general, simplest repair is usually the best repair in exsanguinating trauma patient. If the injury can be repaired with a simple suture – do it. Of course some of the injuries might require a full anastomosis or even an interposition graft.

Venous

Venous haemorrhage is typically best controlled by manual pressure. The IVC and iliac veins can be manually compressed using rolled up sponges on ring forceps (i.e. spongesticks). Small, obvious, holes can be controlled with an Allis clamp. Side-biting of large venous structures with a Satinsky can work, but you must be certain that only one side of the vessel is injured. If a clamp does not provide control – switch to compression. As noted in Table 26.4, most venous structures can be ligated with impunity.

Temporary repair

In damage control situations where a formal vascular repair would be time-consuming and technically difficult, temporary vascular repair might be the best option. The superior mesenteric, common iliac and external iliac arteries are most suited for temporary bypass. A vascular shunt can be used to temporary bypass the flow in these vessels during damage control situations.

Table 26.5 Solid organ management.

Should be fixed (Conservative management)	Can be removed
Liver	Spleen
Head of the pancreas	Kidney
	Distal pancreas

Solid organ injury

The easy way to approach solid organ injuries is to divide them into organs that can or cannot be removed (Table 26.5). The simplest approach is usually the best approach. The art of the trauma laparotomy is expedient and efficient control of bleeding and contamination.

Liver

The first move in dealing with liver injury is discerning a small injury from a large injury and obtaining adequate exposure before getting into trouble. Exposure can be rapidly obtained by mobilising the falciform ligament (this should already be done) and triangular ligament on the side of the injury. If there is a suspicion for retrohepatic IVC injury, do not unroof this haematoma.

Packing

The key to liver packing is pressure from without and within. Packs should be placed both outside of the liver between the parenchyma and the thorax and between the liver and the internal structures, i.e. right retroperitoneum, hepatoduodenal ligament and the stomach (Figure 26.6). In cases where the packs will be left in as part of damage control, we prefer to roll the laparotomy pads or towels in Ioban™ to prevent adherence to the surrounding parenchyma and bowel. This simple technique can prevent undesired removal of clot or deserosalisation of bowel during pack removal at re-operation.

Adjuncts

The argon beam coagulator can be helpful in dealing with liver injuries but is not required. When available it is a nice adjunct to absorbable haemostatic agents. A judiciously placed 'liver stitch' (typically a #1 Vicryl on a large, blunt point needle), will at times help approximate edges of the injured liver parenchyma with either absorbable haemostatic material (Gelfoam® wafer soaked in thrombin) or omental pedicle in the middle of this 'parenchymal sandwich'.

Direct attack

When compression and local haemostasis fails, direct attack by further opening the injured parenchyma and suturing or clipping the bleeding vessels is possible. The Pringle manoeuvre should be used at a minimum prior to undertaking the direct attack. Left lateral sectionectomy and segment VI or VII segmentectomies can be rapidly performed with a stapler if necessary. However, direct attack can be a major undertaking and should not be undertaken without experience. Any hepatorrhaphy or hepatic resection should be accompanied by closed-suction drainage to help detect and possibly control a biliary leak.

Interventional radiology

In those cases where haemorrhage cannot be controlled with packing or local manoeuvre, interventional radiology should be mobilised. After packing the liver and applying a damage control dressing, the patient needs to be rapidly transported to the angiography suite for selective embolisation of a bleeding segment or lobe.

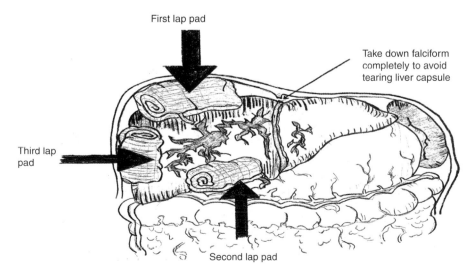

First lap pad

Take down falciform completely to avoid tearing liver capsule

Third lap pad

Second lap pad

Figure 26.6 Proper technique of liver packing: without and within.

Spleen

Recent advances in radiology will guide your management of isolated splenic trauma. It is unlikely that a grade 3 splenic injury without a blush will require a splenectomy. However, if the patient requires a trauma laparotomy for exsanguination, take that same spleen out even if the haemorrhage is likely the result of concomitant liver injury. The key to a trauma splenectomy is quick mobilisation of the injured spleen towards midline.

Taking down the attachments

The spleen has four ligamentous attachments: gastrosplenic, splenorenal, splenocolic and splenophrenic ligaments. All four will need to be divided prior to removal of the spleen, though sometimes the injury has taken down several for you. The key manoeuvre in trauma splenectomy is division of the splenorenal ligament. This allows for mobilisation of the spleen towards the midline, as well as up and into the surgical field. Splenorenal, splenocolic and splenophrenic ligaments can be rapidly divided with either electrocautery or Metzanbaum scissors. Division of the gastrosplenic ligament, however, needs to be more judicious (clips and ties). After all, short gastrics and splenic vessels are contained in this ligament.

Pitfalls and collateral damage

One of the pitfalls of rapid division of gastrosplenic ligament is iatrogenic injury to the tail of the pancreas or the stomach. Pancreatic injury can lead to bleeding as well as a pancreatic leak. Stomach wall injuries can lead to gastric wall necrosis and gastrointestinal leak. Care must be taken to avoid these injuries by not suture ligating (or clipping) too close to the stomach wall. After splenectomy, use a lap-roll method to methodically evaluate the splenic bed for any ongoing bleeding and control these with suture ligatures.

Kidney

The injured kidney is completely retroperitoneal (unless disrupted by severe injury) with its own compression mechanism for haemostasis and rarely requires removal. Grade 1–4 kidney injuries can almost always be managed non-operatively. However, devastating kidney injuries, especially those with rapidly expanding zone 2 haematoma and suspicion for major vascular compromise might require a trauma nephrectomy. In cases of laparotomy without prior abdominal imaging, a good first step is checking the other side for presence of contralateral kidney. In the very rare circumstance where none is present or if it feels atrophied, an attempt at kidney preservation might be entertained, and a urology consultation might be useful.

Similarly to the bleeding spleen, the key to rapid trauma nephrectomy is quick mobilisation of the organ towards midline. A medial visceral rotation to the appropriate side will rapidly expose the kidney. Gerota's fascia can be quickly incised allowing the kidney to be mobilised towards the midline. Adequate medial visceral rotation and mobilisation of the kidney out of the Gerota's fascia will allow isolation of the vascular pedicle. Remember that the renal veins overlay the renal arteries, and that the right renal vein is very short. An injury to the right renal vein is essentially a side hole in the IVC, while the longer left renal vein traverses over the aorta and can be proximally ligated given its collateral drainage. The quickest way to control renal vessels is either with vascular clamps or a vascular stapler. If possible the renal artery and vein should be ligated separately. Do not forget to isolate and ligate the ureter; this is usually performed as distal as possible.

Pancreas

In trauma, the pancreas can be divided into two components based on the location with respect to the surgical neck: 'head and tail'. The 'trauma tail' of the pancreas is the portion extending from the surgical neck distally and includes the anatomic body and tail. This is easily identified as that area to the left of the superior mesenteric artery (SMA) and superior mesenteric vein (SMV). While the 'tail' can be safely and rapidly resected, the head of the pancreas is usually best managed non-operatively.

Exposure

To adequately view the injured pancreas you must be in the lesser sac. The easiest approach to good visualisation is through the gastrocolic omentum. The most fastidious approach is mobilisation of the tail of the pancreas from the left with a distal pancreatectomy with splenectomy. The splenorenal ligament is incised and the spleen is mobilised towards the midline. The spleen is then used as the bucket-handle for mobilising the pancreas from its retroperitoneal attachments.

Distal injury management

In many cases of blunt injury, the proximal transection has already been done. When injury is the result of penetrating trauma, the proximal pancreatic margin can be obtained at the surgical neck with a stapler. Spleen preservation during a distal pancreatectomy is possible, but certainly requires extra time and should not be a part of a trauma laparotomy with exsanguination. After the specimen is removed, a quick attempt can be made to identify the proximal end of the pancreatic duct. If identified, the pancreatic duct can be oversewn with a monofilament suture. Leave a drain in the pancreatic bed to control possible pancreatic leak.

Proximal injury management

When an injury to the pancreatic head is suspected, a full Kocher manoeuvre should be performed, by mobilising the duodenal C-loop from the right towards the midline. Bleeding from the pancreaticoduodenal complex can be usually controlled with judiciously placed monofilament sutures. If pancreatic duct injury is suspected in the head portion, a drain should be left to control possible pancreatic leak. A trauma Whipple should be avoided at nearly all costs. If the injury pattern has performed the resection portion of the pancreaticoduodenectomy, than Whipple reconstruction might be the only option. Regardless, the reconstruction portion of this operation should be performed at re-exploration after damage control and not at the initial trauma laparotomy.

SMA and SMV injury

Injuries to the SMA and the SMV can be associated with pancreatic injury and are usually devastating and difficult to approach. When this injury is suspected, a rapid left and right medial visceral rotation will help optimise exposure. If injury to these vessels remains unidentified, the surgical neck of the pancreas can be divided to provide direct access to these retropancreatic vessels. A simple stitch repair of an identified injury is the best hope for a reasonable patient outcome.

Bowel injury and contamination control

While rapid control of exsanguination is the primary goal of trauma laparotomy, no patient should be transferred back to ICU with ongoing bowel leak. This will only complicate postoperative trauma resuscitation and lead to an uncontrolled systemic inflammatory response (SIRS). Approach to bowel injury depends on the severity of the associated vascular and solid organ injuries and the time remaining on the clock. In cases of damage control, you want to be out of the operating room and in the ICU to resuscitate the patient within one to one and a half hours after incision. However, when cases do not warrant damage control manoeuvres you have more time to perform complete bowel anastomosis.

Rapid control

If you are operating on a patient *in extremis*, then your first priority is stopping the haemorrhage. Just leave the bowel alone and inspect it after the haemorrhage is stopped. If gross spillage is noted, however, these areas of injury can be quickly controlled with umbilical ties proximal and distal to the defect. Once the bleeding is controlled, the whole bowel must be inspected. Run the small bowel first from the ligament of Treitz to the ileocecal valve, or the other way if you prefer. Any injuries can be controlled with Allis or Babcock clamps, or silk suture. Inspect the colon from right to left – from the caecum to the extraperitoneal rectum. Again, control any obvious injury as with small bowel. Do not forget that half of the colon circumference is retroperi-

toneal. If an injury is suspected at any specific location, mobilise the colon and inspect the whole circumference. Control options vary from clamps or quick suture to a formal resection.

Resection

Make sure you inspect the whole bowel before performing any resections. Bowel length should be optimised and conserved; come-up with a resection and reconstruction strategy prior to any cutting or stapling. The easiest and the fastest method for bowel division with spillage control is stapling. Simply create a window in the mesentery and staple along the healthy uninjured bowel just beside the area of injury. The mesentery can then be divided with clamps and ties.

Reconstruction

While there are no set guidelines mandating when to leave the bowel in discontinuity or when to create an anastomosis, simple rules should be applied. If you are planning to close the abdominal fascia, you should establish bowel continuity. If there is an injury to the colon, consider a colostomy. Injuries to the right colon can be more frequently reconstructed with an anastomosis; injuries to the sigmoid and the rectum usually require an ostomy. However, if you are applying damage control techniques, then the bowel should be left in discontinuity. Plans can then be made to re-explore the abdomen within 12–48 hours and reconstruction options should be considered at the next operation.

Stomach, duodenum and rectum

Higher possibility of missed injuries is the reason that these gastrointestinal structures are different from the rest of intra-abdominal bowel. Injury to these structures after blunt trauma is rare; however, injury must be excluded in cases of penetrating injuries.

Stomach

Injury to the back wall of the stomach and to the oesophagogastric junction must be excluded any time there is penetrating injury to the left upper quadrant. The majority of stomach injuries are easy to control with suture or clamp and are usually easy to formally resect with a stapler. Injuries to the oesophagogastric junction and the lesser curvature can be trickier to formally repair and should be done at re-exploration if patient requires damage control closure.

Table 26.6 Factors leading to damage control closure.

Physiologic	Injury pattern
Ongoing hypothermia	Combination of major vascular and bowel injury
Ongoing coagulopathy	Combination of solid organ and vascular and/or bowel injury
Ongoing acidosis	Need for re-exploration for evaluation and/or reconstruction of bowel
Ongoing haemodynamic instability	Multiple cavity injury

Duodenum

Duodenum including the ligament of Treitz should be carefully evaluated every time there is penetrating injury to the pancreaticoduodenal area. Simple suture control and pyloric exclusion (with a stapler) can be entertained at the initial operation; formal repair should almost always be done at re-exploration.

Rectum

The rectum needs to be evaluated after any penetrating injury to the pelvis. At times digital rectal examination alone will reveal an injury. However, if the examination is negative, a rigid proctosigmoidoscopy should be performed to exclude rectal injury. In all cases of rectal injury (i.e. extra- and intraperitoneal) a diverting colostomy is the best treatment option.

Miscellaneous injuries

In this brief section, we will mention a few structures which must be fixed during the first trauma laparotomy and that do not fit into one of the three criteria mentioned above. Specifically, these are the diaphragm and the bladder.

Diaphragm

Both blunt and penetrating injuries can cause diaphragmatic injuries. Higher level of suspicion should exist after any case of penetrating thoracoabdominal trauma. The diaphragm should be visually and manually inspected by both surgeons to exclude an injury. We repair all diaphragmatic injuries with #1 non-absorbable suture. Controlling the corners of diaphragmatic laceration with Allis clamps will help evert the edges of the diaphragm towards you. A large needle will help obtain good purchase on the muscle.

Bladder

Intraperitoneal bladder injuries are usually easily identified by the presence of a urine leak even if the bladder is decompressed by a urinary catheter. A simple one layer repair with #3–0 absorbable suture will usually work; however, some groups advocate a two-layer closure. Data on the duration of mandatory bladder decompression vary; a minimum of 5–7 days and/or a contrast study should be performed before removing the Foley catheter.

Abdominal closure

Shortly after initiating a trauma laparotomy, the surgeon should decide (and voice this decision to the members of the operative team) the closure option that will be performed. In trauma laparotomy there are two choices: primary abdominal fascial closure or an abbreviated laparotomy with application of damage control techniques. A number of factors influence the decision for choosing the damage control option (Table 26.6). In addition to the development of the lethal triad, a combination of major vascular and hollow viscus injuries or exsanguination from numerous structures are best approached as a two-stage procedure. Questionable bowel viability should also be re-examined with a 'second look' laparotomy.

Primary fascial closure

There are many methods to closing abdominal fascia. Running #1 looped polydioxone (PDS II) sutures; one from each side of the incision with a knot just above the umbilicus is a commonly accepted method. The subcutaneous tissues should be irrigated and skin edges re-approximated with staples.

Damage control

Towel clips, running suture and Bogota bag (intravenous fluid bag) have all been described as quick and easy closure methods when employing damage control. Many units prefer the vacuum-pack abdominal closure technique. This is simple and fast.

Once the decision has been made to perform damage control closure, alert the nursing staff to get the appropriate supplies. First layer is a bowel bag ventilated with numerous holes which is generously spread underneath the fascia to protect the intra-abdominal contents. Second layer is a moistened surgical towel tucked just under the fascia edges and overlaid with two flat-fluted Jackson-Pratt® drains which will be placed to suction.

An optional surgical towel can be placed on top of the drains. Lastly an Ioban™ antimicrobial adhesive drape is used to seal the contents of the vacuum-packed abdomen.

A member of the operating team should accompany the anaesthesia team in transporting a critically injured patient with damage control closure to the ICU. A word of caution: all surgical bleeding must be controlled prior to damage con-trol closure. Damage control closure will not stop major vascular exsanguination. Furthermore, all sources of contamination should be controlled to prevent exacerbated SIRS.

Further reading

Feliciano DV, Mattox KL, Moore EE (eds). *Trauma*, 6th edn. McGraw-Hill, New York, 2008.

Hirshberg Λ, Mattox KL. *Top Knife: Art and Craft in Trauma Surgery*. TFM Publishing Ltd., Shropshire, 2005.

Souba WW, Fink MP, Jurkovich GJ, et al. (eds). *ACS Surgery*, 6th edn. American College of Surgeons, New York, 2007.

Operative Management of Thoracic Trauma

Thomas König[1] & Nigel Tai[1,2]

[1]Defence Medical Services, Trauma Clinical Academic Unit, Royal London Hospital, Whitechapel, London, UK
[2]Academic Department of Military Surgery and Trauma, Royal Centre for Defence Medicine, Birmingham, UK

Introduction

Most thoracic injuries can be managed non-operatively or by intercostal tube drainage, but a number of thoracic injuries require operative intervention. Three types of intervention exist:

1 Resuscitative surgery to immediately address exsanguination or cardiac tamponade.

Resuscitative thoracotomy via a left anterolateral or bilateral "clamshell" thoracotomy.

2 Urgent surgery to address significant ongoing haemorrhage, compensated cardiac tamponade or major air leak.

Anterolateral (ipsilateral or bilateral) thoracotomy or median sternotomy

3 Elective surgery to treat the retained haemothorax or to stabilise the chest wall.

As above; video-assisted thoracoscopic surgery (VATS)

Early involvement of cardiothoracic personnel is desirable but absence of cardiothoracic (CT) surgeons and heart bypass facilities should not preclude appropriate interventions when necessary. *However, surgical intervention should only be performed by those who are trained and competent to do so.*

Resuscitative (clamshell) thoracotomy

Background

• Should be performed immediately when required and so can be carried out in the resuscitation room.

• Indications: *In extremis* (actual or near circulatory arrest) patient with **penetrating** trauma to the chest, root of the neck or epigastrium **and** recent (<10 minutes) presence of vital signs (spontaneous movements, pupillary response, eye movement, spontaneous respirations, narrow complex electrical activity by ECG, >40 beats/minute).

• Survival rates are highest in isolated penetrating cardiac injury and lowest in blunt trauma.

Emergency Surgery, 1st edition. Edited by Adam Brooks, Peter F. Mahoney, Bryan A. Cotton and Nigel Tai. © 2010 Blackwell Publishing.

• Resuscitative thoracotomy in blunt trauma patients is controversial and should be confined to patients with ultrasound evidence of pericardial blood and recently present vital signs (as described above).

• Post-survival neurological impairment occurs in 15% of survivors.

Resuscitative thoracotomy procedures

The four manoeuvres that can be accomplished by resuscitative thoracotomy are:

1 Drainage of the pericardium (pericardiotomy) and control of a cardiac laceration.

2 Internal cardiac massage (if no cardiac output).

3 Lung twist or hilar clamp (to control massive pulmonary haemorrhage).

4 Aortic compression or cross clamping (to augment cerebral perfusion).

Equipment

Universal precautions and sterile preparation and equipment when possible

Scalpel no. 22 blade for skin incision

Spencer Wells forceps for separation of intercostal muscles from superior rib surface

Gigli saw and handles or heavy scissors for sternal division

Rib spreader (large)

Forceps (toothed or otherwise) to tent the pericardium

Scissors to open the pericardium

Needle holder

Prolene and pledgets to repair myocardial wounds

Aortic cross-clamping to optimise cerebral and myocardial perfusion and oxygenation

Satinsky clamp (can also be used to clamp the hilum of the lung)

Large gauze swabs and/or portable suction apparatus

Procedure

1 Quick skin preparation from neck to subcostal margin and laterally.

2 Bilateral anterolateral thoracotomies across the midline in the inframammary fold below the nipples.

3 The incision is deepened and the intercostal muscles divided until the pleura is visible. This is then incised and opened with scissors from sternal border to mid axillary line.
4 The pericardium and heart are separated from the posterior surface of the sternum via a digital "sweep".
5 The sternum is divided with scissors or with a saw.
6 The rib spreader is inserted or the superior thoracic wall held open by an assistant.
7 Cardiac tamponade should always be excluded. A longitudinal incision is made in the midline anterior to the phrenic nerve. Clotted blood is removed and the heart is delivered and inspected. Obvious holes are controlled by finger pressure while a suture is mounted and pledgets placed for repair of repairable wounds.
8 Internal cardiac massage should be instigated if there is no return of spontaneous activity.
9 If fibrillating, defibrillation should be carried out internally and resuscitation should continue as per ACLS protocols (10–30 Joules).
10 Manual or instrumental compression of the descending thoracic aorta above the diaphragm can be carried out to maximise myocardial filling and perfusion of the heart and brain.
11 Massive lung parenchyma bleeding or air leak should be immediately controlled by hilar compression. This can be done by clamping or 180° lung twisting after division of the inferior pulmonary ligament.
12 If no thoracic injuries are found and infradiaphragmatic injuries are suspected the aorta should be clamped and fluid replacement should begin (ideally with blood and blood products). If the heart shows signs of activity then further operative intervention in the abdomen is warranted.
13 Closure may be primary or delayed and intercostal drains should be placed in the pericardium and laterally Care should be taken to ensure that the internal mammary arteries – divided during sternal division – have been properly ligated.
14 Primary closure involves approximation of the ribs with interrupted Ethibond sutures, closure of the chest wall musculature with continuous Vicryl and skin staples.
15 Temporary coverage methods include gauze Opsite 'sandwiches' or large saline bags ('Bogota bag') sutured to the skin edges.

Adjuncts to myocardial repair and optimisation of coronary artery pressure

Finger pressure if repair is not possible whilst cardiothoracic help summoned
Foley catheter insertion and inflation (also allows a portal for fluid and drug infusion)
  • This may be either through the myocardial wound or separately into the right atrium. A purse string suture will be required to reduce blood loss from around the catheter and to hold it firmly in place.

Skin stapling devices for rapid closure of ventricular wounds

Pitfalls
• Damage to the myocardium and underlying lung parenchyma due to inexperienced, overly exuberant, rushed incision-making during initial.
• Care should be taken to ensure that the incision is not too low and the diaphragm is not damaged and the abdomen inadvertently entered.
• Nipple injury is to be avoided.
• The 'clamshell' thoracotomy is not ideal when attempting to repair posterior chest wall bleeders or injuries to posterior mediastinal structures.

Median sternotomy

Background
• Useful when dealing with root-of-neck penetrating trauma to gain control of the aortic arch vessels.
• Acceptable for urgent cases where access to the heart is the primary objective and no other hilar/lung injury suspected.

Procedure
Vertical incision in the midline from sternal notch to below the xiphoid process
Bluntly develop the retrosternal plane from above the manubrium and below through the linea alba
A saw should be used to divide the sternum in the midline
Diathermy and bone wax can be used to control bleeding from the bone edges
Open slowly with Finochietto's retractor
Identify the brachiocephalic vein, clamp, divide and ligate it to gain access to anterior arch
Dissect backwards and sloop arch vessels as required (note posterior position of left subclavian)
Closure using steel wires to approximate sternal edges.

Hilar clamping

Background
• Used to gain control of massive air leak and uncontrolled lung haemorrhage.
• Poorly tolerated in shocked patients.

Procedure
Expose lung
Divide inferior pulmonary ligament
Identify the hilum and pulmonary artery, vein and mainstem bronchus
Encircle the hilum between finger and thumb; easier when lung ventilation is stopped
Sling with a tape or clamp with a vascular clamp

Perform rapid repair of lung tissue (tractotomy and non-anatomical resection)

Lung twist allows for rapid control without the need for clamping

Aortic cross-clamping

Background
• Should be performed as distally as possible in the thorax.
• Manual compression against the vertebral column can be carried out prior to instrumentation and is safer.
• An under-filled and pulseless aorta is difficult to locate if inexperienced (have someone pass a nasogastric or orogastric tube to distinguish aorta from oesophagus).
• Aim is to optimise cerebral blood flow and coronary vessel pressure.
• Clamp-time should be minimised to 30 minutes or less to avoid profound visceral ischaemia and reperfusion injury.
• No return of blood pressure after clamping = futile procedure.

Procedure
Retract the left lung anteriorly
Palpate the posterior chest wall from lateral to medial, feeling the ribs as they arch towards the spine
The first tubular structure is the aorta
Open the parietal pleura anterior and posterior to the vessel with scissors
Apply blades of vascular clamp anterior and posterior to aorta and occlude with minimal necessary force
Be very wary of intercostal vessels or injury to the aorta itself

Tracheobronchial repair

Background
• Injury to trachea, right and left main bronchi and bronchioles.
• Can occur in both blunt and penetrating trauma.
• Results in failure of ventilation and oxygenation.
• Indications for surgery include persistent pneumothorax/massive air leak despite multiple intercostal drains, suction and low-volume ventilation strategies.

Procedure
Double lumen endotracheal intubation allows selective ventilation.
Optimal access to the thoracic cavity ('Collar' incision or median sternotomy for tracheal injuries, anterolateral thoracotomy if spine not "cleared"; posterolateral thoracotomy offers a better view of the entire lung (but the lateral patient positioning required is often not feasible in the acute setting).

Operative closure of airway by suture and soft tissue wrapping using intercostal muscle flap.

Pericardiotomy and myocardial repair

Background
• The anteriorly placed right ventricle is the most commonly affected part of the heart.
• Tamponade may occur after a small volume of blood fills the pericardium.
• For best results, surgery and release should occur before cardiac output is lost.
• Indications for surgery include penetrating torso injury and:
  ○ Pericardial effusion on ultrasound examination +/− cardiovascular instability
• Mandatory pre-discharge echocardiography to rule out missed valvular/septal injury after successful repairs.

Procedure (see resuscitative thoracotomy)
Clamshell thoracotomy or median sternotomy according to patient stability.
Visualisation of pericardial surface and generous longitudinal incision anterior to phrenic nerve.
Remove clot
Assess for myocardial injury to the anterior and posterior surfaces, filling state and activity of the heart
Inspect for wounds to the surrounding structures in particular the great vessels
Treat myocardial wounds as found
Atrial injuries:
  Low pressure system
  After digital pressure, forceps or a clamp can be used to gain control
  Over-and-over stitch or purse string suture
Ventricle injuries:
  High pressure system
  Avoid occlusion of coronary vessels
  Horizontal mattress suture with 3/0 prolene, double ended
  Pledgets, either Teflon or pericardium, should be used to augment repair and prevent sutures tearing through

Control and repair of lung injury

Background
• Required when pulmonary puncture, laceration, or contusion results in a massive haemothorax or major air leak.
• Indications for surgery:
  ○ Initial intercostal tube drainage of >1500 mL
  ○ More than 500 mL/hour for 2 consecutive hours

○ Massive air leak manifesting as failure to oxygenate and/or persistent leak and 'bubbling' of air into the underwater drain

○ Cardiovascular instability

Procedure

Extended anterolateral or posterolateral thoracotomy and parenchymal repair

Superficial wounds:

Interrupted Z-mattress 2/0 prolene sutures

Non-viable tissue:

Non-anatomical wedge resection using a linear stapler-cutter or a crushing clamp, resection and over-suture of the lung edge.

Deep wounds:

Avoid simple surface closure and thus avoid air embolism or entrapment of on going intra-parenchymal haemorrhage with resultant abcess formation.

Hilar control should be gained first in exsanguinating haemorrhage.

Uncontrollable haemorrhage, widespread parenchymal damage and non-viable tissue:

Bleeding is commonly from multiple or indeterminate sites and a formal lobectomy or pneumonectomy may be required.

Lobectomy:

After parenchymal dissection, the veins, then artery and bronchus are divided

Pneumonectomy:

Associated with a 50% mortality. This is readily undertaken using a surgical stapler device (eg TA stapler), dividing the hilar structures distal to the stapler before the device is removed and over-sewing the staple line. Pneumonectomy may precipitate right heart failure and necessitate extracorporeal membrane oxygenation (ECMO) support.

Repair of traumatic aortic injury

Background

• Usually occurs just distal to the left subclavian artery.

• Bleeding is constrained by the adventitial layer.

• Beta-blockade aids preoperative control (assuming patient is not in shock from other sources).

• All injuries must be repaired, though intra-abdominal sources of bleeding should be addressed first.

Procedure

Endovascular management:

• Thoracic endovascular aortic repair is finding favour in specialist centres.

• Complications include stent collapse, embolisation or endoleak.

• Lifelong follow-up needed to monitor stent.

• Some patients require revascularisation of left subclavian (covered by stent).

Operative management:

• Posterolateral or extended left anterolateral thoracotomy

• Clamp above and below the transection

• Gott shunt or heparin-bonded shunt from above to below to maintain lower body perfusion

• Direct repair using pledgetted 3/0 prolene or interposition graft

• Full or left-heart bypass can be used to lengthen repair times

Complications include renal failure and paralysis.

Repair of superior mediastinal vascular injuries

Background

• Associated with penetrating injuries to Zone 1 of the neck (see chapter 24).

• Unstable patients require urgent operative intervention with out delay. Stable patients may undergo confirmatory imaging (CTA) first.

• Endovascular stent repair of proximal subclavian artery injury is a favourable technique in the stable patient and avoids a morbid incision.

Procedure

Median sternotomy provides optimal access in order to gain proximal control of the injured subclavian or brachiocephalic vessels.

Distal control of vessels can be gained within the chest or by extending up in to the anterolateral neck (carotid) or laterally via supra- and infraclavicular counter incisions (2nd/3rd part of the subclavian artery respectively).

The second and third parts of the subclavian vessels can be reached via supraclavicular and infraclavicular counter incisions.

Proximal and distal control is required prior to exploration of upper mediastinal haematoma.

Vessels are repaired by direct repair, patch repair, end-to-end repair, vein graft or interposition graft.

Repair of oesophageal injury

Background

• May occur in blunt, penetrating or barotrauma

• Single breaches are most common

• Surgical repair is mandatory

Procedure

Incision depends on location of injury; left anterior border of sternocleidomastoid (neck), thoracotomy or midline laparotomy

One- or two-layer technique (one mucosal and one muscular) with tissue wrapping of the repair

Drainage close to the repair

Nasogastric tube drainage and feeding jejunostomy

Diaphragmatic injury

Background

• Occurs in both blunt and penetrating trauma

• Abdominal visceral herniation into the thorax (more common on the left side) can result in strangulation of bowel with subsequent perforation

• Suspicion may be aroused by a poorly defined hemidiaphragm on chest radiograph, or viscera in the chest on CXR or CT

Procedure

Repair is typically undertaken by laparotomy using interrupted 1-prolene sutures after reduction of abdominal contents into the abdomen.

Video-assisted thoracoscopic surgery

Background

• As a minimally invasive procedure the morbidity and mortality of the procedure is less than open surgery.

• Of little use in the acute setting and in the cardiovascularly unstable patient.

• Retained haemothoraces are at high risk of infection and subsequent empyema formation or formation of a fibrous capsule restricting lung expansion.

Procedure

One lung ventilation is required to allow deflation of the ipsilateral lung

The camera is introduced into the pleural cavity via pre-existing incisions made to site intercostal drains

Further incisions are made over the site of the haemothorax under direct vision to introduce large bore suction/irrigation

Adhesions are broken down and the clot aspirated. Two chest drains are placed

Postoperative chest radiography confirms lung re-inflation and drainage of retained fluid

Pearls and pitfalls

• Preoperative chest radiography with marking of the entrance and exit wounds aids decision making.

• When inserting an intercostal drain, assign someone to monitor the output.

• Be aware that the drain may kink, become blocked or fall out under the draped patient.

• Thoracoabdominal penetrating wounds present difficulties in selecting which body region to enter first:

   ○ Injuries may occur to organs either side of the diaphragm

   ○ Be vigilant and tactically versatile and flexible

   ○ Change your plan and body region quickly if required

   ○ Remember that bleeding may be coming across the diaphragm from injured abdominal viscera particularly the liver

• Gunshot wound Trajectories that cross the midline (particularly with bullets) in hypotensive patients are associated with poorer outcomes and require a damage control approach from the outset.

• Remember that thoracotomy and laparotomy are acceptable as aids to diagnosis in the unstable patient:

   ○ Control bleeding at all costs

   ○ Replace lost fluid with blood and blood products

   ○ Warm the patient during surgery

• Match the surgical intervention to the patient's physiology.

Further reading

Kenneth DB. *Manual of Definitive Surgical Trauma Care*. Arnold Publishers, London, 2003.

Trauma Organisation. www.trauma.org.

28 Abdominal Trauma: Operative and Non-Operative Management

Roland A. Hernández[1], Aviram M. Giladi[2] & Bryan A. Cotton[3]

[1]University of Michigan School of Medicine, Ann Arbor, MI, USA
[2]Department of Surgery, University of Michigan School of Medicine, Ann Arbor, MI, USA
[3]Department of Surgery and The Center for Translational Injury Research, The University of Texas Health Science Center at Houston, Houston, TX, USA

Introduction

When approaching abdominal trauma, it is critical to determine the mechanism of injury. Abdominal trauma is broadly divided into blunt and penetrating injuries, with management guidelines differing accordingly. Rapid evaluation, diagnosis and treatment are key to preventing or lessening the overwhelming potential for morbidity and mortality.

Penetrating abdominal trauma may result from any penetrating injury as high as the nipple line anteriorly and the scapula tip posteriorly, and as low as the buttocks inferiorly. While 80% of all abdominal gunshot wounds (GSWs) require operative intervention, only a third of stab wounds require laparotomy. Antibiotic coverage with extended spectrum penicillin, a second-generation cephalosporin, or metronidazole and an aminoglycoside is often indicated if surgery is required. All patients will need tetanus prophylaxis.

A significant majority of blunt trauma (~80%) is caused by motor vehicle or motorcycle collisions. Other mechanisms include: falls, athletic collisions, bicycle crashes and assaults. Mechanism of injury plays a role in determining potential for intra-abdominal injury. Injury to abdominal viscera in these patients results from shearing, compression, rapid and drastic increases in abdominal pressures, or any combination thereof.

> Patients with blunt mechanism of injury with haemodynamic instability and positive FAST (focused assessment with sonography for trauma) or DPL (diagnostic peritoneal lavage) should undergo immediate laparotomy.

Emergency Surgery, 1st edition. Edited by Adam Brooks, Peter F. Mahoney, Bryan A. Cotton and Nigel Tai. © 2010 Blackwell Publishing.

Distal oesophagus

Injuries to the distal portion of the oesophagus are very rare, and when they do occur they are almost always from penetrating trauma. That being said, 6–10 cm of oesophagus exist in the abdomen, so injury is a possibility. If injury is detected in the vicinity of the oesophagus, it must be evaluated. This may require mobilisation of stomach, spleen and left lobe of liver, rotating the oesophagus through 180° to fully examine. If there is high suspicion but injury is not seen, infusion of normal saline (or methylene blue) into the distal oesophagus with the proximal stomach clamped may define an injury. Alternatively, the surgeon may try infusing air into the oesophagus while the stomach is filled with normal saline to detect an air leak.

Treatment

Decisions on repair depend on time from injury. Injuries less than 6 hours can be repaired primarily with two layers of absorbable sutures and buttressed with pleura. With more complex injuries, or those older than 6 hours, repair may be possible but diversion with a cervical oesophagostomy may be required. All injures should be drained with two or more chest tubes. In addition, a feeding gastrostomy or jejunostomy should be placed.

Complications

Anastomotic leak, empyema, oesophago-cutaneous fistula formation and sepsis are increased with delays in diagnosis. In fact, a delay in diagnosis of as little as 12–16 hours can markedly increase the risk of complications and death. For this reason, many authors would suggest aborting attempts at primary repair and simply debriding and widely draining this population.

Outcomes

Oesophageal injuries carry a fairly high mortality owing to the injuries often associated with trauma to the distal oesophagus. However, the primary determinant of outcome lies in time to diagnosis. Patients who have their injures diagnosed in the first 12 hours and undergo simple repair have a 10–12% mortality rate. Those whose injuries are diagnosed after 12 hours and those requiring debridement and wider drainage have mortalities of 30–40%.

Gastric

Gastric injuries occur in 10–15% of penetrating traumas and in 1–2% of blunt trauma. The stomach has an extensive blood supply provided by the gastric, short gastric and gastroepiploic arteries. Physical examination may demonstrate peritoneal signs or bloody nasogastric aspirate may be observed in up to a third of patients. Injury may also be demonstrated by computed tomography (CT) findings, or DPL returning gastric fluids. Chest X-ray may reveal free sub-diaphragmatic air in less than 50% of blunt gastric rupture.

Treatment
Treatment for gastric injury is usually laparotomy with debridement and repair. Only rarely is gastric resection required. Pyloroplasty may be performed to avoid stenosis. The abdomen should be irrigated to remove spilled gastric contents.

Complications
While outcomes for the gastric injury itself are generally good overall, morbidity and mortality from associated injuries are common. Recent studies have reported a high risk of intra-abdominal infection and sepsis associated with gastric injury. Up to 25% of patients will develop postoperative symptoms after gastric surgery, with 2–4% having debilitating symptoms.

Duodenum

Up to 75% of duodenal injuries are due to penetrating trauma, especially GSWs. These injuries are rarely isolated, with up to 98% having injury to surrounding structures. The second portion of the duodenum (D2) contains the opening of the bile and pancreatic ducts and is the most commonly injured segment. Clinical suspicion should guide diagnosis as signs and symptoms may be subtle. In blunt injuries, the patient may complain of mid-epigastric or RUQ pain, with or without peritoneal signs. Abdominal X-ray may show retroperitoneal air or an obliterated right psoas muscle margin. CT should be performed with water-soluble oral contrast and may show para-duodenal haemorrhage and an air or contrast leak. If CT findings are equivocal, an upper gastrointestinal (UGI) swallow study should next be performed starting with water-soluble contrast. If this is negative, a bar-

ium study should follow. Intramural duodenal haematoma will have a 'coiled-string' appearance on UGI study.

Treatment
Duodenal perforation requires operative repair and this repair is often 'diverted' for protection. Diversion can be done via gastrostomy, jejunostomy or duodenostomy. Repairs may also be protected by pyloric exclusion – closure with suture or staple – which will gradually re-open over a 3-week period. With exclusion procedures, gastric drainage is usually into a loop of jejunum. Rarely, injuries to the duodenum and pancreatic head may require a pancreaticoduodenectomy (Whipple procedure).

Intramural duodenal haematoma occurs more commonly in children, and is managed non-operatively with nasogastric (NG) suction and bowel rest. Follow-up gastrograffin UGI study is performed every 7 days if an obstruction clinically persists. Operative management is usually required if there is no clinical resolution after 7–14 days. If the injury is first found at laparotomy, proper treatment remains controversial. Some advocate evacuation and repair, while others support exploration for perforation and NG decompression if no perforation is found. Regardless, a jejunal feeding tube should be considered for postoperative feeding.

Complications
Almost two-thirds of patients with duodenal injury will develop complications. Almost half of all deaths following duodenal trauma are due to duodenal dehiscence and sepsis. Fistula formation occurs in 10–15% of cases, but is reduced to 2% with retrograde decompression.

Outcomes
The mortality rate approaches 40% if the diagnosis is delayed (after 24 hours), but is reduced to 10% or less if diagnosed in the first 24 hours. Given the significant reduction in complications (especially fistula formation) with retrograde tube decompression, it is not surprising that mortality is reduced dramatically when decompression is employed (19–9%).

> Irrespective of time to diagnosis or type of operative management chosen, duodenal injuries requiring surgical intervention are at a high risk of leak and should be widely drained.

Small bowel

The small bowel (SB) is the most commonly injured organ in penetrating trauma. Blunt SB injuries are less common, comprising 5–15% of all blunt injuries. The SB is supplied by the superior mesenteric artery and drained by the superior mesenteric vein. SB injuries often go undiagnosed on initial presentation, but should be suspected when the patient has evidence of lap belt contusion. Because the SB contents have a neutral pH, the patient is less likely to have peritoneal signs initially. Perforation secondary to blunt injury is most common at the ligament of Treitz, the ileocaecal valve, the mid-jejunum and in areas of abdominal adhesions. Chance fractures of the lumbar spine increase the likelihood of duodenal injury 30–60%.

Treatment

Simple lacerations can be closed transversely if less than 50% SB circumference is involved. Larger defects require resection and anastomosis. Caution should be exercised with mesenteric injury, as there is a risk of significant bleeding. In cases of mesenteric haematomas, the area should be imbricated along the anti-mesenteric wall to rule out occult perforations which can have a delayed presentation.

Complications

Anastomotic leak occurs in 2% of cases. This may manifest as an enterocutaneous fistula, frank peritonitis or intra-abdominal abscess. SB obstruction also occurs in 2% of cases.

Outcomes

Delayed diagnosis contributes significantly to morbidity and mortality. If identified and repaired early, outcomes are generally good.

Colon

Penetrating large bowel injuries occur in 25% of GSW and 5% of stab wounds. The large bowel is injured in 2–5% of all blunt injuries. The rectum is injured in up to 5% of all colon injuries. Blunt rectal perforation is associated with pelvic fractures or concussion injury, or due to de-vascularisation from mesenteric injury. Patients may have peritoneal signs or free intraperitoneal air on imaging. Gross blood demonstrated on rectal examination and occurring in the context of pelvic fracture should lead to prompt proctoscopy. Haemodynamically stable patients may undergo proctoscopy in the OR, whereas unstable patients are first managed with laparotomy. Gross blood on rectal examination with penetrating injury to abdomen, buttocks or pelvic wound is pathognomonic of colorectal injury, even if no defect seen on proctoscopy. Many rectal injuries have concomitant bladder and distal ureter injury.

Treatment

Traditionally, colon injuries were resected and anastomosed or resected and a colostomy created. Currently, however, primary repair should be undertaken if the following criteria are met: (1) minimal faecal spillage, (2) absence of shock (systolic BP >90 mm Hg), (3) minimal associated intra-abdominal injuries, (4) less than 8 hours between diagnosis and treatment and (5) less than 1 L blood loss. Primary repair is contraindicated with extensive intraperitoneal faecal spillage, extensive colonic injury requiring resection and major abdominal wall loss or mesh repair. Colostomy or resection and anastomosis should be performed if primary repair cannot be performed safely.

Rectal injuries involving the intraperitoneal rectum can often be primarily repaired as with the colon. However, those injuries below the peritoneal reflection (extraperitoneal) are often treated with diverting sigmoid colostomy. This is based on the density of bacterial colonisation versus the remaining bowel, adequacy of blood supply and constraints of a low pelvic anastomosis given the acutely altered surgical field.

Complications

Similar to that for small bowel injury, colocutaneous fistulae occur in approximately 2% of patients. Five per cent of patients with colorectal injuries develop an intra-abdominal abscess. This is highest among those undergoing colostomy, in which 15–20% develop abscesses. Fortunately, most are amenable to percutaneous drainage.

Outcomes

Overall morbidity and mortality rates are 5–10%. However, there is less morbidity associated with primary repair performed in a single procedure as compared to an initial laparotomy with colostomy and a later reversal. The mortality for pelvic fracture with rectal perforation is 20%.

> Most colon injures seen in civilian settings can be managed with resection and re-anastomosis.

Liver

The liver is the most commonly injured abdominal organ, with penetrating injury occurring more often than blunt injury. Due to multiple ligamentous attachments, mobilisation/repair of the liver may result in injury to diaphragm, phrenic veins and hepatic veins. The right and left lobes are divided along a sagittal line formed by the IVC and gallbladder fossa – the plane created here is relatively avascular.

Treatment

The majority of hepatic injuries are now managed non-operatively with increasing success (regardless of injury grade). Non-operative management is most successful in patients that are haemodynamically stable and who have no other abdominal organ injuries requiring operative repair. The presence of haemoperitoneum does not mandate surgical intervention. However, higher-grade injuries (IV and V) and those with active contrast extravasation or intra-abdominal pooling by CT are likely to fail conservative management. It is prudent, though, to attempt angioembolisation if there is active bleeding requiring repeat transfusion. Laparotomy should be performed if the patient is unstable, develops peritoneal signs or fails embolisation.

Many common practices in non-operative management are without sound support in literature. There is no clearly shown need for serial haemoglobin/haematocrit, continuous bed rest or prolonged ICU monitoring and care. As well, repeat CT is largely unnecessary. If laparotomy is required, evaluate the need for immediate transfusion of blood and blood products.

Intraoperatively, the liver can tolerate between 60 and 90 minutes of warm ischaemia time. Hepatorrhaphy with individual vessel ligation is preferred to mass parenchymal suturing.

Segmental resection with debridement and direct suture control of vessels/ducts in non-viable tissues is preferred over true anatomic resection. Hypothermia, coagulopathy and continuous haemorrhage necessitate a damage–control intervention with perihepatic packing to control bleeding. Hepatic artery ligation to control intraparenchymal bleeding is a rarely needed but usually survivable technique due to portal blood oxygen delivery. Ligation of the hepatic vein can result in compromise of both liver and bowel.

Outcomes

As most injuries to the liver are grade I and II injuries, overall mortality rates for hepatic injuries are approximately 10%. In those with higher grades, however, associated mortality ranges from 25% for grade III injuries to almost 80% for grade V injuries. The liver has tremendous ability to heal. While not confirmed with controlled trials, the general practice is to observe hepatic injures in the hospital for at least 1 day/injury grade, keep the patient on light activity for at least 1 week/injury grade and restrict from contact sports/high-impact activities for 1 month/injury grade.

Complications

Ongoing bleeding occurs in 5–7% of patients and will require either embolisation or return to the operating theatre. To minimise this, ensure that any hypothermia and coagulopathy are corrected.

Intrahepatic abscesses, perihepatic abscesses and bilomas occur in up to 40% of patients, and can usually be treated with percutaneous drainage. Haemobilia is rare and can present anywhere from days to weeks after initial injury. The classic triad of jaundice, right upper quadrant pain and haemorrhage is seen in only a third of patients. The management of haemobilia centres around angiography and embolisation. This complication may indicate presence of a hepatic artery pseudoaneurysm. A biliary fistula is defined as bile drainage of greater than 50 mL/day for at least 2 weeks. If external drainage is adequate and there is no distal obstruction, most fistulae will resolve without operative intervention. However, when bile leaks exceed 300 mL/day, evaluation with ERCP should be performed. Most will resolve with endoscopic sphincterotomy or transampullary stenting but major ductal injury may require duct stenting to facilitate healing and operative intervention may be required in rare circumstances.

Extrahepatic biliary injury

Injuries to the extrahepatic biliary tree are rare, with gallbladder injury being the most common. When injuries to the duct do occur they may be missed without careful inspection of the porta hepatis. Once injury to the extrahepatic biliary tree is identified, a cholangiogram through the cystic duct stump after cholecystectomy can help define the injury.

Treatment

Gallbladder injury is treated with cholecystectomy. Location and severity of ductal injury determines treatment. Simple bile duct injury with less than 50% circumferential injury can be primarily repaired with suture (transversely). Complex bile duct injury, with more than 50% circumferential injury, may require Roux-en-Y choledochojejunostomy or hepaticojejunostomy. It is not recommended to attempt primary end-to-end anastomosis for repair, as the stricture rate can approach 50%.

Hepatic artery ligation is a rarely needed but survivable technique due to portal blood oxygen delivery. Ligation of the portal vein, however, can result in compromise of both liver and bowel. In patients with porta hepatis injuries, cholecystectomy should be performed to avoid delayed necrosis from compromised blood supply.

Complications

The most common complications of the extrahepatic biliary tree injury are fistula and stricture formation. Strictures may present with cholangitis or biliary cirrhosis. While fistulas may be amenable to percutaneous drainage, strictures will require operative or endoscopic intervention.

Outcomes

Blunt injury to this area, in general, has poorer outcomes than for penetrating injuries; collateral damage/associated injuries versus isolated injury from GSW. However, even outcomes for blunt portal injuries seem to have improved over the past decade with the wider application of damage control principles. Initial reports with portal vein repair had survival at 10% compared to those with ligation yielding survival as high as 80%.

Spleen

The spleen is frequently injured, with blunt injuries far more common than penetrating. These injuries are strongly associated with lower rib fractures – up to 25% of rib 9–12 fractures have associated splenic injury. Splenic injury is the most common cause of haemoperitoneum in trauma. Numerous ligamentous attachments tether the spleen to the stomach, diaphragm, left kidney/adrenal gland, colon and body wall. Angiography can be used for therapeutic embolisation of arterial bleeding, although this appears to be most valuable in mid-grade injuries with an active contrast 'blush'.

Treatment

Non-operative management

Non-operative management is successful in up to 65% of blunt traumatic injuries. Grades I and II are almost always successfully managed non-operatively. Grade III can often be treated non-operatively and angioembolisation can be a useful adjunct in those with a contrast 'blush'. Grades IV and V often present with haemodynamic instability and proceed directly to the operating room. In the patient that is haemodynamically stable, non-operative management with close ICU observation and ready access to emergent OR has been successful. Changes in clinical examination, haemodynamic stability, ongoing fluid requirements or need for transfusion require laparotomy. The failure rate of non-operative management is 5% for grade I, 10% for grade II, 20% for grade III, 33% for grade IV and 75% for grade V. Most failures will occur by 72 hours after injury.

In children, non-operative management is successful in as many as 90% of cases regardless of severity of injury. Risk of failure does not directly correlate with grade of injury. OPSI/S is more common in children. The risk significantly increases with age <5 years, underscoring the importance of conservative management in children. Management will be somewhat guided by injury grade, with higher grades requiring more frequent abdominal examinations, closer haemodynamic monitoring and serial haematology studies.

Operative

Splenectomy in trauma is best approached through a midline incision, packing for haemorrhage and controlling GI spillage first. The gastrosplenic and splenocolic ligaments must be ligated as they contain vascular structures. Ligate these vessels closer to the spleen to prevent risk of gastric necrosis. The short gastric vessels may not be intact as they are often avulsed from the spleen with blunt trauma. The splenorenal and splenophrenic ligaments are avascular. Although rarely an option, attempt spleen-saving manoeuvres with grade I and II injuries in the non-coagulopathic patient. Topical haemostatic agents, argon beam coagulator, suture repair, mesh wrap or even segmental resection with lobular artery ligation have been advocated. One-third of the splenic mass must be functional to maintain immunocompetence. Therefore, the ability to save at least half of the organ is needed to justify splenorrhaphy.

> Splenic bed drains are associated with increased incidence of subphrenic abscess; drains should only be placed if there is concern for injury to the tail of the pancreas.

Complications

Given the association of splenic injury and rib fractures, it is not surprising that the most common complications observed in both operative and non-operative patients are pulmonary in nature. These include atelectasis, left pleural effusion and pneumonia. Left subphrenic abscess occurs in 3–13% of postoperative patients, with an increased risk in patients with concomitant bowel injury and/or drain placement. Thrombocytosis is very common (up to 50%) after splenectomy. The platelet count will often peak by postoperative day 10, and may remain elevated chronically. If platelet counts exceed 1 million/mL, some advocate treatment. Both hydroxyurea and aspirin have been used, without literature to support one modality over another.

Outcomes

Failure of non-operative management approaches 20% in adults (10% in children). Re-bleeding after splenorrhaphy is 1–2%. Due to the risk of overwhelming post-splenectomy infection and sepsis, and its associated mortality of up to 50%, risk of infection with *Haemophilus*, *Streptococcus*, *Staphylococcus* and *Escherichia coli* must not be ignored. Immunisations against the encapsulated organisms *H. influenzae*, *S. pneumoniae* and *N. meningitis* should be given to all patients post-splenectomy and potentially to those with large parenchymal loss post-embolisation. While a few trauma centres administer vaccinations 3–5 days post-injury (because of concerns for lack of adequate follow-up), available evidence would support administering the vaccines at 14 days post-splenectomy. Delaying their administration until this time allows for maximal antibody response without increased risk of infection. Patients must be clearly instructed regarding their increased risk of infection and the importance of informing health care providers of their splenectomy. Bracelets identifying patients as asplenic are strongly recommended.

> Fevers, even if low-grade, must be taken seriously in asplenic patients, with early penicillin therapy often indicated.

Pancreas

Pancreatic injuries are relatively uncommon, comprising less than 10% of abdominal injuries. The majority of these (70–75%) are caused by penetrating injury. Blunt injuries occur more often in children (classic bicycle 'handle-bar' injury). Associated abdominal injuries are seen in over 90% of patients. The most commonly injured organs are liver, spleen, duodenum and small intestine. Major vascular injury is associated with 50–75% of penetrating pancreatic injuries but only 12% of blunt injuries. The pancreas is retroperitoneal, with the head lying right of midline at L2, the body crossing midline and the tail in the splenic hilum. The superior mesenteric artery and vein lie just posterior to the neck of the pancreas.

Treatment

Suspected pancreatic injuries should be surgically explored. Important treatment principles include control of bleeding, debridement, maximal preservation and wide drainage with closed-suction drains. Pancreatic contusion or capsular laceration without ductal injury is treated with wide drainage. Pancreatic transection distal to the superior mesenteric artery is treated with distal pancreatectomy and suction drainage. In cases of pancreatic transection to the right of the artery not involving the ampulla, treatment is controversial. Treatment options include: wide drainage, ligating both ends of the duct and wide drainage and Roux-en-Y jejunostomy. Severe injury to pancreatic head (and duodenum) may require Whipple procedure. Post-injury feeding either nasojejunal or a feeding jejunostomy (or gastrojejunostomy) should be applied liberally to avoid the need for parenteral nutrition.

Complications

Complications following pancreatic trauma approach 40%. The highest risk of complications is among those patients with associated duodenal injuries. Pancreatic fistulae occur in 20–35% of cases, with most of these, fortunately, resolving spontaneously. Intra-abdominal abscesses or wound infections are common, with true pancreatic abscesses occurring at a rate of 5%. Pancreatitis occurs in 10–15% of patients. Pseudocysts are also observed and may be simple or complicated by associated abscess formation. The most serious postoperative complication, however, is haemorrhage. This occurs in 5–10% of patients and will often require re-exploration. Some centres, though, have reported successful angioembolisation in lieu of re-operation.

Outcomes

Vascular injury is responsible for the majority of the immediate deaths. Mortality associated with early haemorrhage requiring re-operation is high as 80%. Early deaths are often due to haemorrhage, with late deaths arising from infection. Endocrine and exocrine functions are preserved clinically as long as 10–20% of the pancreas remains intact.

Diaphragm

Diaphragmatic injuries occur in up to 8% of all blunt injuries, with up to two-thirds occurring on the left side. Associated intra-abdominal injuries are seen in three-quarters of all patients. When one considers that the diaphragm attaches anteriorly to the inferior sternum and the costal margin, posteriorly to the 11th and 12th ribs, and centrally to the pericardium, it is not surprising that diaphragm injury is seen with at least one-third of abdominal GSW. Despite ATLS recommendations, more and more centres are withholding placement of nasogastric tubes on non-intubated patients. As such, many diaphragm injuries are being missed or their diagnoses at least delayed as the classic 'chest nasogastric tube' not likely to be identified.

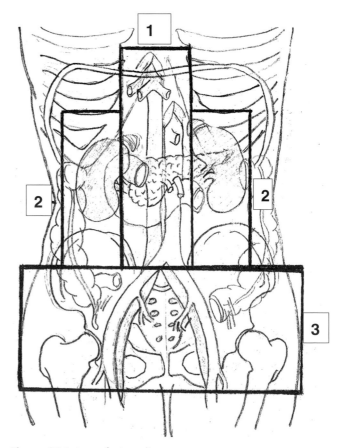

Figure 28.1 Areas of retroperitoneum.

Treatment

Acute injuries are managed via laparotomy with sutured repair. When the central tendon is involved, great care should be taken to prevent inadvertent placement into the pericardium. In cases of intra-abdominal contamination of the pleural cavity, copious irrigation of the chest prior to closure of the diaphragm defect is encouraged. A chest tube will usually be inserted and left in place postoperatively. Thoracotomy is normally performed in delayed diagnoses to facilitate lysis of adhesions between lung and abdominal contents. Expectant management is reserved for select isolated injuries to the right hemidiaphragm.

Complications

While most complications are secondary or attributable to associated injuries, some are related directly to the injury and the repair itself. Suture-line dehiscence, general 'failure' of repair, phrenic nerve injury, empyema and subdiaphragmatic abscesses are seen early after repair. Late complications are typically due to anastomotic breakdown or missed injury (strangulation and perforation of hollow viscus and bowel obstruction).

Outcomes

Morbidity and mortality are mostly due to associated injury, and occur at rates of 80% and 40%, respectively. Morbidity is significantly decreased when recognised and repaired early.

Retroperitoneal haematoma

Management depends largely on mechanism and location of injury (Figure 28.1). All penetrating wounds of the retroperitoneum generally require thorough exploration. Non-expanding perinephric haematoma may be initially managed with observation. If haematoma is large, expanding or proximal to the major retroperitoneal vessels, prox-imal and distal control must be obtained before exploration. Blunt trauma accounts for 80% of retroperitoneal haematomas.

Expanding lesions require exploration. Non-expanding zone II and III lesions almost never require exploration as long as overlying bowel is intact. Zone I haematomas, even if not expanding, require exploration to rule out visceral or vascular injury.

Treatment

Most retroperitoneal vascular injuries can be repaired with a primary repair or simple ligation. If a patch is required, prosthetic material can be used unless colon contents have grossly contaminated the area. In attempting to control ongoing haemorrhage in zone I injuries, the aorta may be occluded above or below the diaphragmatic hiatus. Caution should be exercised to not injure the ureter(s) during this exploration. While this may seem to go without saying, the haemorrhaging retroperitoneum is a difficult field to navigate and ureter injury is not uncommon.

> Prior to unleashing potential haemorrhage from the retroperitoneum, the surgeon should obtain proximal and distal control, both arterial and venous.

Further reading

Gracias VH, Mckenney MG, Reilly PM, Velmahos G. (eds.) *Acute Care Surgery*. McGraw-Hill, New York, 2008.

Hirshberg A, Mattox KL. (eds.) *Top Knife: The Art and Craft of Trauma Surgery*. TFM Publishing Ltd., Shropshire, UK, 2005.

Feliciano DV, Mattox KL, Moore EE, et al. (eds.) *Trauma*, 6th edn. McGraw-Hill, New York, 2003.

Peitzman AB, Rhodes M, Schwab CW, Yealy DM, Fabian TC, (eds.) *The Trauma Manual*, 3rd edn. Lippincott Williams & Wilkins, Philadelphia, PA, 2007.

7 Critical Care

29 Critical Care

Andrew McDonald Johnston

Department of Military Medicine, Birmingham Research Park, Edgbaston, Birmingham, UK

Clinical assessment

The effective management of critically ill emergency surgical patients requires close collaboration between critical care specialists and emergency surgeons. Both must have an understanding of what the other speciality can realistically achieve, what their aims are, and what the indications for and complications of the common procedures are.

Emergency surgical patients are typically physiologically compromised by the time they present to the emergency department. Therefore, a judgment as to whether critical care admission is appropriate for the patient should begin as soon as the emergency department or receiving surgical team are aware of them. The critical care team should be notified as soon as it becomes clear that the patient is likely to require their input. They can then see the patient and plan ahead. This allows treatment of physiologic compromise to be initiated promptly and logistic factors such as the availability of beds and nursing staff to be catered for.

Assessing critically ill patients

It is important that the principle of 'physiology first' is adhered to whilst assessing the patient. Measures are taken to correct any physiological abnormalities as they are found, working through key systems in a systematic fashion, with attention to detail. Ideally several staff members will carry out interventions simultaneously, with one managing airway, one venous access, and so on, with one team member having an overview and formulating a diagnosis and plan. Various systems exist for assessing the critically ill patient. A schema which covers some of the factors relevant when assessing the critically ill patient is given in Figure 29.1.

A well organised, rapid but comprehensive approach to assessing the patient is essential to avoid missing key signs.

Emergency Surgery, 1st edition. Edited by Adam Brooks, Peter F. Mahoney, Bryan A. Cotton and Nigel Tai. © 2010 Blackwell Publishing.

Often critically ill patients deteriorate extremely quickly, so treating physiologic disturbances before a diagnosis is secure is not uncommon. Young or physically fit patients are typically able to compensate for haemorrhagic or septic shock for longer than older patients, but may deteriorate very suddenly and rapidly when compensatory mechanisms fail. Older patients may present atypically and may not develop the expected symptoms or signs. Patients who are taking cardiac medications such as beta-blockers may not develop a tachycardia in the face of acute surgical conditions.

Admission to critical care

The operative procedure the patient will be having should be taken into consideration. How will it influence the patient's recovery and requirement for critical care? Factors such as the anaesthetic and operative techniques required, the patient's injuries, co-morbidities, the likely morbidity resulting from the operative incision, postoperative pain and other factors including likely fluid losses from drains, stomas or burned skin should all be assessed. These factors will determine in part whether postoperative care in a high dependency unit (HDU) or in an intensive therapy unit (ITU) is required. Anaesthetic complications such as difficult intubation, hypothermia or prolonged paralysis due to neuromuscular blockade may require unplanned critical care admission.

Patients with conditions which do not require surgery should be transferred to the ITU as soon as they are stable. The transfer should be prompt, as delay worsens outcome. Patients who need urgent but not immediate surgery and have physiological disturbances such as hypothermia, dehydration or anaemia will benefit from a period of admission to ITU or management by the critical care team prior to surgery. Patients who undergo damage control surgery often spend a period of time on the ITU after their life saving surgery to allow stabilisation before the performance of definitive interventions.

Assessing the critically ill patient

Do you need additional help or resources? e.g. in the Emergency Department or on the ward

Airway and breathing

Is oxygen being administered at an appropriate concentration?
Does the patient need intubation due to reduced conscious level?
Is respiratory failure present?
Is an immediately remediable cause present (tension pneumothorax)?

Record respiratory rate and oxygen saturation

Circulation

Is the patient shocked? Is shock imminent?
Are they responding to fluid boluses?
Is transfusion of blood products required?
Are vasopressors required?

Record heart rate and blood pressure

Disability

Does the patient have an altered conscious level?
Is there neurotrauma, neurological disease or drug ingestion? Are they hypoglycaemic?
Are they suffering from delirium?
Are they in pain?
Are they oversedated?

Record conscious level

Exposure

Is there pathology elsewhere (secondary survey)?
Is there skin infection? (necrotising fasciitis, wound infection)
Is there an intra-abdominal emergency?
Is there overt blood loss?
Are there signs of occult bleeding?
Is there fever or hypothermia?

Record temperature

Host defence/Microbiology
Does the patient have signs or symptoms of infection? Is there proven infection?
Are there any positive or pending microbiology results?
Is the patient septic? Are antibiotics needed immediately?
Do they need urgent control of the source of infection (abscesses, infected lines)?

Renal/Metabolic/Endocrine
How much urine is the patient passing?
How much fluid has been administered?
Are they losing fluid through drains, stomas or burns?
Is there an electrolyte disturbance or renal failure?
Is there an acid–base disturbance?
Is there an endocrine disorder?

Differential diagnosis

Is there a clear diagnosis?
Are further diagnostic tests or a definitive surgical procedure required?
Is senior or expert advice required?

Management plan
Treat physiological disturbances
Aim for early definitive treatment where possible
Communicate plan to patient, team members, nursing staff and relatives
Record assessment clearly and contemporaneously in case notes
Review patient to ensure interventions are successful

Figure 29.1 Assessing the critically ill patient. This gives some of the factors to consider when assessing the critically ill patient.

Critical care admission is not an entirely benign intervention. Patients admitted to the ITU are at risk of many complications of their disease or operation; worsening of co-morbid conditions; drug reactions; medical error; complications of intensive care procedures such as central line insertion or tracheostomy; hospital acquired infection; psychological problems including acute delirium and chronic post-traumatic stress disorder; thromboembolism; critical illness myoneuropathy; and numerous other problems. Many ITU patients are left with scars from line insertion, tracheostomy and other interventions.

Postoperative problems

Return to theatre for complications such as bleeding is more difficult in the intubated ITU patient, particularly if they have multiple infusions of sedative and vasoactive drugs.

Internal medical complications occurring in the days immediately after surgery include perioperative myocardial ischaemia or infarction, postoperative pneumonia, pulmonary oedema, cardiac arrhythmias such as atrial fibrillation or supraventricular tachycardia. Sometimes these complications will mandate admission to the HDU or ITU, but often early recognition and treatment of complications will be sufficient to stabilise the patient and avoid admission.

Monitoring

The monitoring required by an individual patient is determined by the severity of their critical illness and their co-morbidities.

Minimally invasive monitoring includes recording physiological variables such as pulse rate and blood pressure. Urinary output gives a good idea of end-organ perfusion, with a minimum target of 0.5 mL/kg body weight/hour. Invasive arterial pressure monitoring allows beat-to-beat recording of blood pressure, and is used in shocked patients and those requiring vasoactive drugs. Central venous access via a multi-lumen catheter allows measurement of central venous pressure (CVP) and the administration of vasoactive drugs. CVP, and the response to fluid boluses can give an indication of intravascular volume.

Numerous forms of non-invasive and invasive cardiac output monitoring are available. These include oesophageal doppler, dye or lithium dilution techniques and thermodilution techniques (as well as pulse contour analysis and electrical impedence methods). These provide physiological information about the patient, which most intensivists find helpful in guiding treatment decisions, particularly about fluid administration and vasoactive drug use. It should be noted that the evidence that invasive monitoring improves patient outcomes is largely lacking, with a few exceptions. In emergency department patients with septic shock there is evidence that early goal directed therapy using invasive monitoring of CVPs and mixed venous oxygen saturation improves survival. There is also evidence that fluid administration guided by invasive monitoring prior to surgery (preoptimisation), or early after ITU admission (postoptimisation) may reduce mortality and length of stay on the ITU. If fluid and vasoactive drug administration is given late in the disease course, it seems to increase mortality.

Vasopressor and inotropic drugs

Vasopressor drugs in common use on the ITU include norepinephrine, dopamine, epinephrine and vasopressin. These drugs are used to treat hypotension and low cardiac output states. The particular drug used in an individual patient will depend on various factors, including the aetiology of their shock. The evidence for use of vasopressor agents is perhaps best studied in septic shock and is discussed in more detail in the Surviving Sepsis Campaign (SSC) guidelines. Norepinephrine and dopamine are the vasopressors of choice in sepsis. A fixed, low dose of vasopressin may be used with norepinephrine. Epinephrine may be effective if the patient is resistant to the initial drug. In septic patients whose hypotension does not respond to fluid loading and vasopressors intravenous corticosteroids may be beneficial in restoring vasopressor responsiveness. It should be noted that the use of 'low-dose' or 'renal-dose' dopamine to protect the kidneys is ineffective. In patients with low cardiac output states dobutamine is used as an inotropic agent.

Sedation and paralysis

Various different sedative drugs are used, the commonest including combinations of opiates and either benzodiazepines or the anaesthetic agent propofol.

In some patients these drugs may accumulate either by distribution into fat, or due to renal impairment and impaired excretion. This leads to delayed waking once the drug is stopped. Daily interruption of sedation reduces the chance that sedatives will accumulate to this extent. Daily interruption of sedation may not be appropriate in patients who are difficult to ventilate or require further operations.

Paralysing agents act by causing neuromuscular blockade, and are used to make intubation and ventilation easier. Most patients do not require prolonged paralysis, with exceptions being patients who are difficult to ventilate due to poor lung compliance or patient–ventilator dyssynchrony. The use of neuromuscular blocking agents is associated with critical illness myoneuropathy.

Organ failure

Patients with one organ failure may be managed on the HDU rather than the ITU, unless they have respiratory failure requiring invasive ventilation. The greater the number of organs that fail, the greater the risk of the ITU patient dying. Various physiology scores exist such as the Sequential Organ Failure Assessment score (SOFA) and the Acute Physiology And Chronic Health Evaluation 2 score (APACHE 2). These scoring systems allow calculation of the mortality that a population of patients with a particular score will have, but are not always helpful in the individual patient.

Renal support

Many patients admitted to the ITU develop renal failure, often from prolonged hypotension during the resuscitative phase of their care. Other factors that may contribute to renal failure include radiocontrast nephropathy and pre-existing renal impairment.

Renal support on the ITU is typically carried out using venovenous or arteriovenous haemofiltration or haemodialysis. Continuous venovenous haemofiltration (CVVH) involves the use of a large bore double lumen venous catheter which allows the extraction and return of large volumes of blood from a central vein (internal jugular, subclavian or femoral). This blood is passed through a circuit allowing filtration and replacement of a variable volume of fluid. In continuous venovenous haemodialysis (CVVHD) fluid is passed in the opposite direction against the flow of filtrate. The volume of dialysis fluid administered can be adjusted to allow replacement of intravascular volume.

Renal replacement therapy also allows correction of acid–base and electrolyte abnormalities. Pitfalls associated with its use include hypotension, loss of blood volume when the haemofiltration machine circuit clots and the complications of obtaining large bore vascular access.

Sepsis

Sepsis is the combination of systemic inflammation and infection. Sepsis manifests as some or all of tachycardia, hypotension, temperature dysregulation (fever or hypothermia) and immune dysregulation (raised or lowered white blood count). Important sources of infection in emergency surgical patients include intra-abdominal abscess, faecal peritonitis, anastomotic leak, necrotising fasciitis, hospital acquired pneumonia and line infections. The SSC guidelines cover the management of sepsis in depth. Some of the key SSC interventions are listed in Figure 29.2. Interventions such as the early administration of antibiotics are straight-

forward – once hypotension is present mortality rises dramatically with delay in antibiotic administration. In patients who have septic shock with hypotension due to an intra-abdominal abscess following bowel surgery, a period of critical care 'stabilisation' may seem reasonable, when in fact the most important intervention is drainage of the abscess either percutaneously or at laparotomy. In this setting resuscitation and circulatory support are aimed at getting the patient to the point where they are fit for the 'source control' intervention. Delay in source control clearly increases the risk of death.

Daily review

Systematic daily review is carried out by the critical care team who set parameters for acceptable physiologic variables. They also identify short-term and longer-term goals. These range from scheduled central line changes to weaning and discharge plans. A close working relationship with the critical care nurses and good communication skills are required.

Another key part of the daily routine on the ITU, and one of the most important, is liaison with the critical care outreach team. This team comprises experienced critical care nurses and often critical care doctors as well. Their role includes reviewing patients who may require critical care. These patients are identified by general ward staff using a medical early warning score (MEWS) or similar. The outreach staff also review patients who have been discharged from ITU and who may not yet be fully recovered from their illness.

Other medical and paramedical staff are also be involved in the management of ITU patients, including physiotherapists with expertise in respiratory management and rehabilitation. The hospital microbiologists perform regular ward rounds on the critical care unit, reviewing positive microbiology results and antibiotic usage.

The emergency surgical team should review their critical care patients daily or more frequently, and the senior surgeon and intensivist should discuss what management changes they feel are appropriate. If radiological imaging or diagnostic tests are required, it should be clear who is responsible for ordering and reviewing them. Clear, contemporaneous notes are mandatory, and any change in management must be both documented and discussed with a senior member of the critical care team, usually a consultant or senior trainee.

Ventilation

Ventilation is required when a patient has respiratory failure due to their disease or the disordered physiology resulting

Key points in the acute management of sepsis

From Surviving Sepsis Campaign Guidelines 2008

Resuscitation (first 6 Hours)

In a shocked patient or with a raised lactate (>4 mmol/L) don't delay resuscitation until admitted to ITU
Aim for CVP of 8–12 mm Hg (>12 mm Hg if ventilated), Urine output of 0.5 m L/kg/min, MAP of ≥ 65 mm Hg
Aim for central venous oxygen saturation of ≥ 70% or mixed venous of ≥ 65%
If O_2 saturation not achieved consider further fluid, transfusion or inotrope use
Use boluses of crystalloid (1000 mL) or colloid (3–500 mL) over 30 minutes

---

Diagnosis and antibiotic therapy

Obtain cultures prior to antibiotic use as long as this doesn't introduce significant delay
Arrange early imaging to confirm and sample sources of infection
Begin antibiotics early, always within first hour of recognising severe sepsis or septic shock
Use one or more broad-spectrum drugs with appropriate coverage and penetration

---

Source control

Look for a focus of infection suitable for drainage/debridement
Identify site of infection within 6 hours of presentation
Choose least invasive but most effective method of source control
Remove lines if they may be infected

Vasopressors and inotropes

Maintain MAP ≥ 65 mm Hg monitored by arterial line
Use norepinephrine or dopamine by central line
Don't use epinephrine, phenylephrine or vasopressin first line
Don't use low dose dopamine for renal protection
Dobutamine is the inotrope of choice – but avoid supranormal cardiac index
Consider hydrocortisone if patient has resistant hypotension

Other

Consider recombinant human activated protein C in selected patients with high risk of death and no
contraindications
Transfuse to restrictive target of Hb 7–9
Don't use fresh frozen plasma unless patient is bleeding or invasive procedures are needed
Use lung-protective ventilation
Avoid oversedation and neuromuscular blockade

Consider thromboprophylaxis
Prescribe stress ulcer prophylaxis

Figure 29.2 Key points from the Surviving Sepsis Campaign guidelines. This is a summary of the SSC guidelines.

from it. There are numerous ventilatory modalities that may be used to treat a critically ill patient.

Continuous positive airway pressure (CPAP) use involves the use of a tight fitting face mask allowing the application of a variable oxygen concentration at 5–10 cm H_2O pressure. It is of use in patients with pulmonary oedema and may be used in other patients as a temporising measure prior to ITU admission.

Non-invasive ventilation (NIV) is ventilation using a tight fitting face mask (or occasionally a nasal mask, full face mask or a plastic helmet). A ventilator that can automatically compensate for any air leak around the mask is required. NIV may be helpful in some patients, and may prevent the need for invasive ventilation. However, it requires an awake patient who is not confused, and intensive nursing supervision to prevent removal of the mask. Many patients find mask ventilation very claustrophobic. In patients who are likely to have a prolonged period of respiratory failure, for example following major abdominal surgery, NIV may not be the best option, and intubation and invasive ventilation may be more appropriate.

Invasive ventilation involves ventilation via an endotracheal tube. Nasotracheal tubes are rarely used on the ITU because of the risk of sinusitis, and laryngeal mask airways are not used because they do not prevent aspiration of secretions, with a concomitant risk of aspiration pneumonia.

Various different modes of ventilation are available, the terminology of which varies to some extent dependent on ventilator manufacturer. The mechanical ventilator can be set to deliver varying levels of support to the patient, from fully machine delivered breaths to minimal support breaths initiated by the patient, dependent on the patient's condition. Many aspects of ventilation are modifiable, including the fraction of inspired oxygen (FIO_2), the tidal volume and the peak airway pressure.

Ventilation of patients who are critically ill aims to achieve a minimum PaO_2 of 8 kPa in patients without significant cardiac or neurological disease. In patients with ischaemic heart disease, neurotrauma or neurological conditions a PaO_2 target of 10–13 kPa is the goal.

In patients in whom ventilation or oxygenation proves difficult due to diseases such as pulmonary contusions from chest trauma, the presence of a large arteriovenous shunt, or coexisting chest disease other special ventilatory modalities may be used. These include high frequency oscillatory ventilation (HFOV), jet ventilation, extracorporeal membrane oxygenation (ECMO) and extracorporeal carbon dioxide removal. Ventilating the patient in the prone position may also be used. These ventilatory modalities do not currently have evidence of superiority over standard modes of ventilation, but may be helpful in the individual patient in whom standard ventilation is failing.

Invasive ventilation is associated with ventilator-associated pneumonia (VAP). VAP is though to be due in part to aspiration of small volumes of secretions past the inflated cuff of the endotracheal tube or bacterial biofilm formation on the tube.

It is not uncommon for patients who have undergone major surgery or major trauma to develop acute lung injury (ALI). There is convincing evidence that ventilating patients with tidal volumes above 6–8 mL/kg increases the risk of lung injury, and is associated with an increased risk of renal failure and multi-organ failure. ALI is associated with a much higher mortality. ALI may recover, or may progress to the acute respiratory distress syndrome (ARDS). The factors associated with the development of ALI and ARDS are still incompletely understood, but the combination of mechanical ventilation with injury elsewhere or endotoxinaemia has been shown to markedly increase the risk of ALI/ARDS in animal models.

Tracheostomy

A tracheostomy is an artificial airway inserted through the trachea typically between the first and second tracheal rings. This is much less uncomfortable for the patient, and often allows a rapid reduction in the amount of sedation they require. There is some evidence it allows earlier liberation from the ventilator (or weaning), and that it may reduce the incidence of VAP. Tracheostomies may be inserted surgically or using one of several percutaneous techniques, usually on the ITU. There appears to be little difference between surgical and percutaneous techniques in terms of complications. However, these complications may be life-threatening, and include puncture of the mediastinal vessels, tension pneumothorax and tracheal tear or transection. Therefore, tracheostomy should only be performed by those who are appropriately trained in the technique or with senior supervision. Some patients, particularly those with short necks or marked obesity may be anatomically unsuitable for percutaneous tracheostomy, although surgical tracheostomy may still be possible.

The tracheostomy facilitates both ventilation and the removal of secretions, but initially at least prevents the patient from talking. Many patients find this distressing, and this inability to make themselves understood may contribute to ITU delirium. Tracheostomy tubes with speaking valves are available, and may be inserted once the track from insertion is well established, and the weaning process is well underway. The tracheostomy tube is removed once the patient is breathing a low FIO_2, without support from the ventilator, and is able to cough with sufficient force to propel any respiratory secretions into the mouth. The timing of tracheostomy removal is not always straightforward, and requires the expertise of critical care doctors, respiratory physiotherapists, respiratory specialists or rehabilitation specialists.

Patients with a tracheostomy who are discharged from the ITU to a ward with a lower level of nursing support are at risk of various problems. The tracheostomy tube may become displaced. If this occurs a member of staff with expertise in tracheostomy care may attempt to replace it through the same track. This requires that the tracheostomy has been in place for sufficient time for a clear track to form. There is a risk of creating a false lumen in the pretracheal fascia, and obstructing the existing track with an associated risk of hypoxia. If positive pressure ventilation is reinstituted whilst the tube is incorrectly sited air may be forced into the mediastinum or pleural cavities, causing tension pneumothoraces and possibly death. The alternative to replacing the tracheostomy tube is to support the patient's ventilation via a face mask, and occlude the tracheostomy stoma. If intubation is required in an acutely unwell patient with a displaced tracheostomy the standard route of oral intubation may be the safest.

Tracheostomy tubes not infrequently become blocked with hardened, dried secretions. In this situation the inner tube of the tracheostomy (assuming one is fitted) should be removed to restore a patent outer tube. This complication can be prevented or lessened by the use of humidified oxygen.

After removal the tracheostomy site is covered with an occlusive dressing. In most patients it gradually heals to leave a scar. Rarely sutures may be required.

Weaning

Weaning is the process of liberation from the ventilator. The ideal weaning strategy is not entirely clear, and prediction of when a patient will be able to manage without the ventilator is an imprecise science. One of the most effective ways to determine if the patient is likely to manage without ventilatory support is to carry out a spontaneous breathing trial (SBT). This involves the patient breathing without the support of the ventilator for 30–120 minutes.

Prior to carrying out an SBT the patient must be stable both physically and psychologically.

Some patients who initially appear to tolerate breathing without the ventilator will later tire and require ventilation again. Strategies to attempt to avoid reintubation such as the use of non-invasive ventilation have not been proven to work.

Transfer for diagnostic tests

Transferring an intubated patient out of the ITU for tests such as CT or MRI is not a minor undertaking, and there is a small but real risk to the patient from doing so. The risk includes equipment failure, from infusion pumps, ventilators or oxygen supply. If a complication such as cardiorespiratory arrest, massive haemorrhage or unplanned extubation occurs in an unfamiliar part of the hospital it may be more difficult or impossible to deal with in a timely fashion.

Equipment used for transferring patients for diagnostic tests should be checked for usability at least daily, and clinical areas such as the CT scanner where ITU patients are regularly taken should have appropriate resuscitation equipment including oxygen supply and working suction.

Critical illness myopathy and neuropathy

The commonest cause of weakness found in ITU patients, this debilitating condition is associated with the use of steroids or neuromuscular blockade. Critical illness myopathy/neuropathy (CIM) doubles the length of time on the ventilator, prolongs weaning and lengthens hospital stay. Some patients with CIM may not recover normal function.

Care bundles

Care bundles are a combination of interventions that individually have been shown to be effective, packaged together to simplify their use. For example, a ventilator bundle may be made up of several interventions shown individually to reduce pulmonary complications. These include positioning the patient with a 30–45° head up tilt to reduce aspiration pneumonia; carrying out a daily sedation hold and considering weaning; initiating peptic ulcer prophylaxis; and initiating deep venous thrombosis prophylaxis.

Nutrition

Adequate nutrition is a key part of critical care. Enteral nutrition is superior to parenteral, and also provides other benefits, such as more rapid healing of gut anastomoses and a reduction in the risk of gastrointestinal ulceration. Various nutritional supplements have been subjected to trials in critically ill patients, but none have a convincing evidence of benefit at present. Some critical care patients, particularly those with a prolonged illness prior to surgery or ITU admission (e.g. Crohn's disease and alcoholism) are at risk of the refeeding syndrome. Refeeding syndrome is a consequence of prolonged malnutrition followed by rapid refeeding. Refeeding causes a severe drop in phosphate levels, along with calcium. There may also be profound thiamine depletion. It manifests as confusion, weakness, coma and convulsions and if untreated may lead to death.

Stress ulcers may occur in critically ill patients. Where GI tract failure or surgical considerations prevent early institution of feeding the patient should be treated with ulcer prophylaxis, usually with a H_2 receptor antagonist.

Communication

Discussion of the patient's progress and prognosis with their family is an important part of their care. If the patient is likely to die despite treatment this should be discussed, and where appropriate the patient's wishes should be taken into account to allow planning of limits to interventions. It is important both to prevent misunderstandings and to allay fears that regular conversations with family members take place. Where possible discussion should also occur with the patients themselves. Communication with patients' relatives is not always easy, and requires time, empathy and the avoidance of medical jargon. It is important that the likely outcome is discussed, without being unduly pessimistic or inappropriately optimistic. If the patient is certain to die, consideration should be given to treating them palliatively. Communication within the critical care team is also of paramount importance, and is reinforced by ward rounds attended by all team members on duty, and clear hand-over rounds at shift changes.

Discharge from critical care

Discharging patients from critical care requires planning, usually days in advance. For some patients, for example those with significant fluid losses from stomas, open abdom-inal wounds or those requiring ongoing specialist care discharge from ITU to a specialty HDU, e.g. surgical HDU or neurosurgical HDU will be appropriate for a period of time prior to discharge to a surgical or rehabilitation ward.

There are certain pitfalls in discharging patients from ITU. Patients discharged at a weekend or at night may be at greater risk of adverse outcomes. Patients who have had a prolonged ITU admission are likely to require a prolonged period of ongoing care on a surgical ward. Occasionally, these patients may require readmission due to physiological instability following repeat surgery or intercurrent infection.

Further reading

Chalfin DB, Trzeciak S, Likourezos A, Baumann BM, Dellinger RP, for DELAY-ED Study Group. Impact of delayed transfer of critically ill patients from the emergency department to the intensive care unit. *Crit Care Med* 2007;**35**:1477–1483.

Dellinger R, Levy M, Carlet J, et al. Surviving sepsis campaign: international guidelines for management of severe sepsis and septic shock: 2008. *Crit Care Med* 2008;**36**(1):296–327. Available online at www.survivingsepsis.org.

Pinsky MR. Hemodynamic evaluation and monitoring in the ICU. *Chest* 2007;**132**:2020–2029.

Rivers E, Nguyen B, Havstad S, et al. Early goal-directed therapy in the treatment of severe sepsis and septic shock. *N Engl J Med* 2001;**345**:1368–1377.

The Acute Respiratory Distress Syndrome Network. Ventilation with lower tidal volumes as compared with traditional tidal volumes for acute lung injury and the acute respiratory distress syndrome. *N Engl J Med* 2000;**342**:1301–1308.

Winters BD, Pham JC, Hunt EA, Guallar E, Berenholtz S, Pronovost PJ. Rapid response systems: a systematic review. *Crit Care Med* 2007;**35**:1238–1243.

30 Postoperative Complications

Abeed Chowdhury & Adam Brooks

Department of Surgery, Queen's Medical Centre, Nottingham, UK

Introduction

A postoperative complication is defined as 'any undesirable and unexpected result of an operation affecting the patient'. Although postoperative complications are relatively common, the majority of complications lead only to minor consequences for patient outcomes; rarely complications can have dramatic effects and lead to significant morbidity or even mortality. Complications are usually classified as either early or late or by the affected system. Below is a list of common complications, some of which are detailed further in the following sections.

Early complications

Cardiovascular – hypotension; myocardial infarction; arrhythmia (particularly atrial fibrillation); haemorrhage; deep vein thrombosis and pulmonary embolus (DVT/PE)

Respiratory – atelectasis; pneumonia (including aspiration pneumonia); pulmonary collapse; pneumothorax

Gastrointestinal – postoperative nausea and vomiting (PONV); ileus; obstruction; anastomotic leak; malnutrition; abscess; duodenal ulceration; diarrhoea (*C. difficile*); constipation; acute gastric dilatation

Urogenital – oliguria; anuria; urinary retention; urinary tract infection; acute renal failure (ARF)

Neurological – neuropraxia; transient ischaemic attack (TIA); stroke; confusion; pain

General – wound infection; wound dehiscence; pressure sores; cannula site infection; sepsis; psychological

Late complications

Scarring (including hypertrophic and keloid formation); adhesions and bowel obstruction; infection; recurrence of pathology; hernias; chronic pain; fistulae; disability; psychosexual/psychological dysfunction.

Pyrexia

Pyrexia occurs commonly in the postoperative period. There are numerous causes of pyrexia and the timing of its onset often gives an indication as to its origin. Some common causes of postoperative pyrexia are detailed in Figure 30.1.

Pyrexia developing in the first 24 hours frequently is a response to surgical trauma and only in a minority of cases there is a specific aetiological factor. Pyrexia within 48 hours of surgery can be caused by pulmonary atelectasis. This is usually secondary to poor inspiration due to postoperative pain and is commonly seen after laparotomy with a midline incision. Between 48 hours and 5 days, pyrexia may be the result of thrombophlebitis caused by reaction to intravenous cannulae or infection of the urinary tract or the chest, and more than 5 days after surgery, a wound infection or anastomotic breakdown should be suspected. A detailed history and clinical examination should be carried out to establish a possible source. Treatment with antibiotics should be started only after specimens have been collected for microscopy culture and sensitivity. These would usually include sputum, urine, wound swabs and blood depending on the suspected site of sepsis. Rarer causes of pyrexia, such as reactions to drugs or blood products should be suspected if there is no obvious infective cause.

Wound complications

Problems with wound healing can lead to a variety of postoperative complications and can involve differing tissues. The consequences of aberrant wound healing lead to incisional hernias, poor cosmetic appearance of skin, keloid and hypertrophic scarring, anastomotic breakdown and wound dehiscence.

Emergency Surgery, 1st edition. Edited by Adam Brooks, Peter F. Mahoney, Bryan A. Cotton and Nigel Tai. © 2010 Blackwell Publishing.

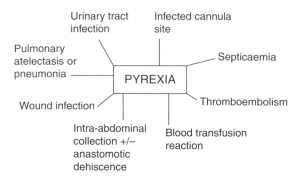

Figure 30.1 Common causes of pyrexia.

Risk factors for wound complications

Wound healing can be affected by systemic and local factors and some of these are listed below:

Systemic	Local
Malnutrition	Contamination
Chronic disease	Trauma
Shock	Irradiation
Age	Malignancy

Nutritional status, age and the presence of underlying chronic disease are determinants in successful wound healing. The presence of diabetes, jaundice or immunodeficiency affects wound strength and higher incidences of wound infection are observed in patients with these conditions.

Contamination and infection of wounds are major risk factors for complications in wound healing; this is especially the case in wounds with uncontrolled levels of bacterial contamination and associated local tissue injury, such as that occurring with gunshot injuries involving the gastrointestinal tract or severe burns. Higher levels of tissue necrosis frequently seen in these types of wound lead to propagation of bacteria and subsequently defective wound repair.

Patients undergoing emergency surgery and enduring periods of systemic hypotension have a higher incidence of wound complications. This is secondary to tissue hypoperfusion which can also be aggravated by local tissue factors such as peripheral vascular disease, oedema and irradiated tissue.

Wound infections

Wound infections are manifested by pain, discharge, odour, wound failure and the features of inflammation. Superficial wound infections can be managed with adequate drainage of collections. The addition of systemic antimicrobial therapy may be indicated in patients with signs of a systemic inflammatory response after sufficient microbial cultures have been obtained.

Wound dehiscence

Wound dehiscence is the breakdown, either partial or complete, of some or all the layers of an operative wound. Dehiscence can occur in many types of wound but has significant consequences when associated with the myofascial layer of the abdominal wall. The reported incidence of myofascial dehiscence ranges from 0.25 to 3%. It arises primarily due to technical failure of wound closure or due to patient-related factors. Common aetiologies include wound infection, haematoma, abdominal distension, malnutrition, obesity, steroids, chemo- or radiotherapy and cardiopulmonary disease.

Myofascial dehiscence presents commonly around 7–10 days postoperatively. The patient may feel something 'give' in the wound and there may be the appearance of a serosanguinous discharge. The dehiscence may range from superficial to partial or to deep, with protrusion of bowel loops and a distressed patient.

Assessment

If a defect is visible, its extent should be determined. This can be achieved using a microbiology swab as a wound probe, with a sample of fluid being sent for microscopy, culture and sensitivity where appropriate. In the majority of fascial dehiscences a polymicrobial infection is present.

Resuscitation and management

Restoration of abdominal wall integrity is vital. Superficial dehiscence can be managed conservatively with secondary intention healing and antibiotics; surgical closure of all or some of the abdominal wall layers; split-thickness skin grafts over granulated bowel, local or regional tissue flaps and vacuum assisted closure devices. If there is fascial involvement, delayed primary closure may be employed with or without prosthetic mesh placement and/or local tissue flap construction.

Full depth dehiscence, with visible bowel is a surgical emergency with a mortality of up to 30% more related to the patient's physiological status than the anatomical defect. Patients require expeditious return to theatre; covering the bowel with warm, wet saline packs and a suitable adherent dressing overlying the packs.

In theatre having reopened the entire wound, bacteriological swabs should be taken, with subsequent resuturing of the fascial layers. Primary closure is the most preferable form of definitive closure, provided undue tension is not present – which may increase the risk of an abdominal compartment syndrome. The use of deep tension sutures remains controversial and many surgeons believe that the adverse effects of trauma and ischaemia on the skin caused by deep tension sutures outweigh the limited reduction in the incidence of secondary fascial dehiscence.

Alternative closure methods include a Bogota (IV fluid) bag, non-adherent plastic drape or mesh placement sutured to the surrounding skin or fascia, allowing wound closure by granulation or delayed suturing. Vacuum drains or systems such as vacuum-assisted closure (VAC) can also be applied over the wound/dressing applying negative pressure to facilitate wound closure. The sutures should remain for at least 14 days; and antibiotics commenced perioperatively should be continued until course completion. Often definitive fascial and/or cutaneous reconstructions have to be delayed due to the wound or the patient's condition. A number of long-term sequelae of myofascial dehiscence are possible and some of these are outlined below.

Complications
- Enterocutaneous fistula following bowel exposure
- Incisional herniae
- Poor cosmesis

Anastomotic leak

Any anastomosis is at risk of breakdown, particularly those involving the rectum, oesophagus or pancreas. Local and systemic factors are responsible for the maintenance of anastomotic integrity, in particular, blood supply, lack of tension, good apposition and tissue quality. Leaks can be classed as major or minor; radiological or clinical.

Clinical
Anastomotic leaks tend to present 3–7 days postoperatively and depending on the degree of leakage, resultant peritonitis can be localised or generalised. It can present with faecal or purulent wound or drain discharge; abscess or sepsis (hypotension, tachycardia and pyrexia); persistent ileus or with fistulae. In addition, anastomotic leaks are often heralded by cardiac rhythm abnormalities, such as atrial fibrillation or tachycardias.

Assessment
Patients with contrast imaging demonstrating anastomotic leaks but lacking the symptoms and signs of sepsis may be classed as having a radiological leak. These patients may be managed with close observation, intravenous broad-spectrum antibiotics and bowel rest. Worsening of clinical parameters or failure to improve would provide a firm indication for exploration with laparotomy. Patients with major clinical leaks with or without systemic sepsis warrant urgent assessment and management. The extent of contamination determines the surgery and supplementary antimicrobial therapy with broad-spectrum antibiotics are usually indicated in this setting. This can be determined from clinical examination combined with radiological imaging.

Investigation
Imaging, such as computed tomography, contrast enemas and swallows may aid diagnosis and the presence of concurrent abscesses, collections or fistulae. Definitive diagnosis is often made at laparotomy.

Management
Patients with major leaks and associated generalised peritonitis require aggressive resuscitation and input pre- or postoperatively in a HDU or ITU environment. This allows close monitoring, rationalisation of intravenous fluid therapy and inotropic support.

Surgical repair is indicated for major leaks, especially with concurrent dehiscence. The anastomosis can either be revised, repaired (in the case of proximal small bowel anastomoses) or taken down to allow faecal diversion. The decision to repair or take down an anastomosis should take into account local and systemic factors which may impact on outcome, such as level of contamination and the comorbid or nutritional status of the patient. Repair can be achieved either by refashioning the anastomosis or by the use of a patch involving either the omentum or a segment of jejunum (serosa-to-serosa patch). The peritoneal cavity subsequently requires a thorough lavage and the placement of surgical drains. Temporary proximal defunctioning of an anastomosis to prevent the consequences of a further leak is warranted.

Patients who develop anastomotic leaks often have nutritional deficits in the postoperative period and therefore require thorough nutritional assessment and supplementation where necessary.

Complications
Complications are dependent on the site of the leak, the presence of fistulae or abscesses and therefore increase the risk of systemic sepsis. Minor leaks can result in septic complications such as pelvic abscesses; urinary and respiratory tract infections and prolonged ileus. Major leaks are associated with systemic sepsis, confusion, CVA, cardiorespiratory complications and multisystem failure.

Surgical site infections

Postoperative surgical site infections (SSIs) remain a major cause of morbidity and rarely mortality and are defined as occurring in either surgical incisions or organ space. Infection rates vary according to the operation performed (due to variable levels of perioperative contamination), but occur in surgical incisions with a frequency ranging from 1 to 40%. Nearly 60% of these infections occur in patients following hospital discharge.

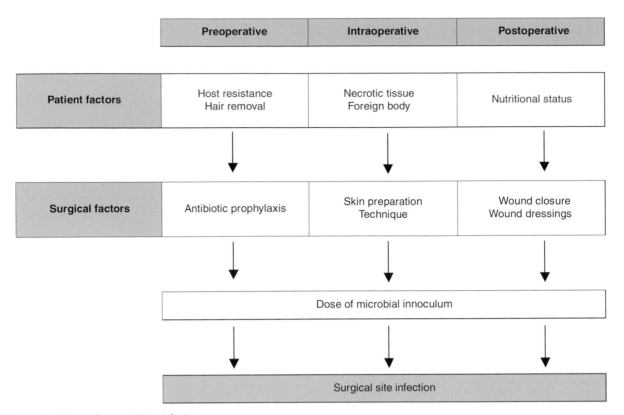

Figure 30.2 Risk factors for surgical site infections.

SSIs involving surgical incisions are usually classed as either superficial (skin and subcutaneous tissues) or deep (fascia or muscle). Organ space SSIs, involving viscera or perivisceral spaces occur with less frequency than superficial SSIs but may require intervention and examples would include abscesses or fluid collections.

Risk factors

A number of factors are involved in creating a wound at risk of infection (Figure 30.2). The type of organism and the extent of microbial inoculum within a wound can influence the likelihood of infection. Other features of the wound such as the presence of necrotic tissue or foreign material as well as patient factors such as immunodeficiency, diabetes and the use of tobacco might increase the risk of infection.

Clinical

The majority of SSIs usually present in the first week postoperatively but the presentation can be occasionally delayed some weeks later. Patients typically describe increasing wound pain and are generally unwell with malaise, nausea or vomiting and anorexia. Clinical examination may reveal tenderness, with other cardinal signs of inflammation; calor, rubor, swelling and possible fluctuance. Pyrexia with swinging fluctuations can indicate an organ space infection typi-

cally associated with systemic features of infection and leucocytosis.

Assessment

All wounds should be examined to establish the extent of infection and presence of cellulitis but in particular following synthetic graft placement. This is usually indicated by erythema and margins should be marked to allow detection of progression or improvement. Fluid collections usually exhibit fluctuance or discharge of pus and will require drainage. Organ space infections are suspected with the presence of systemic features of infection and require radiological evaluation to determine suitability for drainage. Other sources of pyrexia, such as the urinary or respiratory tracts should be examined if overt evidence of an SSI is absent.

Investigation

Inflammatory markers are frequently elevated in patients with SSIs, in particular the leucocyte count. Longstanding or chronic infection may lead to a fall in the serum albumin. Pus specimens should be obtained and sent for microscopy, culture and antimicrobial sensitivity. Radiological imaging including computed tomography or magnetic resonance can be useful if deep collections are suspected.

Table 30.1 Risk factors for venous thromboembolism.

	Low risk	Intermediate risk	High risk
Patient factors	Age ≤45 years	Age >45 years BMI ≥ 30	Age >60 years Previous DVT Malignancy Thrombophilia
Surgical factors	Minor surgery	Gynaecological surgery Laparoscopic abdominal surgery Postoperative immobility	Elective hip/knee surgery Hip trauma surgery Neurosurgery Lower limb embolectomy

Resuscitation

Patients presenting with features of septic shock require urgent assessment and management. Clinical features such as oliguria, confusion or decreased conscious level and hypotension should raise the suspicion of systemic sepsis. Laboratory investigation should include arterial blood gas sampling and serum lactate levels in order to determine the severity of acidosis. Fluid resuscitation may need to be aggressive and antibiotics, either empirical or directed are indicated. Further management in a high dependency or intensive care setting may be indicated to allow accurate physiological monitoring and organ support.

Management

Any collection needs drainage, either percutaneously (with or without radiological assistance) or operatively. Superficial wound collections can be drained by removing selected stitches or clips and gentle probing to allow drainage of pus. Wounds should then be allowed to heal by secondary intention, with regular dressings. In some cases, debridement may be necessary and appropriate dressings may be applied. Wounds undergoing sharp debridement require regular evaluation to assess the progression or improvement of tissue necrosis. Antibiotics should be administered if spreading cellulitis or systemic illness is noted.

Complications

Deep collections, persistent discharge from sinuses and fistulae are a major risk if superficial infections are left untreated or do not respond to initial management. Collections can be subphrenic, perihepatic, paracolic, inter-bowel loop or pelvic.

Cardiovascular complications

Deep vein thrombosis and pulmonary embolus

If no prophylaxis is initiated, 25% of general surgical patients may suffer a DVT. This proportion is doubled for those patients undergoing major pelvic or abdominal surgery and even greater in hip and knee replacement surgery. Of those patients with a DVT, 20% are at risk of developing a PE.

Risk factors

Prophylaxis and identifying patients with risks are important (Table 30.1)

The use of compression hosiery, intraoperative calf pumps, heparin (commonly low molecular weight heparin), as well as earlier mobilisation reduce the risk of venous thromboembolism.

Clinical

DVT characteristically presents with a continual tachycardia and low-grade persistent pyrexia. Other signs depend on the site of the thrombus, with tissue oedema and tenderness frequently occurring distal to the thrombosis and pain localised over the involved vein. Pulmonary embolism usually presents with pleuritic chest pain, persistent tachycardia (often with sinus rhythm, but classically S1, Q3, T3 on ECG), possible haemoptysis and shortness of breath. Frequently, however, there are no chest signs.

A life-threatening PE can result in a raised JVP (indicating right ventricular strain), gallop rhythm and hypotension with potential acute circulatory collapse and cardiac arrest.

Investigation

Duplex scan is the preferred method of investigation for a DVT. Other tests include venograms and assay of D-dimers (although this also rises in infection). Arterial blood gases, an ECG and chest X-ray can be performed to aid diagnosis of a PE, in particular to exclude consolidation or congestive cardiac causes.

The gold standard investigation is a CT pulmonary angiogram. Some centres also offer ventilation–perfusion (V–Q) scans, which report the probability of an embolus based on the matching of areas of ventilation and perfusion defects. The reliability of this test, however, is reduced in patients with concurrent chest consolidation.

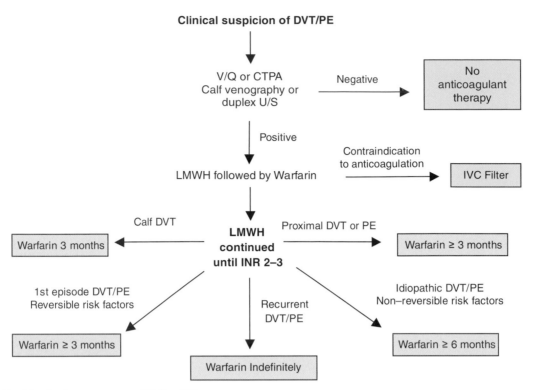

Figure 30.3 Algorithm for the management of DVT and PE.

Management

If venous thrombosis is confirmed, full anticoagulation with intravenous unfractionated heparin or subcutaneous low molecular weight heparin, followed by oral warfarin therapy is advised. The duration of anticoagulation is dependent on the site of thrombosis and reversibility of causative risk factors. An algorithm for the management of PE is given in Figure 30.3.

Haemorrhage

Postoperative haemorrhage is an important cause of early morbidity and mortality following emergency surgery.

Clinical

Bleeding from wounds becomes immediately apparent postoperatively with soaking of dressings. Bleeding subcutaneously results in haematoma which may cause significant discolouration and discomfort. Intra-abdominal bleeding may initially cause few abdominal symptoms and signs.

Patients sustaining a large postoperative haemorrhage usually display clinical signs of hypovolaemia and these are due to decreased organ perfusion ultimately resulting in a cascade of neuroendocrine responses. Tachycardia is present when intravascular volume has been depleted by 15%. Sys-temic vascular resistance is increased in order to maintain blood flow to vital organs and results in cold peripheries. This also leads to the first physiological change observed after significant bleeding which is a decrease in the pulse pressure. This is due to an increase in systemic vascular resistance in response to a decreased preload and predominantly affects the diastolic component of the cardiac cycle. Tachypnoea and changes in mental status also ensue.

Patients who are young, athletes or taking beta-blocking medications may not display the normal physiological elevation in heart rate in response to hypovolaemia (Table 30.2).

Assessment

Bleeding is relatively common as an early complication following surgery and requires urgent assessment and management. Obtaining an accurate history and details of the operative procedure are vital to identifying possible sources. In addition, other causes of shock should be considered in any patient undergoing recent ventilation such as pneumothorax and cardiac tamponade in cardiothoracic patients.

Postoperative haemorrhage can be classified as:

- Primary – perioperative bleeding from uncontrolled vessels.
- Reactionary – within 24 hours postoperative. Usually occurs as blood pressure rises and vasospasm from uncontrolled vessels ceases and from increased venous pressure after moving and coughing.

Table 30.2 Classification of hypovolaemia.

	Class I	Class II	Class III	Class IV
Loss of circulating volume (%)	>15	15–30	>40	>30–40
Heart rate (bpm)	<100	Tachycardia	Tachycardia	Marked tachycardia
Pulse pressure	Normal	Narrowed	Narrowed	Very narrow
Systolic BP	Normal	Minimal decrease	Decrease	Significant decrease
Urine output/hour	≥0.5 mL/kg	≤0.5 mL/kg	<0.5 mL/kg	Minimal
Mental status	Normal	Anxiety	Confused	Depression/lethargy

– Secondary – usually presents 7–14 days postoperatively, due to the reopening of a blood vessel, either from erosion following infection or thrombus separation. This can be preceded by a 'herald' minor bleed.

Resuscitation

In shocked patients, restoration of adequate tissue perfusion and control of bleeding are the ultimate objectives. Manoeuvres to secure airway patency and adequate ventilation are vital prior to addressing circulatory disturbances. If obvious sources of haemorrhage are identified, efforts to control these with compression should be attempted. Large bore cannulae should be inserted into large peripheral veins and intravenous fluid therapy initiated. Blood samples for assay of haemoglobin and for cross-match of blood type in preparation for transfusion should be sent. Appropriate monitoring of tissue perfusion including acid–base status and accurate evaluation of urine output is useful to guide fluid therapy.

Management

Postoperative patients with hypovolaemic shock require operative intervention with control of haemorrhage. Intra-abdominal bleeding requires urgent laparotomy. If the source of bleeding is unknown a systematic method of examining the peritoneal cavity should be employed. Four quadrant gauze swab packing with sequential examination allows for controlled assessment. Once a source of bleeding has been identified, means with which to obtain control should be attempted. Smaller vessels may be cauterised with diathermy; however, if larger vessels have been injured, control should first be obtained with vascular slings and clamps prior to definitive control with ligation or repair of vessel wall defects.

Complications

Immediate complications from bleeding include risk of cardiac arrest, pain, haematoma, infection and changes in mental status. Complications of large volume blood transfusion include coagulopathies and platelet deficiency. Bleeding into the abdominal cavity may predispose to peritoneal adhesions in the long term.

Renal complications

Common renal tract complications occurring in the postoperative period include urinary tract infections, urinary retention secondary to pain or anaesthesia and ARF. Of these complications ARF is the most serious and will be discussed further.

ARF is defined as an abrupt loss and sustained decline in glomerular filtration rate. An increase in the serum creatinine concentration of over 50% above the baseline combined with a urine output of less than 400 mL/day (oliguria) or less than 50 mL/day (anuria) indicate the severity of ARF. Surgery is a common cause for ARF and accounts for figures in the region of 20–50% of hospital-acquired cases. In addition, 2% of patients receiving intravenous contrast for computed tomography or angiography develop ARF. Mortality from ARF can be up to 40% in severe cases.

Risk factors

The risk factors are summarised in Table 30.3. Pre-existing renal insufficiency and diabetes are the most important risk factors for the development of postoperative ARF. Use of nephrotoxic drugs and intravenous contrast agents are also significant aggravating factors in patients who already have pre-existing renal insufficiency.

The incidence of developing ARF in the postoperative diabetic patient is 7% but this figure may increase threefold in the presence of sepsis or hypovolaemia. Patients who have abdominal compartment syndrome are at risk of severe ARF. Normal abdominal pressure ranges from 0 to 12 mm Hg but can be elevated in conditions such as trauma,

Table 30.3 Risk factors for the development of ARF.

Pre-existing renal insufficiency	Jaundice
Diabetes mellitus	LVF
Increased age	Increased inra-abdominal pressure
Male gender	Chronic disease
Use of nephrotoxic drugs	Sepsis

ARF, acute renal failure; LVF, left ventricular failure.

Table 30.4 Differential diagnosis of ARF in surgical patients.

Prerenal ARF	Renal ARF	Postrenal ARF
Hypovolaemia	Drugs	Ureteric obstruction or injury (calculi, surgery and trauma)
Cardiac failure	Rhabdomyolysis	Urethral obstruction or injury (BPH, malignancy and trauma)
Sepsis	Pyelonephritis	Bladder dysfunction or injury (anaesthesia and nerve injury)
ACE inhibitors Abdominal compartment syndrome	Pre-existing renal disease	

ARF, acute renal failure; ACE, angiotensin-converting enzyme.

intra-abdominal bleeding, burns, pancreatitis and ascites. When pressures exceed 30 mm Hg patients may become anuric and emergency decompression with laparotomy is indicated.

During emergency abdominal surgery it is possible to damage the renal collecting system through iatrogenic injury. If a procedure carries a high risk of ureteric injury (determined preoperatively), ureteric stents can be placed to help prevent inadvertent division.

Clinical

ARF becomes evident clinically with a fall in hourly urine output; however, other causes should also be explored. A common cause of a sudden drop in urine output is a blocked urinary catheter. If flushing or replacing the catheter does not resolve the problem, then hypovolaemia should be suspected even if blood pressure and pulse rate are normal. A fluid challenge of 250 mL of crystalloid or colloid fluid over 30 minutes should increase the urine output if this is a result of hypovolaemia. Monitoring of central venous pressure aids in directing intravenous fluid therapy and is advisable especially in patients with sepsis or heart disease. In a hypovolaemic patient, there should be a slight rise in central venous pressure after fluid challenge. If the volume deficit has been corrected and urine output does not improve, then a small dose of diuretic may be appropriate (e.g. 20 mg or 40 mg of frusemide given intravenously).

Assessment

To prevent further decline in renal function it is vital to establish the precipitating factors and potential reversibility. Progressive renal failure may result in life-threatening hyperkalaemia and therefore patients require urgent assessment and management. Causes of ARF are classed as prerenal, renal or postrenal and identification of precipitating factors will aid treatment. The differential diagnoses of these are given in Table 30.4.

Investigation

A thorough history and examination should be carried out in order to exclude possible exposure to nephrotoxic drugs or contrast agents. Laboratory tests should include urea and electrolytes, urinalysis, urine samples for microscopy, culture and sensitivity and urine osmolality. If sepsis is suspected, samples of blood should be sent for culture before starting antibiotics. Renal ultrasound demonstrating hydronephrosis may indicate a postrenal cause for ARF.

Resuscitation

Patients with oliguria in the postoperative period usually reflect hypovolaemia and respond to replacement of circulating volume. Patients should be managed with an input/output chart and strict evaluation of fluid lost perioperatively and insensible losses should be calculated in order to guide replacement. The primary hazard in ARF results from severe hyperkalaemia. This can result in cardiotoxicity and also manifest changes on the ECG. Administration of calcium gluconate (10 mL of 10% intravenously over 60 seconds) can be cardioprotective. Reduction in plasma potassium can be achieved by giving dextrose and insulin and nebulised salbutamol. Medications likely to increase plasma potassium such as ACE inhibitors should be discontinued. Central venous catheterisation is indicated, allowing rationalisation of fluid therapy, access for fluids, haemofiltration and therapeutic medications.

Management

Maintaining adequate intravascular volume and the exclusion of nephrotoxic agents is the mainstay of treatment. Patients with worsening renal function despite these measures may require renal replacement therapy. The indications for dialysis are volume overload that cannot be managed with fluid restriction or diuretics, hyperkalaemia and severe acidosis. Patients need to be managed by the intensive care team in the HDU or ITU setting.

Complications

Most patients who suffer from ARF in the postoperative period recover some of the renal function but 17% will go on to develop chronic renal impairment requiring dialysis. Overall mortality in severe cases ranges from 40 to 60%.

Further reading

Carmichael P. Acute renal failure in the surgical setting. *ANZ J Surg* 2003;**73**(3):144–153.

Heller L, Levin SL, Butler CE. Management of abdominal wound dehiscence using vacuum assisted closure in patients with compromised healing. *Am J Surg* 2006;**191**:165–172.

Thromboembolic Risk Factors (THRIFT) Consensus Group. Risk of and prophylaxis for venous thromboembolism in hospital patients. *BMJ* 1992;**305**:567–574.

Tytherleigh MG, Bokey L, Chapuis PH, et al. Is a minor clinical anastamotic leak clinically significant after resection of colorectal cancer? *J Am Coll Surg* 2007;**205**:648–653.

Index

Note: Italicized b, f and t refer to boxes, figures and tables

Index